What You Need to Know Right Now!

HOW TO
SURVIVE
PANCREATIC
CANCER

VITAL INFORMATION FROM DOCTORS, SURVIVORS,
AND LISA STOUGH'S PERSONAL JOURNEY

LISA & ROBIN STOUGH

The authors are not medical doctors, and this book is not intended as a substitute for medical advice from licensed medical doctors. The reader should regularly consult a licensed medical doctor in all matters relating to his or her health, and particularly in respect to any symptoms that may require diagnosis, treatment, or medical attention.

Email address: PancreaticCancerBook@gmail.com

Printed in the United States of America.

ISBN: 979-8-8782-6909-4

First Trade paperback edition in 2024.

Author Consultant and Editing: Company 614 Enterprises, LLC.
Cover Design: Saheran Shoukat and Rick Soldin
Text Design and Composition: Rick Soldin
Photos from Lisa and Robin Stough Family Collection and used with permission.
Authors' Photo by Cindy Hammond with permission.

All trademarks, service marks, and company names are the property of their respective owners. This includes but not limited to the registered trademarks of Actonel, Adrucil, ALOXI, Ativan, Bard PowerPort, Benadryl, Bexsero, Carafate, CaringBridge, ChronoFlex, CINVANTI, Compazine, CREON, Decadron, Dermabond, Duramorph, Ensure, Forteo, Fosamax, Gas-X, Hibiclens, Keytruda, Life Alert, Lovenox, LYNPARZA, Maalox, Marinol, Menactra, Neulasta, Pancreatic Cancer Action Network, PedvaxHIB, Pepcid AC, Pneumovax, Prevnar 13, Prilosec, Protonix, Pulsar, PurpleStride, Queasy Drops, Reglan, Sancuso, Tigan, Toujeo, Tums, Tylenol, Versed, Xarelto, Xeloda, ZENPEP, Zofran.

This is a book with true events. Some characters' names have been changed. Some event sequencing, locations, and dialogue have been changed or created to tell this story better. Some real-life participants have been excluded, and some characters have been combined or created.

This book is dedicated to every patient and caregiver fighting pancreatic cancer. May God grant you the wisdom, strength, courage, and determination to beat this awful disease.

—Lisa and Robin Stough

Contents

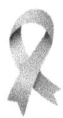

Introduction

"YOU HAVE PANCREATIC CANCER."

These are the four most devastating words I'd ever heard, and it started a terrible time in my life. Instantly, my husband and I were scared to death as fear and loneliness invaded every corner of our bodies. With mortality staring me in the face, how do I handle this deadly diagnosis? Where do I turn for help? And what is the next step in getting the best care out there?

For me, I had just entered the frightening, unfamiliar, and confusing world of pancreatic cancer. This is the story of my journey through that world.

At the time, Robin, my husband, grabbed every book he could find. Yet none of them put everything together in one place. We had to piecemeal information from various sources and books. And we promised ourselves if I could survive this, we'd write something that would become a resource for this challenging disease. This book is it. Although every pancreatic cancer journey is different, we hope some of this information will help you with yours.

We have created three distinct sections. Each one can be resourced and read separately. First is the story of our journey. It details the moment of diagnosis and continues through chemo, radiation, surgery, chemo again, and survival. This section will give you a glimpse of what you might face.

The next section contains interviews with doctors who diagnose and treat pancreatic cancer. Each one provides vital information about current treatments and promising looks into the future. These medical professionals cannot be thanked enough for their participation and for sharing invaluable information.

Finally, we have a complete section of survivor's stories. Each one traveled a different path while enduring various treatments. We believe their stories will not only educate you about different options out there but provide you with hope.

As a bonus, there's an epilogue detailing my experience with a clinical trial. I also included my CA 19-9 readings and a photo section so you can identify with us. I hope you find this helpful.

Speaking of hope, on January 17, 2024, the American Cancer Society updated the five-year survival rate for pancreatic cancer. It has increased to 13%, up for the third straight year. Just a decade earlier, it was only 6%. This increase signals essential progress in the pancreatic field, with more patients living longer.

Like all cancers, early detection of pancreatic cancer is critical. Unfortunately, there is no established way or test to find pancreatic cancer early. Fortunately, research is underway that focuses on blood tests, tumor markers, improved imaging, and artificial intelligence. It can't come soon enough.

Now it's time for the legal disclaimer. While we have tried very hard to describe all the technical aspects in this book accurately, we are not doctors. Thus, one must always seek medical advice rather than rely on this book.

Due in part to the relatively small number of patients diagnosed each year, pancreatic cancer research is underfunded. As a small part of giving back, proceeds from our book will be used to fund pancreatic cancer research.

As you read our book, certain themes are evident. Be a strong advocate for yourself or have a strong advocate on your behalf. Be in charge of your journey. Solicit second and third opinions. Be treated at a high-volume facility that has a lot of pancreatic cancer experience and expertise. And don't forget the caregivers. Having them break down can be just as devastating as some of the treatments.

Finally, our thoughts and prayers are with every pancreatic cancer patient and those touched by this disease. We pray this book will provide you with important information and hope. Just don't give up.

—Lisa Stough

Are You a Cancer Survivor?

An individual is considered a cancer survivor from the time of diagnosis through the rest of life.
~ National Cancer Institute

Anyone who has ever been diagnosed with cancer no matter where they are in the course of their disease.
~ American Cancer Society

A survivor is anyone living with a history of cancer—from the moment of diagnosis through the remainder of life.
~ National Cancer Survivors Day Foundation

You became a survivor on the day you were diagnosed.
~ MD Anderson Cancer Center

Every pancreatic cancer journey is a fight for survival, a life-defining challenge. Still, it's important to remember you became a survivor from the moment of diagnosis through the remainder of life.

Regardless of the stage of your disease or situation, you are a survivor. Don't ever give up!

—Robin Stough

Chapter One

Lisa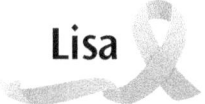

For as long as I could remember, my life rolled on without much drama. A wonderful husband. A nice home. Friends. Family. Travel. Not much to complain about.

At 61 years old, I was healthy and worked out at the gym two to three times a week. Sure, I had smoked a little back in college but stopped after a few years. Really, I had no health problems. Then one day, I felt a twinge in my back on the lower left side. I was pretty sure I'd tweaked it by lifting weights. As always, I kept moving, certain it would eventually disappear.

It didn't.

Before long, the pain became intense. It came at night when I lay on my left side but went away when I rolled onto my right side. That helped me sleep.

Around this time, the University of Pittsburgh had a basketball game against North Carolina. My husband Robin was a Pitt graduate, and we both supported Pitt's teams. We even had season tickets to the basketball games. One day, we left Dallas and flew to our hometown of Pittsburgh to see the game and visit friends.

The first night we were there, we went out and had a nice dinner, then returned to our hotel and went to bed. All night long, I experienced intense indigestion. There was nothing I could do, so I just suffered with it.

The following week, we went on vacation to Cabo San Lucas, Mexico. I had never been there and looked forward to the trip. Incredibly, the first night brought me complete relief. The pain in my left side disappeared. Problem solved.

But the second night, the pain returned. Whatever this was, it was maddening because I never knew if or when it would show up.

When we returned home to Dallas, I called Dr. Philip Aronoff, who had been my primary care physician for over thirty years. He's practically part of the family. I set an appointment and put it out of my mind, confident he'd sort it out.

The day before my appointment, I finally told my husband about what I had been enduring. I had been silently suffering from this pain for about a month without telling him. I laid out everything I'd been going through and he listened intently.

"Are you sure you need a doctor?" he asked. "I have all kinds of aches and pains."

"No, this is a bad, bad pain, and it's not going away."

He nodded and agreed that seeing Dr. Aronoff was the right thing to do.

⸻

ON TUESDAY, FEBRUARY 11, 2020, I saw Dr. Aronoff. After examining me, he said, "I have no idea what's causing your pain. Do you want to have a CT scan?"

"Yes," I replied.

The scan was scheduled for Friday, February 14—Valentine's Day. It was a day I'll never forget. That morning, I had the CT scan, then drove to my job at Marsh, a large insurance broker located in downtown Dallas. I'd been in the insurance industry for thirty-eight years, with twenty-three of them at Marsh. They'd been very good to me and I felt blessed to have the job.

It was a busy day with lots to do. I enjoyed lunch with my coworkers and discussed what we were doing that night for Valentine's Day. Afterward, we returned to work and resumed our day.

Around 2 p.m., I was away from my desk, but when I returned, I noticed Dr. Aronoff had called my cell phone. Before I could listen to the message, Robin called and said, "Hey, Dr. Aronoff's office left a message on our home answering machine. He said you need to call them right away. He's been trying to get in touch with you."

My heart sank. The doctor's office had never tried to reach me like this. Instantly, I knew something was wrong. Pieces started fitting into place.

Just two months earlier, we'd traveled to Columbia, South Carolina, to spend Christmas with Robin's mother. Robin had five siblings, and his entire family had gotten together for the first time in decades. I remembered thinking that this gathering signaled something terrible was going to happen. It just felt like someone wouldn't be around by next Christmas. Suddenly, I realized that person might be me.

At Marsh, having personal calls in the office was not a problem, but even so, I grabbed my cell phone and took the elevator to the lobby. I didn't want to be around my coworkers if the news was bad.

I reached the lobby and found a quiet, private spot. With a shaking finger, I pressed the button and called my doctor. It took only seconds to get him on the phone—another sign of trouble.

"Lisa," he said, his voice dark and serious, "something is showing on your pancreas and we need to jump on this right away."

In over thirty years, I'd never heard Dr. Aronoff sound like this. He'd always been calm, professional, and in control. He was like an angel, making you feel like nothing would happen as long as he was around. Yet the shock and urgency in his voice were unmistakable. I held the phone away from my face while I decided if I would pass out, cry, or scream. I did none of these and instead took a deep breath and collected myself.

Dr. Aronoff set up a meeting with a gastroenterologist on Monday to review the CT scan. Once we'd hung up, I called Robin. I told him what Dr. Aronoff had said, the tone of his voice, and that I was scheduled to have additional tests. Robin was concerned but calmed me down. "Let's wait and see what the tests show," he said.

He was right. There wasn't anything I could do right now except go back to work. But on the elevator, another image hit me—the Purple-Stride Walk in support of pancreatic cancer research. I had recently seen a promotion for it on TV and couldn't get it out of my mind. Every time they showed it, I stopped what I was doing and watched it.

Also, there was the *People* magazine article on Alex Trebek's pancreatic cancer diagnosis I had just read. I felt it speaking to me. And the *Daily Bread* someone had set out in my gym's locker room, reigniting interest in my faith. Then the Christmas family get-together in South Carolina. Plus, I had been searching on the internet for causes of back and side pain. One reply kept showing up. Deep down in my heart, it all made sense. *I don't need a biopsy to tell me I have pancreatic cancer.*

The only thing I knew about the disease was that it was a death sentence. My husband would soon be a widower, and I'd be in the ground. My life was ending and there was nothing I could do about it.

———————————————

But it was still Valentine's Day and Robin had arranged dinner at Cool River Café, an upscale steak restaurant in Las Colinas, a suburb of Dallas. So we went to dinner. We needed something to take our minds off this news. Besides, it might be the last Valentine's Day with my husband of forty years. I needed to soak up every bit of humanity I could.

I don't drink much, but I had two glasses of wine that night. It was a lot for me because I'm a small person, about 115 pounds. I didn't care.

The rest of the meal was a blur.

Back home, we slid into bed and I reached over, grabbing Robin's hand. *How many more times will I be able to do this? Will there be a night when he reaches over and I'm not there?*

I found it hard to sleep. I felt like someone had pulled out a kitchen timer and set it on my nightstand, counting down the minutes to our final day together. Each tick weighed heavier and heavier on my shoulders.

Is there a way to survive pancreatic cancer?

Alex Trebek was still alive. Maybe I could survive too.

Chapter Two

Robin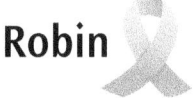

DAY 1 – FRIDAY, FEBRUARY 14, 2020 – I sat in my office, holding an unopened packet from our lawyer. Lisa and I had been redoing our wills. Since we had no children, I thought the estate planning would be easy. It wasn't. I needed to review this material and get it back to him. This was as good a time as any to sort through it. Then the phone rang.

"Hey, have you spoken to Aronoff?" I asked Lisa when I answered the phone.

"Yes," she replied. "He said the scan found something on my pancreas."

The pancreas, I thought. *The pancreas!*

My body turned to jelly.

I quickly gathered my thoughts. "We need to wait for the next round of testing. Let's not panic," I reassured her. We ended the call and Lisa went back to work.

I sat back and thought about all this. *Wait!* I told myself. *Sure, Dr. Aronoff is worried, but he hasn't mentioned anything about pancreatic cancer. Or even cancer. We need to stop all this worrying and wait for the tests. We'll find out soon enough what we're dealing with.*

I put down the estate planning packet and picked up a photo from our early days. Suddenly, I was back in 1979. I had just walked into the Loft, a hangout bar in Greensburg, Pennsylvania. It was Friday night. The place was packed.

I spotted my buddies standing together in a corner. As I joined them, I learned that one of them knew a group of girls at the end of the bar. Like a school of fish, we weaved and darted through the crowd, making our way over so introductions could be made. After surveying the lovely ladies, I settled onto a barstool next to this petite beauty who was smiling at me.

"Lisa," she said as I shook her hand. Of course, I was smitten. Years later, I'd put a ring on her other hand.

The memories brought a smile to my face. I pulled the keyboard over and searched for other causes of lower back pain and spots on the pancreas. *Maybe this isn't cancer.*

DAY 2 – SATURDAY, FEBRUARY 15, 2020 – The dinner at Cool River had gone as well as possible. We talked things over and agreed not to worry about it.

Now it was Saturday morning. I went to play golf while Lisa joined some friends for lunch. We tried to keep our schedules normal. In reality, it was the calm before the storm.

After golf, I sat down at my desk and continued researching the pancreas on my computer. I wanted to learn as much as possible to understand whatever the doctors might tell us. Lisa and I were a team, and I was determined to live up to my responsibilities to her.

DAY 4 – MONDAY, FEBRUARY 17, 2020 – Weeks earlier, I had made an appointment with our attorney and CPA for today. It was in one hour. I watched as Lisa put on some nice clothes. When she finished, I studied her appearance. The clothes were baggy and loose-fitting.

"You've lost some weight," I told her.

"Yeah, I have," she replied.

"Do you think it's some kind of symptom or stress?"

"I don't know," she said, her voice trailing off. "I just wish this pain would go away."

We climbed into my car and took off for the meeting. In a mental fog, I drove to the attorney's office and listened as he reviewed our estate plans. I was 64, and Lisa was 61. Having a solid estate plan was important to us. But now, it took on even more significance.

Lisa was mostly out of it because of the intense pain. It had been getting worse each day, and the pain was no longer confined to sleeping on her left side at night. It was constant.

Truthfully, with her condition, it was hard to concentrate. We were both stressed and anxious about the upcoming doctor's appointment.

As soon as we finished, I drove straight to Dr. Lamani Finau's office, a gastroenterologist specializing in endoscopies that take biopsies of growths on the pancreas. (Note: We did not get the gastroenterologist's permission to include him in this book, so we have created a name for him.) Almost immediately, Dr. Finau told us that the CT scan likely confirmed pancreatic cancer. He wasn't positive, but he was pretty sure.

Pretty sure!

His words hit me hard as he pulled up the CT scan and showed us the tumor's location. The pancreas is an elongated, tapered organ located in the abdomen, tucked behind the stomach and surrounded by the small intestine, liver, spleen, and gallbladder. Technically, it's both an organ and a gland and is roughly six inches long. It's shaped somewhat like a tadpole, fat at one end and slender at the other. The wide end of the pancreas on the right side of the body is called the head. The tapered left side extends slightly upward. These middle sections are referred to as the neck and body of the pancreas. The thin end of the pancreas on the left side of the body is called the tail and ends near the spleen. Lisa's growth was on the body of the pancreas.

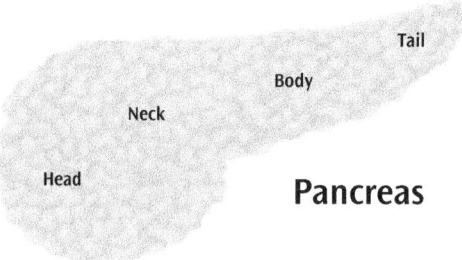

Dr. Finau said he would perform an endoscopy with a fine needle aspiration (EUS–FNA) in a few days. After putting Lisa under anesthesia, he would slide a miniature camera attached to a tube through her mouth down the esophagus into the stomach. Once there, he would use Doppler ultrasound technology to "see" through the stomach wall and find the pancreas. After locating it, he would insert a tiny needle down the tube and penetrate her stomach wall to take a tumor sample. At any other time, I would've marveled over this incredible technology. But for now, I was just happy we had it available to help confirm what Lisa had growing on her pancreas.

Dr. Finau ended our meeting with a firm date for him to perform the EUS–FNA and a referral to a surgeon, Dr. Betam. (Note: We did not get the surgeon's permission to include him in this book, so we have created a name for him.) If surgery was an option, we needed to get Dr. Betam on the team right away.

As Lisa and I left, we held hands. Whatever this was on her pancreas, we would go through it together. But no matter what, I was determined to find her the best health care available. Anything less was not an option.

Chapter Three

Lisa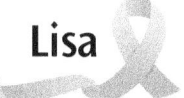

DAY 4 – MONDAY, FEBRUARY 17, 2020 – After first learning about the growth on my pancreas, I texted two dear friends, Teresa and Sallie, both of whom I'd met at work more than thirty years earlier. Despite our moves between different insurance brokers, we were still close friends. Of course, they were crushed to hear about my condition. They called each other and cried on the phone. I'm glad I wasn't on because it would've been rough for me.

Over the next several days, Sallie and Teresa texted me emoji hugs and kisses. I tried to smile each time I read their texts, but I had too much hanging over me.

On Wednesday, February 19, we met with Dr. Betam, who explained that the lesion was about two centimeters in diameter and involved the superior mesenteric artery, vital for bringing oxygen and nutrients to the intestines and pancreas. If this artery was covered with cancer (encased), surgery may not be an option. That meant chemo and radiation treatments would be used to shrink the tumor and hopefully allow for an r0 resection or, in other words, clean margins around the tumor.

Dr. Betam told us he had conducted over 2,000 pancreatic surgeries. Robin and I sat in stone silence as he said that my level of pancreatic cancer growth was categorized as locally advanced or Stage 3A. Later, we read in Dr. Finau's report that it was classified as T4, essentially the same thing as Stage 3A. Then Betam explained that surgery was not an option based on the tumor's proximity to the mesenteric artery.

From our research, Robin and I knew surgery was my best chance at beating this cancer. Without surgery, the odds of survival were low, if not impossible.

Dr. Betam also taught us about a pancreatic cancer marker called CA 19-9. Carbohydrate antigen (CA) 19-9 is a substance pancreatic cancer cells release. A blood sample is taken from the patient and then sent to a lab for testing to find the level of CA 19-9 in the blood. In many patients, the CA 19-9 number rises as cancer spreads. Hopefully, the number will decrease once chemo or radiation hits the tumor. A normal CA 19-9 is anywhere between 0 and 38. My initial reading was 48—just another confirmation of the cancer growing inside me.

Then the final bomb went off. Dr. Betam said my life expectancy was about six months to two years. Because I was healthy, I would be on the higher edge of that range. Robin and I tried to hold back our emotions. It was like being hit in the face. We took notes like robots, just trying to get through the visit. I didn't remember much else.

Outside, Robin and I hugged each other and cried. I felt like I'd just been handed a death sentence. There was nothing left to do but go home and die. It was a terrible time.

DAY 7 – THURSDAY, FEBRUARY 20, 2020 – I had gone without food or water for ten hours. By the time I arrived at the endoscopy center, I was ready for sedation. But all too soon, I came out of it and learned the results.

Dr. Finau confirmed what we already knew. A two-centimeter mass surrounded the superior mesenteric artery and splenic vein on the neck and body of the pancreas. Dr. Betam was present during the endoscopy and studied the images. After careful analysis, he decided that perhaps I could have surgery, but first, I'd have to endure some hard chemo. "We need to shrink the tumor to make it possible for surgery, get it away from that artery."

Robin and I both forced a smile. At least that was something.

Dr. Finau told us that the cancer had not spread to my liver, stomach, or intestines. Again, more good news.

Back in the car, I was still woozy. I tried to process all this as Robin drove. *How many more times will my husband drive me around like this to appointments, surgeries, and treatments?*

I tried not to think about this mess, but it was next to impossible.

Chapter Four

Robin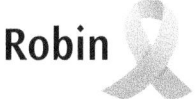

DAY 7 – THURSDAY, FEBRUARY 20, 2020 – The day of Lisa's endoscopy had been a disturbing one for both of us.

She had been sedated for the EUS–FNA. Once the procedure was over, she was wheeled to the recovery room to allow the anesthesia to wear off. As soon as she was barely conscious, she sat up and cried. It was horrifying to watch, so I started crying too. The reaction was shocking, especially since the samples had not yet been sent to a pathologist, so we didn't even have an official diagnosis.

The staff was right there with Lisa. So were the two doctors, Betam and Finau. Everyone was concerned and overwhelmed by her reaction. They tried to calm her down. It was like Lisa had heard what they'd said in the operating room and already knew the preliminary diagnosis.

After she calmed down, the doctors told us once again it was likely pancreatic cancer, but it would have to be confirmed by a pathologist. And Dr. Betam now thought surgery might be an option. That was good news.

At home, I helped Lisa into bed. She fell asleep quickly. I went to my home office and thought back to a few days earlier when we had called my mother.

"What's the matter?" Mom had asked, hearing the distress in my voice.

"Lisa has a growth on her pancreas," I'd said, hesitating as I tried not to cry.

Silence.

"Okay," she said. "Are you still there?"

"Yes, Mom, we're both here. The d-doctor said she has six m-months to two years to live." Stammering, I could no longer hold it back. I just let go and cried. Mom cried with me and so did Lisa. We hardly said another word.

After I'd collected myself and returned to the present moment, I confirmed Lisa's appointment with Dr. Stamply (not his real name), an oncologist recommended to us. Supposedly, he was experienced.

Continuing my online research, I found the Pancreatic Cancer Action Network or PanCAN. I called them and talked with a representative, whom we later learned was a microbiologist. He was very helpful. He even followed it up with an email.

> We discussed that for eligible patients, surgery is the best option for long-term survival of pancreatic cancer. Data shows high-volume surgeons at high-volume hospitals have higher success rates and fewer complications. Although 20 percent of pancreatic cancer patients may be eligible for surgery, data shows that up to half of those patients are told they are ineligible. The Pancreatic Cancer Action Network strongly recommends you see a surgeon who performs a high volume of pancreatic surgeries (more than 15 per year) to determine eligibility.

That got my attention: "… data shows that up to half of those patients are told they are ineligible." Initially, Dr. Betam wasn't sure Lisa could have surgery. Now he thought it might be possible. Was Lisa part of that 50 percent?

I asked the PanCAN rep about Dr. Betam. The rep stated that PanCAN knew him to be a high-volume pancreatic specialist. Dr. Betam had already told us he had performed over 2,000 surgeries on the pancreas, so this matched up. I felt good about our doctor, even though he thought surgery was iffy.

Next, PanCAN discussed having chemo before surgery.

> Since your wife could be a candidate for surgery, and the doctor mentioned treatment before any surgery, I have included the standard of care treatment options for your wife's current stage.
>
> When pancreatic cancer involves nearby blood vessels/ lymph nodes, or has spread beyond the pancreas but

not to another organ, it is referred to as *locally advanced.* The treatment of locally advanced pancreatic adenocarcinoma (the most common type of pancreatic cancer) can vary greatly from person to person depending on the exact location of the cancer and whether or not it can be removed by surgery.

If a surgeon determines at diagnosis the cancer is borderline resectable, treatments may be used to possibly shrink the cancer or move it away from blood vessels so it is more easily removed during surgery. This type of treatment used before surgery is called *neoadjuvant therapy.* Neoadjuvant therapy may involve the use of chemotherapy, targeted therapy and/or radiation therapy.

I had already learned that "resectable" meant something that could be removed by surgery. And "neoadjuvant" meant any treatment occurring before surgery. In this case, it would be chemo or radiation.

Finally, he stated:

Research studies have resulted in conflicting information on the best neoadjuvant therapy for pancreatic cancer. Therefore, there is no definitive standard treatment for borderline resectable pancreatic cancer. However, there are several commonly used treatments for borderline resectable pancreatic adenocarcinoma. These include the following treatments:

- Clinical Trials
- Gemzar® (gemcitabine) and ABRAXANE® (albumin-bound paclitaxel)
- FOLFIRINOX®
- Radiation Therapy

The PanCAN rep then explained some of the existing clinical trials, which were basically experiments to test new drugs and treatments. Every treatment used today began as a clinical trial and the advantage of a trial would be having access to cutting-edge treatments. However, for every clinical trial success, there were many failures. The PanCAN rep offered to run a search of potential clinical trials for Lisa.

The next subject was off-label treatments. This involved drugs used to treat different cancers but which have shown promise in treating pancreatic cancer. The FDA did not approve these drugs for treating pancreatic cancer, but a clinical trial might be available to Lisa as doctors tested them out.

We also discussed supplements. He said most patients took pancreatic enzyme products. This helped improve digestion and the absorption of food.

Finally, the rep spoke about the future of cancer treatment with something called "molecular profiling."

> You asked if there was anything else you should be aware of for your wife. I mentioned that as she is considering treatment options, it would be useful to have her tumor tested for any biomarkers that could be present in her cancer.
>
> Precision medicine, also known as molecular profiling, is an emerging field in cancer treatment. Rather than basing treatment decisions on the cancer type, precision medicine can provide information about a patient's particular tumor to help guide treatment decisions. By analyzing a sample of tumor tissue, molecular profiling can identify specific genetic mutations or biomarkers (measurable substances that can be found in blood or tissue), which oncologists can use to determine if there are therapies to target that patient's tumor.

Essentially, they could examine samples from the tumor and create a treatment to specifically target Lisa's tumor. It was like a tailored suit that only she could wear. That interested me.

By the time I hung up, I realized that PanCAN was a fire hydrant of information. All I had to do was pick up the hose and turn it on.

Chapter Five

Lisa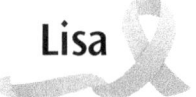

D AY 9 – Saturday, February 22, 2020 – Two days ago, Robin's oldest sister and brother-in-law, Ann and Bill Edwards, sent me an excellent book titled *Anti-Cancer: A New Way of Life* by David Servan-Schreiber, MD, Ph.D. The tagline got my attention: *All of us have cancer cells, but not all of us will develop cancer.* I started reading it and found some great information. I appreciated them thinking of me.

Speaking of family, we knew it was time to notify my father about my diagnosis. I had already told my brother Paul, who insisted on being with Dad when I broke the news. Dad was in poor health and news like this might cause a heart event. Since it was a Saturday and Paul had driven to be with Dad, now was the time to make that call.

The phone rang and Dad picked it up. After we exchanged greetings, I got down to business. Without beating around the bush or trying to soften the blow, I simply said, "Dad, I've been diagnosed with pancreatic cancer."

Silence.

"Dad?"

"Yes, I'm here. I don't know what to say."

"I don't either," I said, fighting back tears.

He told me everything would be all right and promised to call me every day. He lived up to that commitment, phoning every afternoon.

After hearing my diagnosis, I knew Dad was hurting. But he came from a generation that had been through World War II, plus he'd served in the Korean War. They couldn't afford to let themselves become depressed because they'd spent most of their time just surviving. Dad said he loved me; I returned the sentiment and we hung up. It was done.

That night, I was in bed while Robin worked in his study upstairs, researching pancreatic cancer. He constantly did that, wading through the tsunami of available information, determined to save me.

I had my eyes closed but had not yet fallen asleep. Suddenly, I heard a door shut, yet there was no one downstairs. *How did that happen?*

Instantly, I felt the presence of my deceased mother. It was as if she was checking on me. The same thing happened two weeks after Mom died. Robin and I had both been asleep when I woke up because I felt someone sitting at the end of our bed, their weight pushing the mattress down. I was sure this was Mom again. Maybe she would help me through this disease.

DAY 18 – MONDAY, MARCH 2, 2020 – It was a rainy, dreary day, the kind when you feel like rolling over and sleeping for another hour. But not today. I needed to have a port placed in my upper left chest so I could receive chemo and start shrinking this tumor.

Robin drove me to the hospital, where Dr. Betam waited. He wanted to place it himself so nothing went wrong. From what I'd read and been told, the port would be implanted under my skin with a flexible catheter inserted into one of my veins. If everything worked, the chemo nurse could snap in a needle and deliver my medicine.

The oncologist and Dr. Betam had already discussed my situation. I would receive FOLFIRINOX—a combination of drugs: fluorouracil (5-FU), leucovorin (derivative of folic acid), irinotecan, and oxaliplatin. Since the first goal was to shrink the tumor away from the artery, the two doctors wanted to administer the most powerful chemotherapy possible. The hope was that I could handle it.

I slipped into a surgical gown and kissed Robin goodbye as they took me back to surgery. The next thing I knew, I was awake. Then the nausea hit me. For some reason, I had a very bad reaction to the anesthesia drug combo.

I had been knocked out before during colonoscopies, wisdom teeth extractions, and the recent EUS–FNA, so I couldn't understand why this happened. But at least I wasn't crying or emotional as I had been eleven days earlier.

Instead of going home, I had to be monitored in the hospital for eight hours until the nausea was under control. After checking on me several times, Dr. Betam finally felt comfortable discharging me. Once he signed the release papers, Robin and I went home, and I went straight to bed. I soon discovered that sleeping would be a huge part of fighting this disease. Robin had even read about a pancreatic cancer survivor who said she felt like all she did for one entire year was sleep.

Still nauseous, I fluffed up my pillow and buried my face in it. Then I let the dreams take me away.

⸻ ❋❋❋ ⸻

DAY 19 – TUESDAY, MARCH 3, 2020 – With my port in place, we traveled back to the oncology center for an orientation class on chemo. I met with the oncologist, who inspected my port. Satisfied, he let me attend a thirty-minute class where they explained how chemo worked and the side effects. An oncology nurse covered nausea and the drugs they would prescribe if I experienced it. They also said tingling or numbness in the hands and feet were possible side effects. Infection from lowered immunity was another issue. Little did I know this class was not preparing me for the horrific effects of chemo and how hard it would be to simply crawl out of bed. My body and soul were about to go through hell. If I wanted to beat cancer, I'd first have to survive chemotherapy.

⸻ ❋❋❋ ⸻

DAY 20 – WEDNESDAY, MARCH 4, 2020 – Chemo Day finally arrived. Robin had spent a lot of time talking about maintaining a positive attitude. There was so much negativity about chemo that I wanted to take the high road. And it would all start with this first treatment. Nothing would stop me from being thankful I had access to such life-saving medicine.

That said, I was scared out of my mind. Fear of the unknown is a powerful force. It does strange things to you.

I glanced around at the infusion clinic community room and the people in it. Many of the patients looked like they'd been through hell. Missing hair with facial features sunk deep into skulls. It was bad. Closing my eyes, I tried to relax in the chemo chair as the oncology nurse unsheathed the needle and inserted it into my port.

"Okay," she said, "I'm going to start with a bag of saline to help with hydration. This will be done first during all your chemo sessions."

She handed me a schedule of everything I'd receive. Adding it up meant I'd be there for five and a half hours. This would be a grind. I watched as the liquid snaked through the clear tubing and into my body. Suddenly, I felt a sharp pain on the left side of my chest, causing me to wince, and I shrieked.

"What's wrong?" she asked.

"That was painful. It hurts right here!" I replied, pointing to the spot.

"Well, it shouldn't hurt," she said.

The nurse removed the needle and reinserted it. When she let the saline run again, the pain returned. I mean, it really hurt.

"We need to stop this right now," Robin said. "Something's wrong. Have you seen this before?"

The nurse shook her head. "Not really, although sometimes a blood clot will develop."

Again, she removed the needle and left to talk to the oncologist. Ten minutes later, she returned. "The doctor said it might be a blood clot. Let me put something in there to dissolve the clot."

She injected a solution into my port and had me sit still for thirty minutes.

"Okay, let's try it again," she said, starting the process over.

The pain returned. When I complained loudly, Robin became upset and the nurse immediately went back to the oncologist. We waited and waited until she returned. "Something's wrong with your port," she said. That was an understatement. "We can't do the chemo today, so you can return home. We've called Dr. Betam's office and they're going to call you this afternoon."

"Hold on," Robin said. "That's not going to work. We're going up to his office right now!"

Disgusted, annoyed, and in shock, we began walking out of the oncology center. Before we could clear the door, one of the oncology nurses said, "What's the matter? No poison for you today?"

We ignored her and kept on walking. It was like being in the *Twilight Zone*.

When we got to the car, Robin gunned the engine and took off, driving the few hundred yards to the building where Dr. Betam had an office. He parked and said, "Let's go," as he helped me out of the car.

We took an elevator to Betam's office and told his nurse what had happened. I could tell they had already heard from the oncology center.

"We need you to go downstairs to the radiology department," the nurse told me. "They'll take X-rays of your port."

We went down and waited an hour before they could squeeze us in. An interventional radiologist came and took us back to our room. As we entered, I noticed a massive screen mounted high up on the wall. It was very high-tech.

The radiologist had me lie on the table and injected some die into my port, taking several images. He immediately diagnosed the problem. "The port catheter tip is in the azygos vein," he said. "That's the wrong one because it's too small. See this larger one? That's where it should be. I'm surprised about all this because after they place the catheter in there, they're supposed to check and make sure it's in the right vein."

Just as he finished that sentence, Dr. Betam appeared. The radiologist showed him what he'd found.

"Yeah, it's in the wrong vein," Dr. Betam admitted.

This was terrible. Not only could I not receive chemo, but I'd have to endure another surgery to fix the port. I tried to hold back the tears as I felt my tumor growing with every second wasted. *Why am I facing so many obstacles?*

Chapter Six

Robin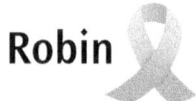

Day 20 – Wednesday, March 4, 2020 – Initially, I was very enthusiastic about Dr. Betam. His insistence on putting the port in himself was refreshing. He could have pawned it off on a less-experienced surgeon but wanted to do it himself. But now, this screw-up had cost us precious time.

"Let me go get an operating room ready," Dr. Betam said before disappearing.

Within minutes, they whisked Lisa away to surgery and put her under light anesthesia. The interventional radiologist performed the corrective procedure, which I was happy about. It took about thirty minutes before I could see Lisa. This time, she woke from a different combo of sedation with no problem.

After the procedure, Dr. Betam and the interventional radiologist came out to talk to me. I had already questioned Betam about why he'd put the port on Lisa's left side since most ports are on the upper right chest. (Later, I learned surgeons are more inclined to place it there.) With his years of experience in this field, I assumed he knew what he was doing. But now, I was distraught. After all, Dr. Betam had insisted we jump on this right away. "Time is our enemy," he'd proclaimed. "We need to get going fast."

I decided to question him about this error. "What happened here?"

"The catheter must have slipped into the wrong vein. It was an accident, but we fixed it. It's not a big deal."

I felt my rocket ignite. "I'm concerned about this because time is of the essence. She needs to start chemo right away—*tomorrow*."

"Weeks or days, it's not going to matter." His voice was conciliatory, trying to calm me down, but I wasn't having any of it.

"No! That's not what you said the other day. *'We don't have a moment to lose.'*" I let that hang in the air for a few moments. "Can we do chemo tomorrow?" I asked.

The radiologist piped up. "She needs a little bit of time to recover before chemo, plus we can't get an appointment at the oncology center in the next two days. Then there's the weekend when they aren't open."

This meant that Monday, five days from now, was the best we could do. What a disappointment. I frowned and held my tongue. I still needed these guys.

As Dr. Betam left, I turned to the interventional radiologist because I could no longer remain silent. "I'm not impressed with your superstar surgeon. The wrong vein? This seems like a rookie mistake." He just smiled and disappeared, too.

When I got Lisa home and into bed, I quietly closed her door and stood there, unable to move. I was deeply troubled. Finally, I went to my study and started looking through my notes, sending emails to friends and family about what was happening.

I looked back through Lisa's medical records. I had gotten them from Dr. Betam and the hospital to build a comprehensive file. This allowed me to see what *had* happened, what *was* happening, and what *might* happen in the future. All this information was vital to me.

One document I studied read, "Unfortunately, her clinical presentation, splanchnic nerve referred pain, and imaging is very consistent with pancreatic adenocarcinoma." Another read, "She is not resectable with the goal of an r0 margin now and will likely not become so in the future." Then a pathology report sent to her from her primary care physician, Dr. Philip Aronoff, read, "This does look like it could be an aggressive tumor and I recommend treatment ASAP." It was depressing to read that, but I refused to think that Lisa faced a death sentence.

Another medical record talked about staging. For pancreatic cancer, I learned that doctors needed three pieces of information to establish a stage. The first was the location and size of the tumor, including knowing whether it had grown into nearby blood vessels, and the second dealt with nearby lymph nodes. Had the cancer spread to them, and if so, how many? The third factor dealt with spread. Had the cancer spread to distant lymph nodes, organs, or bones? After looking at Lisa's records,

Betam determined she had Stage 3A pancreatic cancer. That was much better than Stage 4.

I picked up the pathology report from the biopsies taken during the EUS–FNA. An email attached reiterated what I'd already read: "It looks like it could be an aggressive tumor and I recommend treatment ASAP." That made me even angrier about the port screw-up. I hadn't decided to take Lisa elsewhere, but I'd been working hard to see what options were available. And even before the port problem, I'd consulted with Dr. Aronoff about seeking other opinions. He gave us his thoughts and guided us on how to retrieve our records so we could visit other doctors. Now, I needed to put that into action and see if we could upgrade from coach to first class.

I called many people and places—cancer centers I knew through reputation, some of the names PanCAN had given me, and others from my sister Amy, a doctor in South Carolina. I had conversations with Johns Hopkins in Baltimore. I called MD Anderson in Houston. And I talked to folks at UT Southwestern Medical Center in Dallas.

At MD Anderson, I learned that the earliest appointment would be at the end of April—two months away. That was distressing. The MD Anderson staff recommended local treatment in Dallas until we could see them. With the pandemic just starting and everything in lockdown, I wrote them off. There was no way I'd let Lisa wait that long to see a doctor, not with pancreatic cancer.

Johns Hopkins was more available to talk. They asked me to send them Lisa's records and I did. I spoke with their head pancreatic cancer nurse, an extremely knowledgeable professional. She told me that if we visited now, there was an 80 to 90 percent likelihood they would recommend the same drug and treatment plan we currently had in place. She emphasized that, while she was only a nurse, she did specialize in pancreatic cancer. She also recommended chemotherapy at our local facility instead of flying to Baltimore every two weeks.

The nurse checked the schedule and said we could get an appointment within a week, but we agreed that there was too much in motion to take that appointment, so we set it for a later date. We would wait until later to see if we still needed it.

Another great referral came from Heather Lyke, the athletic director at the University of Pittsburgh. I'm a supporter of Pitt Athletics, and she'd learned of Lisa's diagnosis through conversations I'd had with friends at the university. She called me to offer support and express her concern. Then she suggested I call Dr. Stanley Marks, chairman and chief medical officer of Hillman Cancer Center at the University of Pittsburgh Medical Center (UPMC). She set up the introduction for me.

Dr. Marks had personally treated Pitt and NFL star James Conner for Hodgkin's lymphoma. I spoke with Marks, who was very willing to give me his time and thoughts. He also confirmed our treatment path would be exactly what his team would recommend, except they did *six* neoadjuvant chemo cycles instead of *four*. Johns Hopkins had also told me they recommended six cycles. Betam and his crew had talked about four neoadjuvant cycles, so I wondered if they had the correct protocol.

We discussed radiation, clinical trials, a core biopsy for molecular profiling, immunotherapy, and other subjects. He confirmed that "reducing the tumor and having surgery" was the proper order of events.

Dr. Marks gave me the names of other doctors in Dallas and elsewhere and offered to help me connect. I looked over the list and one stood out: Dr. Herbert Zeh at UT Southwestern Medical Center in Dallas. Dr. Marks told me Dr. Zeh pioneered robotic surgery for pancreatic cancer and was renowned for his surgical work. He was very highly thought of at UPMC.

Dr. Marks explained that Dr. Zeh had left UPMC two years earlier to take the chair of surgery position at UT Southwestern. They hated to see him go because "he put us on the map up here. He's a good guy, someone you should check out."

When I read one of Lisa's medical records that detailed how our current oncologist had called UT Southwestern for advice regarding her treatment plan, I wondered why we weren't with UT Southwestern, especially since it was part of the University of Texas Health System, which owned MD Anderson. They were like sister hospitals. Really, I felt the stars align. So I put in more calls to UT Southwestern to see what I could find out.

DAY 21 – Thursday, March 5, 2020 – The day after Lisa's port redo, UT Southwestern scheduled us to visit them and see their facilities. Very interested, we hopped in the car and drove toward downtown Dallas. Upon arrival, we were met by a nurse navigator. Behind her stood a dietician, chaplain, and social worker. Although somewhat ominous, it was an impressive welcome.

The group walked us through the entire cancer center, including the lab where the blood work was drawn and analyzed. We heard the term "tumor board" and learned a little about that. We saw the meeting areas and exam rooms and reviewed the backgrounds of their pancreatic cancer team. It was first-class.

Around lunchtime, they brought in food from Jason's Deli. As we sat at a table and ate, they introduced us to Stephen Tanit, a volunteer and pancreatic cancer survivor. He represented PanCAN. We listened to his story and couldn't believe it. (Reader's note: Stephen's full story is in the Survivor section at the end of this book. It's definitely worth reading!)

After lunch, we met with an oncologist, Dr. Beg. He said the neo-adjuvant chemo at UT Southwestern would be six cycles over twelve weeks, not the four cycles over eight weeks our current hospital had planned. This protocol matched up with what I'd heard from Johns Hopkins and UPMC.

During our meeting, we told Dr. Beg we wanted Dr. Zeh to perform the surgery. He set up a surgical consultation for us and provided the date. It was so easy!

Next up was a tour of the infusion clinic. The navigator explained that we would have a private room and showed us what it looked like. Lisa and I glanced at each other and smiled. This was too good to be true.

The navigator talked about genetic testing. When we explained we wanted it, a technician met with us and explained how it worked. He looked at Lisa's records and said some of the tests may overlap with those she'd taken at our current hospital. "You might have to pay out-of-pocket for some of them," he said.

"Give her every test you can provide and let me worry about that," I told him. He nodded and went to work.

One of the blood tests they performed on Lisa was the CA 19-9 tumor marker. The score was 71.0. This was down from 78.1 on Day 13 but still higher than 48.0 on Day 6. Later we would learn about different machines and labs and how the readings could have variances. Still, 71.0 was high since the upper limit of normal was 38.0.

By the time we left, Lisa and I realized two things: (1) UT Southwestern was recruiting us, and (2) we would transfer our care to them. We knew there would be a transition, but it was time to start making the switch. We both felt very certain UT Southwestern was the right place to be.

DAY 22 – FRIDAY, MARCH 6, 2020 – I consider myself an open-minded person. I'll listen to an idea and sort it out. So when a good friend recommended a holistic healer, someone he'd had success with, I decided to check it out.

One morning, Lisa and I drove to a house. Several cars were scattered in a small parking area in front. As we opened the door and stepped over the threshold, it was like entering another world. The inside looked like a futuristic movie, where the world had been destroyed and people were trying to rebuild Earth. There was a stove with pots of food and liquids gurgling. A sickly man sat in a corner, sucking oxygen from a tank. Several ragged folks sat in chairs in what may have been the dining room. Some of them appeared to be living in this place. They all looked to be fighting death.

We announced our presence, and Dr. June Meymand appeared. After paying her $400, she took us into a small room and conducted an interview, scribbling notes and studying Lisa. When the interview was over, Dr. Meymand explained everything she could do for Lisa, from selling us some special supplements, discussing the best nutrition and diet, and instilling in us a positive attitude. She assured us she knew all the oncologists at UT Southwestern and gave us opinions on each one. She said she'd work with our oncologist to provide Lisa with the best care possible. "I'll take these notes and create a report—*a game plan*—of my findings and recommendations. Then I'll send it to you and we can begin your treatment."

Lisa and I exited and quickly climbed into our car. The entire experience freaked us out. As we stared at the odd house, we promised each other that we'd never go back. And we never heard from Dr. June. We also never received her report. But it's only been four years. Maybe it's stuck in the mail. At least she still has our $400.

Chapter Seven

Lisa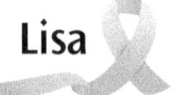

DAY 25 – Monday, March 9, 2020 – It had been five days since the port redo. I was back at the original oncology center for what I hoped would be an actual chemo session—my first time receiving drugs.

For some reason, I kept saying to Robin, "Oh, this will be horrible," to which he'd reply, "Nah, it's not going to be that bad. You'll be good. You're going to do great. You're in good health. This will be fine." I hoped he was right.

We arrived at 7:30 a.m. First up was a visit to the lab. They took some blood and told me to head to the waiting area for the results. Only if my blood work looked "good" could I receive chemo. This would be part of my routine before each new chemotherapy cycle. About an hour later my lab work was completed and the nurse confirmed I was good to begin. She led me to the infusion area to pick out a seat.

As I sat in the chemo chair by the window, I took in the scene. Like the first time, it was horrible. Patients dotted the chairs, mostly looking like survivors from a concentration camp. The only difference was the lack of hair. Really, each patient seemed like they had weeks, if not days, left on Earth. Would I soon look like that? This was a terrible and unfamiliar world I had entered.

I took a deep breath and touched Robin's hand as he sat next to me. We had been worried about whether we were moving quickly enough. With the port screwup, I'd lost five days. Would that be fatal to my outcome? Only God knew.

The room was freezing. I noticed the other patients wrapped in blankets, wearing earplugs or headphones. I assumed they were listening to music and podcasts or watching movies. When the nurse provided me with a blanket, I gladly took it and wrapped myself up. I was already cold and hadn't even started the chemo.

Still apprehensive about the readiness of my port redo, I held my breath as the nurse started me on a saline drip to help with hydration. I watched closely as the fluid made its way toward my body. No pain. It worked! What a relief. My chemo treatments had begun.

Once the saline ran dry, I received some side-effect preventative drugs, including anti-nausea medication. Finally, she hung a chemo bag, and the fun began. Over the next four to five hours, I received bag after bag of different chemicals. It was even a bit boring as I sat there, the liquid drip… drip… drip… falling down the long, clear tubing into my port and then my vein, to be spread throughout my body and, hopefully, to my growing tumor.

Early on in the process, I got hungry. Robin went to a deli in one of the nearby buildings and bought me a sandwich, chips, and a cookie. I heartily ate the small meal and enjoyed it.

As the process continued, the nurse hung a bag of irinotecan. Within a few minutes, my eyelids began twitching. We called the nurse and she explained it was something that sometimes happens. "I'll give you some Benadryl."

After a few hours, I needed to use the bathroom but thankfully my IV pole had wheels just for this purpose. I stood up, rolled it to the bathroom, and took care of business.

"Everything okay?" Robin asked when I returned.

"Floating greasy stools," I replied. I didn't need to tell him what we both knew: Floating greasy stools are another sign of pancreatic cancer. *Is the tumor spreading fast, or is this the result of chemo?* I could tell Robin was worried about it.

Around 1 p.m., with bag after bag drained flat, the nurse told me it was time for the 5-FU. This meant 5-fluorouracil, the last drug in the FOLFIRINOX treatment. Why it's named 5-FU and not 5FL, I have no idea. But it's a fitting name.

I received twenty minutes of this drug and got up to leave, but I had a surprise in store. The nurse brought out a fanny pack containing a rubber bladder, inside of which was more 5-FU. She hooked it up to my port and turned it on. For the next forty-six hours, I would live with the pack as it slowly injected the drug into my body. I would have to sleep and shower with this pack on.

Once in the car, Robin and I looked at each other. My first trip to the infusion clinic was over. It had been long and depressing. Now all I had to do was survive these drugs and pray they shrunk the tumor so I could have surgery.

———————— ⬥⬥⬥⬥ ————————

DAY 27 – Wednesday, March 11, 2020 – I was scheduled this morning for my first visit with radiation oncologist Dr. Aguilera, but was too sick to make the appointment. By the afternoon, I was able to walk into the chemo infusion center even though I felt terrible. It looked exactly as I had left it forty-six hours earlier. The sickly patients had been switched out with other sickly patients. After checking in, I took a seat and waited for the pump's alarm on the bag of 5-FU to go off. We had timed it so I'd be at the center when the audible beep sounded.

As the nurse removed the pack, I told her how nauseous I felt. The drugs were really hitting me.

"Just take your anti-nausea drugs," she said. "I can give you a bag of fluids, but it will take another hour."

I shook my head. "No, I just want to go home."

Robin helped me to my feet and out to the car. At home, I crawled into bed and went to sleep. Again!

Chapter Eight

Robin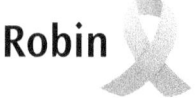

D AY 27 – WEDNESDAY, MARCH 11, 2020 – I awoke before Lisa even stirred, which was getting to be normal. She slept all the time. But I wanted to be ready because today would be a big one. We had an introductory appointment scheduled with Dr. Todd Aguilera, the radiation oncologist at UT Southwestern. After that, we had to be at the oncology center to have Lisa's 5-FU pack removed. I dressed and ate breakfast, giving Lisa plenty of time to get ready. While waiting, I went to my study and picked up a $6,900 invoice for genetic testing. I had ordered all these tests and now it was time for me to figure out how much I actually had to pay.

I gathered my thoughts and started typing emails. When I was done, I glanced at my watch and saw it was almost time to leave. I walked back into the bedroom and found Lisa still in bed.

"Lisa, we have to go soon. Can you get up and get dressed?"

"No," she moaned. "I'm too sick."

Her words slapped me in the face. I knew she felt terrible, but we hadn't been at this chemo thing for even forty-eight hours. We still had eleven and a half weeks to go. How would she make it when we couldn't get off the starting line?

I made sure she had plenty of fluids before I hopped in the car and drove downtown to see Dr. Aguilera myself. I parked the car and hustled to his office. When I checked in, they informed me that without Lisa present, the doctor would not see me. I had just wasted my time.

When I got home, Lisa was still sick, but I got her moving so we could at least make the afternoon appointment at the oncology center. The 5-FU bladder was removed and we headed back home. But Lisa seemed to be getting sicker by the minute.

I sat at my desk and checked some emails. One of them was from my youngest sister, Mimi Holman. Here's what she wrote:

> *Every single experience Moses encountered for seventy-nine years was simply God's way of preparing Moses for what He wanted Moses to do at age eighty. No experiences in life are wasted. Whatever has happened to you in the past is all a part of God's preparing you to serve Him today. And whatever is happening to you now is all His way of preparing you to serve Him in the future. And think of everything that happens to us in this life—it's just God's way of preparing us to serve Him in eternity, for the Bible teaches that in heaven "His servants shall serve Him." (Revelation 22:3 KJV). God has a way of preparing us for what He wants us to do.*

I read the email several times before I responded.

> *Thanks for that Bible verse. There have been a lot of eerie things happening since this began, from dreams to other coincidental things. It all began when Lisa started crying and telling me she thought something very bad was going to happen to her. That was before she had her first doctor appointment and had just very minor pain! It seems like she had some sort of sixth sense. Maybe my imagination is just going wild.*

I sat by myself, thinking about our approach so far. In business, I had played for high stakes. Yet, with Lisa's life on the line, these were the highest stakes possible. So far, we had made good decisions and moved as expeditiously as possible. We now needed to continue building and upgrading our medical care team and support network so we could have the top talent and resources available to us. This would help us continue to make good decisions going forward.

After working at the computer for hours, I checked on Lisa; she was still sick. I went to bed and prayed she would be better in the morning.

DAY 28 – THURSDAY, MARCH 12, 2020 – Once again, we awoke for another doctor's appointment, this time with Dr. Zeh at UT Southwestern.

Lisa could not get out of bed. She seemed worse than last night. I stood over her, pondering this situation. She was very sick and I was worried. I had to do something.

I picked up the phone and called UT Southwestern. The oncology nurse was willing to help. "I don't care what you have to do, carry her yourself, but get her here. We'll administer anti-nausea drugs and fluids and get her back on her feet."

By 10 a.m., I had Lisa at UT Southwestern. The nurse showed us to a private room and began pumping her full of anti-nausea drugs, saline, and nutrients. We spent all day there, but sure enough, she was back to eating and drinking.

While we were there, Dr. Zeh stuck his head in and introduced himself. By then, he knew Lisa was too sick to make our official appointment. As he and his physician assistant came into the room, the first words out of his mouth were, "She's eligible for surgery. We will be doing surgery. I've already looked at her scans and reports. She was always resectable."

The confidence in Dr. Zeh's voice gave us a tremendous boost. Finally, we'd found someone to give us hope. *Maybe this is going to be okay.*

He continued. "I want to consider radiation after chemo and before surgery. We'll evaluate this in more detail later, as sometimes the scans after chemo can be misleading. What looks like a tumor can actually be scar tissue. We'll look at all our markers before we make the call."

That got me thinking again. At one point, Betam had suggested radiation *after* surgery. I thought we wanted to do everything before the surgery to ensure the best outcome. Radiation before surgery made more sense because getting her to surgery was our first goal.

We both noticed a Pittsburgh Steelers lanyard hanging from his neck. "How long have you been in Dallas?" I asked.

"Two years," he replied.

They told us if we moved our care to UT Southwestern, we'd have the team we wanted. Dr. Herbert Zeh as surgeon, Dr. Muhammad Shaalan Beg as oncologist, and Dr. Todd Aguilera as radiation oncologist. They even assigned a dietician to us so we could discuss pancreatic enzymes, food choices, and other issues with her. By the time we left that day, we had decided to formally make the change to UT Southwestern. It was an easy choice.

I put Lisa to bed and went back to work fighting the insurance and administrative wars. First on my list was applying for Lisa to receive disability social security. Along with other information, I needed a letter from a doctor documenting her diagnosis. This would allow the government to review and approve it. Still, this took time and effort on both our parts.

Before I turned in, I saw a CNN story on Alex Trebek. Somehow, he was still beating Stage 4 pancreatic cancer. Alex talked about how brutal the chemo was and that he sometimes thought the chemo would kill him instead of the cancer. Yet there he was, living proof that a person could beat the odds.

Chapter Nine

Lisa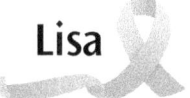

DAY 30 – SATURDAY, MARCH 14, 2020 – The first round of chemo lasted from Monday through Wednesday, ending only when I finished the 5-FU. By Saturday, I was down physically and mentally, fighting nausea with every breath. To make matters worse, my taste buds were messed up. I couldn't take in the food I had always liked or find anything that tasted good. It was very frustrating and depressing.

As I lay in bed, my neck felt weird, like something was pressing on it, but I didn't pay much attention to it and put my head back down on the pillow. Robin came in to check on me and was immediately distracted. "What's this red spot on your arm?" he asked.

I stared at the reddish area. "I don't know. It just showed up."

"It doesn't look like swelling," Robin said.

"There's no pain or discomfort either."

"Let's watch it and see if it gets worse."

It did. As morning turned into afternoon, the discoloration started at the port and went down my left arm. We thought an infection was taking root as the arm swelled and turned a deeper shade of red. Robin sent photos to his sister Amy, the doctor. She had just sent me a beautifully framed needlepoint purple ribbon for encouragement. It was a sweet thing to do and something that instantly lifted my spirits. But that arrived yesterday and today she was worried about my condition. She feared it was a blood clot. She urged Robin to get me to the ER immediately.

Robin contacted UT Southwestern and was told it may be best to call my current hospital and doctor since they had put in the port and our transfer paperwork had not yet become official. Robin called them and heard the same thing Amy had said: Get her to their ER fast!

By now, the pandemic had broken loose. Everything was in lock-down, a first for our modern society. It was after dark when we walked into the hospital and found it completely empty. The eerie atmosphere made me feel worse.

We found the ER and discovered something much different: full-fledged craziness. Sick people littered the area, coughing and hacking, no doubt spreading COVID-19 everywhere. We all had to mask up and sit far apart, staring at each other to see who'd be treated first. It was a memory I wouldn't soon forget.

We waited for several hours before they brought me back. As I passed through the double doors, I heard a three-year-old child screaming hysterically behind a curtain. Next to her was a woman on a gurney with a massive bloody gash on her head. One bay over was a man having a heart attack. It truly looked like the end of the world.

The ER doctor was good. He ordered infection and blood clot testing. It took hours, but the blood work showed high D-dimer levels, indicating a possible blood clot. With that in hand, he ordered an ultra-sound, which pinpointed the issue.

"It's a clot," the doctor confirmed, "right there in your neck and arm." My heart sank. I immediately thought I'd have to have my port redone.

"What caused it?" Robin asked.

"The port, the chemotherapy, and the cancer. Maybe in that order. Or it could've been the chemotherapy, the port, and the cancer, in that order. Or maybe it was the cancer, the chemo, and the port. The fact that your port was put in twice? Maybe that increased the odds. Who knows?"

"What happens now?" I asked sullenly.

"We'll give you a shot of Lovenox in your stomach. It's a blood thinner. Then we'll teach you how to do it yourself at home. You'll have to do that until the port is removed."

I dropped my head. *What else will I need to do to survive this cancer?*

It was after midnight when they released me. As we walked past the moaning and screaming victims, I turned to Robin and said, "Get me out of here." He nodded and hurried me to the car, where we breathed a deep sigh of relief.

DAY 32 – Monday, March 16, 2020 – I was too sick, so Robin went alone to see my primary care physician, Dr. Aronoff. After reviewing my records and talking to Robin, he took me off Lovenox and put me on oral Xarelto instead, 15 mg twice daily for three weeks, followed by 20 mg once a day for 3 months. I only had to stick my stomach with Lovenox a few times before switching to the pills. Eliminating that was a blessing.

Dr. Aronoff also wanted me to monitor my glucose levels and take Toujeo (insulin) if the fasting sugar was consistently over 160. He said I needed to increase my ZENPEP if I experienced diarrhea and found oil floating in the water. ZENPEP is a pancreatic enzyme that aids digestion. Dr. Aronoff also gave Robin a glucose monitoring device and a supply of Xarelto. As we transitioned to UT Southwestern, Dr. Aronoff gave us solid guidance and advice. He was appreciated.

During a rare moment when I felt better, I perused PanCAN.org and found this:

"When you have cancer and a blood clot, it's called 'Cancer-Associated Thrombosis' – or CAT for short. You may be offered medication to prevent blood clots and thin the blood. Clots can occur anywhere in the body. It is likely that the affected area will cause you pain. You can also reduce the chances of a blood clot by taking regular short walks, drinking lots of water, and doing chair or bed exercises (marching, shoulder rolls, etc.). A physiotherapist may be able to advise on some exercise to suit you depending on your activity levels."

Hopefully, this guidance would help me avoid any further blood clots.

───────────────◇◇◇◇───────────────

DAY 36 – Friday, March 20, 2020 – I finally found the strength to write a few emails and texts to friends and relatives. One of them went to Adrienne Irwin, Robin's aunt by marriage. She had sent me such beautiful texts with encouraging messages and a photo of a flower or tree blooming. Each morning, I awoke to find the text waiting for me. I soon learned that she took the photos herself. I also discovered Adrienne had quite a story.

Her mother, Sally, had been a retired registered nurse who had worked in geriatric nursing homes. Sally had always told Adrienne that she hoped she was doing her penance on Earth by caring for patients at the end of life. She prayed the dear Lord would look down upon her and spare her from ending her days in a nursing home. Unfortunately, ovarian cancer ensured Sally would not die in a nursing home.

Sally was diagnosed in 1990. At the time, Adrienne was pregnant. Sally wanted to hang on until the baby was born and took chemo to keep herself alive. Once the baby was born, Sally stopped chemo and, surprisingly, had an energy boost.

One day, Sally, Adrienne, and the baby went grocery shopping. Sally wanted strawberries but couldn't afford them. Adrienne tried to buy some for her but Sally refused. (Later, a neighbor heard about this and bought some strawberries for her.)

At the grocery store, Sally saw a woman she'd known for a long time and called out to her. The woman took one look at Sally and walked away. The cancer and chemo had caused Cachexia, a complex metabolic condition affecting up to 80 percent of people with late-stage cancer. Those with upper gastrointestinal and pancreatic cancers have the highest frequency. Cachexia happens when tumor cells release substances that reduce appetite, which in turn causes poor nutrition. Plus, the cancer itself uses a lot of energy. And the treatments can cause nausea. All this works together to eat away at the soft tissue on the face and make one's features sharper, different. Seeing the woman turn away from her, Sally realized she was so sick that she wasn't recognizable, even to longtime friends. This is one of the terrible psychological, emotional, and social impacts of cancer.

Without chemo, Sally became worse quicker than Adrienne had expected. In her last days, four months after Adrienne's baby was born, Sally awoke and asked Adrienne about her baby. For a brief moment, she was back. Then she waited for her son to visit and talk with her a little bit so she could die. And she did at just 68 years old.

Adrienne attended the funeral with her baby. One life ended as another began—the cycle of life.

Later, Adrienne had a friend, Anna, from Croatia. Anna came down with breast cancer and was bedridden. Since Anna's husband and boys couldn't cook, Adrienne stepped in and took care of their meals until she got better. But Anna grew depressed because she didn't have a sound support system. Within a short time, five of her six sisters contracted breast cancer as well. No one knows for sure, but her entire family may have been affected by the Chernobyl disaster. Eight years after her diagnosis, Anna died.

When yet another friend became sick, Adrienne began sending cards and notes. Whenever her friend felt bad, she'd pull out those cards and notes and look at them. That's why she texted me. She had learned from losing so many people close to her that a daily boost was not only appreciated but needed. Adrienne is a very special person.

Chapter Ten

Robin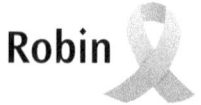

DAY 39 – MONDAY, MARCH 23, 2020 – After the apocalyptic experience of our trip to the ER for Lisa's blood clot, I felt ready for anything. Still, it was hard to fully comprehend driving toward downtown Dallas to UT Southwestern for Lisa's second chemo session (first at UT Southwestern) and seeing the normally traffic-congested freeways utterly vacant. The pandemic had shut everyone in, leaving the roads bare. It seemed like the end of the world.

Lisa and I said little as I navigated the empty Monday morning streets. We'd recently received some additional news: the germline BRCA gene test results came in and she was negative. This had been expected. The BRCA germline mutation is only seen in 5 to 7 percent of pancreatic cancer patients. Those who tested positive could be eligible for targeted therapy, which was the primary reason for the test. But Lisa was not eligible.

In the afternoon, though, we got a bit of good news: she was eligible for full Social Security disability payments. Most pancreatic cancer patients find they are eligible after they've submitted the qualifying medical records. Since the majority of Social Security employees were working from home because of the pandemic, I had to call my congressman to prompt a response, but it had finally been approved. We also considered ourselves blessed because UT Southwestern was still willing to provide chemo when so many others were being denied cancer treatment due to pandemic staff shortages.

We arrived at UT Southwestern and surprisingly found they were still providing valet parking. Pandemic guidelines were just being established, and shortly after this visit, valet parking was stopped.

Since this was our second time at this, we were figuring out the routine. At 7:30 a.m., Lisa's blood was drawn and the samples were taken to the lab, then we waited for the results. Waiting was the main activity when undergoing chemo—lots of waiting.

At 8:30, Dr. Beg appeared with his nurse practitioner. Since this was our first treatment at UT Southwestern, he wanted to personally discuss everything and ensure we were on the right path. After looking at the blood results, he found the white blood cell count a little low but within acceptable levels. The remainder of her lab work returned quickly and was acceptable, clearing Lisa to start her chemo.

Dr. Beg had previously told us her chemo length was being extended from four to six months. She would receive twelve weeks on the front end, then most likely radiation, followed by surgery, and endure another twelve weeks on the back end. He also approved a full FOLFIRINOX regimen. Through my research, I'd learned that some cancer patients taking FOLFIRINOX had to be hospitalized. Other patients—40 percent—are forced to change their FOLFIRINOX regimen because it is too harsh. Even though Lisa had been walloped by the first cycle, she was still standing... barely.

Before Dr. Beg disappeared, I insisted he evaluate Lisa's blood clots and ensure the port and catheter were properly placed. He conducted a physical exam and ordered an X-ray. This took longer, but I was satisfied when he said everything looked good. And he approved the oral blood thinner Xarelto Lisa was already taking. That was more good news.

Finally, at 10 a.m., the chemo started—or actually, the saline push. This was followed by anti-nausea drugs. Suddenly, I saw Lisa grow tired and fall asleep. Apparently, the anti-nausea drugs caused that reaction.

To pass the time, I read things on my phone and searched the internet. Lisa had material to read but she was too fatigued. Luckily, she slept well in this private infusion room. Seeing my wife asleep, I thought of everything we'd been through.

I had grown up in middle-class Jeannette, Pennsylvania, about thirty miles east of Pittsburgh. I was the oldest of six children—four sisters and a brother. Father was an engineer for Westinghouse and Mother a homemaker.

At one time, Jeannette was called the Glass City because it had at least seven glass factories. Plenty of tough, blue-collar residents helped build its reputation as a legendary football town. During my college summers off from the University of Pittsburgh, I worked in one of those factories, Jeannette Glass. It manufactured beer mugs, punch bowls, coffee mugs, and similar items. It was a hot and difficult job, especially since the melting point of glass is higher than steel.

With Jeannette's reputation for tough kids, Lisa's mother discouraged her from coming to the city. Thankfully, she ignored her mother's advice. She grew up in Irwin, Pennsylvania, about ten miles from Jeannette. Irwin was generally regarded as a "nicer" place. She lived in a middle-class neighborhood with her two younger brothers, Paul and Dan. During her teenage years, she worked summers at nearby Lincoln Hills Country Club as a bus girl while her mother worked as a telephone operator. Her father worked in a glass factory in Jeannette called the Window House, manufacturing plate glass for commercial and residential windows. The plates were massive and sometimes moved by workers using large suction cups. It was a dangerous job, as one dropped pane might slice off a foot or break up and slash the workers.

When I met Lisa, she was attending Westmoreland County Community College while working part-time as a salesperson at a local mall department store. Ultimately, she earned an associate's degree in retail management.

After college, I worked at American International Group (AIG) in downtown Pittsburgh. One day they told me I was being promoted to Dallas, Texas. The next thing I knew, I was loading up my car. At the time, I was 24 and living with my parents. I had $2,000 in the bank and a car payment on a brand-new white Monte Carlo, into which I loaded all my earthly possessions. I talked Lisa into coming to Dallas with me for one week to help set up my apartment. We stopped the first night in Memphis to tour Graceland. The next day, we arrived in Dallas and worked on my apartment. At the end of the week, I sent her back to Pennsylvania on a plane. We both knew it could be the end of our relationship, but that Christmas, I flew home and asked her to marry me. She said yes. The only problem was money: I had none of it. Lisa solved the problem by selling her car for $5,000 and using the money to buy a wedding ring. Maybe a little unconventional, but I wanted her to have a nice ring, even though she had to pay for it!

Back in Dallas, we had a justice of the peace marry us. I wore a nice suit for the occasion, and Lisa, who was almost 23, looked gorgeous in her wedding dress as she stood beside me in the courtroom.

Suddenly, we were man and wife. But it was April 1, so when we called our family, they thought it was an April Fool's joke. The rest of the details were fuzzy, but I remembered clearly promising to take care of her in sickness and health. Now, sitting in the infusion room, I thought of all the sacrifices she had made for my career by picking up and moving to some new town. She had also backed me both times when I invested our life savings to start two wholesale insurance brokerages from scratch. Those were two huge risks that eventually paid off. But we're never guaranteed a fairy tale. With this sickness invading my lovely wife, it was time for me to step up and affirm that commitment to take care of her no matter what.

The hours ticked by as the bags of medicine kept coming, dripping slowly down the long, clear tube into Lisa's body. The place was quiet. Being in a private room now, there was no interaction with other patients. At her first chemo session, I'd talked to a couple while Lisa was in the bathroom. The woman told me she had been on a two-week cruise and suffered indigestion but no pain. She had eaten everything in sight but lost weight. She knew something was wrong. When she returned to Dallas, she was diagnosed with pancreatic cancer, and Betam was her surgeon. I wondered how she was doing now.

Mercifully, this chemo session ended. The assistant strapped on the 5-FU brick and ensured it was working. However, it made a noticeable clicking sound when it injected the drug into Lisa. The first one had been mostly silent.

"Do you feel anything when it pumps the fluid?" I asked, concerned about this clicking sound.

"No, not at all," Lisa replied. That was good news.

Like that first time, they sent us home with a biohazard bag. "If this unit comes loose and the needle pulls out, use this biohazard bag to seal up the unit. You must prevent these chemicals from leaking onto you or someone else," the nurse warned us.

I shook my head. *You've got to be kidding me. This stuff will pollute the environment and possibly burn holes in my skin or the bedsheets, yet it's safe to go inside my wife?*

By 5 p.m., I had her back home and in bed. The powerful drugs and the time it took to administer the infusion had taken a real toll. It was difficult to watch.

———————————— ◈◈◈◈ ▮————————————

DAY 41 – WEDNESDAY, MARCH 25, 2020 – The 5-FU pack started beeping as we sat in the infusion room at UT Southwestern. The nurse removed the pack and gave Lisa one hour of IV fluids and more anti-nausea drugs. Just as we were getting ready to leave, the nurse stopped us. "I have to put on your Neulasta."

We had forgotten about that. The previous hospital didn't do it, but UT Southwestern wanted Lisa to have it. The Neulasta helped increase her white blood cell count so she could continue receiving this industrial-strength chemo.

The nurse brought over a small device and attached it to Lisa's abdomen using adhesive strips. "The Neulasta injector will deliver the drug into your abdomen twenty-seven hours from now. When you see the lights flashing and hear alarms beeping, you need to lie down flat and be still as the needle injects Neulasta into your abdomen. The injection process will take forty-five minutes. After it turns green and the level indicator shows empty, you can carefully remove the injector and place it in the biohazard bag. Bring it back to us for disposal."

I thought hard about this. The chemo lowered the white blood cell count, and this device raised it back. This whole chemo process was like lighting your house on fire and then walking inside with a fire extinguisher to save a special piece of furniture. I had no idea how Lisa would make it through all this, especially since we had just started and she felt so nauseous.

The nurse turned on the unit and soon a needle jabbed Lisa in the stomach. "What did it feel like?" I asked.

"Like someone snapping a rubber band on my stomach."

I guess that was somewhat bearable.

We returned home, and as usual, Lisa went straight to bed. I made sure she was comfortable and went upstairs to my office. I started searching on the internet and found the PDF from a presentation Dr. Zeh had made on the PanCAN.org site. It was called *Surgery for Pancreatic Cancer: Who? When? How?* I clicked on the document and got a clearer picture of what we faced. Ultimately, Lisa's surgery was defined as a modified Appleby procedure, similar to the Distal Pancreatectomy but with a Celiac Axis Resection (DP CAR). I could see the organs in color with an easy-to-understand explanation from the surgeon's point of view. I can't say I felt better, just more informed.

Chapter Eleven

Lisa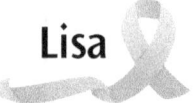

DAY 50 – FRIDAY, APRIL 3, 2020 – It was Friday and thankfully I felt halfway decent. I had learned that after a chemo session, days three through eight were the worst—constant nausea and fatigue. I was past that and didn't have another chemo session for two more days. I wanted to enjoy this time as best I could.

The pandemic had made video calls the norm, and yesterday, Robin and I had one with Dr. Zeh. We had sent in pages of questions beforehand and were thrilled that not only had Dr. Zeh read each page, but he had all the answers. It was as if he enjoyed the challenge of being tested.

During our conversation, we received a lot of information. My last CA 19-9 score was 71, which he said was not that high. He told me, "After the first three months of chemo, I want to cut your score in half. I want you to be under 38, in the normal range. I also want to see a good scan so we can proceed to surgery. But I won't do it unless I'm certain I can achieve an r0 margin." He reiterated that surgery was the best chance at my long-term survival.

We asked him about the length of chemo and he reconfirmed the six-month plan: six sessions every two weeks over three months before and after surgery. "There will be some radiation before surgery, maybe three to five treatments." We mentioned that we had recently been on a Zoom call with a doctor at the Texas Center for Proton Therapy. Dr. Zeh said, "I have no experience doing surgery after proton radiation therapy, so I'm recommending stereotactic radiation." We agreed. Robin and I didn't feel comfortable with proton radiation therapy, which seemed untested when dealing with pancreatic cancer. And we felt it made sense to keep our treatments in-house.

We learned Dr. Zeh had performed over 1,000 robotic surgeries and over 2,000 other surgeries. He reassured us that no residents would be involved. "It will be a two-person operation with Dr. Patricio Polanco assisting me." Like him, he told us that Dr. Polanco had trained at the University of Pittsburgh.

We asked him how long I would be in the hospital. "Five to seven days with no time in the ICU, hopefully. Then four to six weeks of recovery at home." Being home so quickly from the hospital sounded good. I could handle that.

Dr. Zeh explained that 60 to 70 percent of my pancreas would be removed. "The surgery shouldn't cause you to be on insulin or change your diet in any meaningful way. And the pancreas will drain enzymes after surgery, so I may send you home with a temporary tube."

Before we finished, he said I didn't need to store up blood in advance. "And with the biopsy of lymph nodes during surgery plus how the CA 19-9 behaves afterward, these will be important indicators that predict long-term survival. Of course, a low CA 19-9 and a resectable tumor are what we're shooting for."

It may be hard to believe, but we felt pretty good when we hung up. Robin typed it up and sent a mass email to friends and family. The only negative Robin added to the email was how hard the FOLFIRINOX had been on me—hair loss and thinning, bowel movement problems, debilitating nausea with vomiting, extreme fatigue, blood clots, and sensitivity to cold, not to mention that I had lost weight fast. Other than that, life was wonderful.

DAY 54 – TUESDAY, APRIL 7, 2020 – It was dark outside as I lay in bed. The last few days had been a whirlwind. On Sunday, Robin stopped by the Central Market grocery store and encountered lines of masked patrons stretched outside, spaced six feet apart. There were markers on the concrete indicating where you could stand. Workers feverishly sprayed and sanitized carts. It was surreal. Customers were being limited, so it took forever to get inside. He sent me photos from his cell phone. With the pandemic raging and me feeling so bad, I stayed inside until my next infusion or doctor appointment. There was no reason to leave the house.

On Monday, I had chemo session three. It started at 7 a.m., and I was back home in bed at 4 p.m. Of course, I slept through most of it except for the involuntary facial twitching and frozen mouth caused by the irinotecan portion of FOLFIRINOX. That was strange.

The private infusion room was nice because the nurse could monitor me better for side effects and problems. Thank you, UT Southwestern.

Then, this morning, I woke up to two gifts from Sue Thorsen, Robin's second oldest sister and her husband, Rick. They live in North Carolina. The first was a purple comfy blanket. The second was a bell. Her note said to ring it whenever I needed Robin to help me. I chuckled when I read that and, for sure, started ringing the bell. I was certain it would come in handy. Thank you, Sue and Rick!

Next up was a wooden box from Bill Edwards, Robin's brother-in-law. Bill has been battling prostate cancer for over a decade. He's a woodworker in his spare time. Apparently, this box had come from a unique piece of wood he'd been holding for just the right person. I guess he thought I was that person. It was a beautiful little box, exquisitely built. To receive something so personal and personally made was incredible. Thanks, Bill!

I thought of everything so far and how blessed I was, especially waking up every morning and reaching for my phone to see Adrienne's text waiting for me. But despite the love I felt from everyone, life was very hard.

———————————◈◈◈◈▮—————————

It was nighttime and I was in bed again. I had to lie on my back to keep the 5-FU pack from smashing into my stomach. But tomorrow afternoon, it would come off. I couldn't wait.

Suddenly, an alarm went off. It sounded like a smoke alarm when a battery died, but it was coming from my 5-FU pack. I crawled out of bed and went upstairs to Robin's office. "Hey, my pump is beeping."

He looked at it and rebooted the pack without resetting the time. They had given us instructions about this. The beeping stopped, and I went back to bed. Robin joined me shortly afterward.

Around 1 a.m., it started beeping again. I couldn't believe it.

This time, the reboot didn't stop it. Robin called a 1-800 number on the pack and talked to a tech. He had us check the tubes to make sure they weren't kinked. Then he told us to open the back of the unit, remove the batteries, and put them back in. We did, but it kept beeping. Nothing worked. Finally, he gave us instructions on how to shut off the device.

"Remember when I asked them why they used a different unit than we had at the first oncology center?" Robin asked me.

"Yeah," I replied. "They said they had so many problems with that model they switched to this one."

"Exactly. And now this one seems like a piece of junk. I'm calling the after-hours doctor at UT Southwestern."

Robin talked to the doctor and explained the situation. He instructed us on how to clamp down all the lines and said to come in first thing in the morning. He reminded us that 5-FU is meant to be delivered slowly. It scared us when he emphasized how fluid could quickly back up into my port if we didn't have this done. We tried to get back to sleep, but once again, it was stressful and hard.

DAY 55 – WEDNESDAY, APRIL 8, 2020 – We arrived back at the infusion room at 6:30 a.m. The place was vacant. Robin reminded me that last night the doctor had said he didn't think this little glitch would cause the 5-FU delivery to be ineffective but added, "There are no studies on it."

Research hospitals! Everything's a study.

At 6:45 a.m., our assigned nurse arrived, surprised to see us. She immediately punched in and began helping me. "How are you feeling?" she asked.

"I feel terrible and almost threw up on the way over," I told her.

"I'm so sorry. I'll check with the oncologist's nurse practitioner and find out the protocol for an interrupted treatment."

It turned out that I had received only 30.5 hours of 5-FU. They pulled out a new pack and set it to deliver another 15.5 hours. Then they gave me more IV fluids and anti-nausea medication. A few hours later, we were back home, knowing that tonight, at 1 a.m., the pack would beep, signaling it was done. We planned to shut it off and be back here again at 7 a.m. to disconnect the pack and receive the Neulasta injector. What a grind.

DAY 58 – Saturday, April 11, 2020 – My birthday finally arrived. I was greeted with the news that the Simmons Cancer Center at UT Southwestern was shutting out visitors due to the pandemic. That meant Robin would not be able to attend chemo sessions with me. This depressed me.

The sun rose, but I stayed in bed. I felt terrible. The nausea was always with me. Forget even looking at a birthday cake. And I was beginning to doubt my ability to make it through six full sessions of FOLFIRINOX.

To take my mind off it, I thought about how Robin had wanted to get married on my birthday so he could always remember our anniversary. I had put my foot down because I didn't want to be cheated out of receiving two separate presents, which likely would've happened. Thinking about it now, it all seems so silly. Then there was our unique marriage ceremony. The downtown judge who'd married us had just finished a racquetball game and his hair was wet from showering. That had stuck in my mind all these years.

Dallas had been great for us as young people. We had lots of fun living in an apartment in the Village. The area was trendy and happening, with plenty of young people hanging out by the pools. We had a wonderful time.

My mind snapped back to reality as I heard Robin cleaning a toilet. Just another depressing thought. Like all marriages, we had made a silent bargain—an unwritten contract—about dividing up responsibilities. He handled the finances and yardwork—anything outside. I took care of everything inside. Since chemo had started, I spent most of every day and night in bed listening to Robin doing the laundry, cooking, and cleaning, all the things I used to do. When he came in to ask which button to press on the washing machine, I could feel his frustration. Watching him do all this work made me feel guilty, which added to my misery.

Before the diagnosis, we had plans for me to retire and do some traveling. Now all that seemed out the window. Even though I didn't feel I'd done anything to cause my cancer, I still felt deep guilt. And I couldn't help but think Robin might soon have to plan my funeral. Then he'd be alone doing all the household chores while answering a constantly ringing doorbell from a line of single women holding casserole dishes.

I thought back to my father and mother. Having endured the Great Depression and World War II rationing, Mom and Dad both worked and never called in sick. They never complained or cried about the straws of life they'd drawn. They just rolled out of bed at the crack of dawn and did what had to be done, surviving each day only to wake up and have to survive the next one. They spent their lives honoring that silent bargain because they had no choice.

Then, one day in 1979, Mom was sitting in the kitchen and passed out. Luckily, one of the neighbors was there having coffee. They rushed Mom to the hospital, where the doctors found a spot on her brain. They wanted to keep an eye on it and do occasional scans. In 1985, it started to grow, and they admitted her so they could take a sample with a biopsy. My father went to pick her up the next morning. When he arrived at the hospital, he learned she had just suffered a massive stroke. She never talked after that day and could barely walk. Suddenly, Dad was left to care for Mom while holding down a full-time job.

I was 27 and living in Dallas, so I couldn't do much. My younger siblings and neighbors pitched in to help. Dad took a night shift so he could be home to care for Mom all day. He had to keep his job because they needed his weekly paycheck to survive.

It was confirmed she had brain cancer, so they put Mom through radiation and chemo. I recall Dad commenting that all this would not have a happy ending. He was right. Two years later, God took Mom away. She was only 56.

At the time, I had imagined what it would be like to be in bed next to your spouse, knowing she couldn't talk or care for herself, just lying there suffering until she died. That's what I felt Robin would have to go through, and that scared me. All I could do was cry every night and pray to God I'd make it.

Chapter Twelve

Robin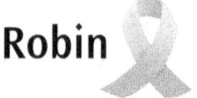

DAY 60 – MONDAY, APRIL 13, 2020 – Lisa was crashing. She gagged and threw up after eating anything, even half a popsicle. She drank very little water, which came back up most of the time. She was suffering from extreme nausea and debilitating fatigue, and she rarely got out of bed. This FOLFIRINOX was literally killing her. I had to do something.

Lisa's manager, Hartwell Lewis, sent a video to encourage her. He had been on FOLFIRINOX for colon cancer but was forced to change the formula due to liver damage. I got Lisa into the car and once again drove her to the UT Southwestern Cancer Center for emergency treatment. Once there, they pumped bags of fluids with anti-nausea medication into her for two hours. After Lisa looked somewhat revived, the nurse discussed whether she could continue on FOLFIRINOX. I was leaning toward no. Lisa didn't answer. Instead, we silently drove home.

———— ⬥⬥⬥⬥ ————

DAY 64 – FRIDAY, APRIL 17, 2020 – A lot had happened in the last four days and Lisa was still ill with diarrhea and vomiting. She was down to 103 pounds and withering away. A new regimen of anti-nausea drugs was basically worthless. We had to do something.

The morning after our UT Southwestern emergency visit, Lisa was marginally better, although she still couldn't get out of bed. I was certain she needed to go back for another infusion of fluids, so I called the nurse, who had me take her blood pressure and pulse. Both were normal. We agreed to have Lisa attempt to eat and drink something small every thirty minutes. Still, it was hard for her to do that without throwing up. With the nausea and weight loss, Lisa grew depressed. Things were spiraling out of control.

Lisa was scheduled to start her fourth chemo session on the 20th but I knew she couldn't make it. After discussing her case with his team, Dr. Beg agreed she needed a week off from the chemo regimen. He told us he would make a dose modification for her next chemo session, which was rescheduled for April 27.

We told him we were sending Lisa's records to Johns Hopkins for their thoughts. Dr. Beg was on board with that. Then he shifted to Lisa's deteriorating condition. He said the choices were simple: (1) stay the course, which didn't seem possible, (2) reduce each drug by a certain percentage, (3) eliminate one drug, or (4) switch to gemcitabine. Dr. Beg was worried about her weight loss because she couldn't have surgery if she lost too much. We discussed the tradeoffs and pros and cons. We didn't want to switch to gemcitabine because we needed to keep that in reserve as a second-line chemo drug. Dr. Beg said he would choose to eliminate oxaliplatin. It's the roughest on patients and can contribute to nausea. The resulting cocktail, FOLFIRI, was still potent. "We need to get her eating and functioning again," Dr. Beg said. "Eliminating this drug is our best chance for that."

After discussing this strategy, Lisa agreed. It was a very traumatic moment during her treatment. She was on a full dose of FOLFIRINOX because it gave her the best chance for survival. Once we abandoned that, how did the survival rate look? We were all concerned, but it was clear there was no way she could continue like this.

I called Johns Hopkins and ran all this by them. They agreed with the changes. When I asked them if they knew our surgeon, Dr. Zeh, they said, "Oh yes, we know Herbie. You're in good hands." Dr. Zeh had spent eight years at Johns Hopkins and was still remembered in a positive light. I felt great hearing that.

During that stressful time, three UT Southwestern nurses called to check in with Lisa. We were impressed with all the first-class service.

***

DAY 67 – MONDAY, APRIL 20, 2020 – Although Lisa was up and around some, there was no possible way she could have endured her scheduled chemo treatment. She was still very weak and fatigued and spent a lot of time in bed. In addition to her normal anti-nausea medications, such as

Compazine, Zofran, Ativan, and the Sancuso patch (there were many more along the way), we put raw peppermint oil on cotton balls and had her sniff it. It helped her nausea a little bit.

As I watched her inhale the peppermint oil, a thought struck me. All the torture she'd endured had nothing to do with her cancer. It was from the chemo. We were fighting the cure and not the disease.

Huh.

———————————————— ⊕⊕⊕⊕ ————————————————

DAY 74 – MONDAY, APRIL 27, 2020 – Once again, we headed to UT Southwestern, this time for Lisa's fourth chemo session. I wasn't able to accompany her inside because of the pandemic. This upset both of us. After everything she'd been through, I wanted to be with her. Instead, we communicated through FaceTime during her lab work and oncology visit. Once she began her infusion, I wasn't able to communicate with her. Apparently the walls of her private room were lined with lead because it used to be part of a radiology lab, so this blocked all calls. Left with no choice, I sat in the park across the street and waited for her treatment to end.

We were very concerned the treatment was less effective without oxaliplatin, although no study was available to support that. The good news was that this past Monday (the day of her canceled chemo session), Lisa had not thrown up for the first time in almost a week. And she was up and around most of the day. She ate some small bland meals and took her anti-nausea medicine. The nurses wanted her to keep something in her stomach but not get full.

Since Lisa was now receiving chemo on the 27th, we had to cancel our previously scheduled scan for that day. Due to the pandemic, it took some work to get it rescheduled. We also tried to set up a Zoom call with Johns Hopkins, but the laws of Maryland and Texas did not allow doctors to perform telemedicine between them. I never understood that. It was nuts! My unofficial conversations with Johns Hopkins were about to come to an end.

By now, the medical bills were rolling in. I learned that the health-care industry is the only industry that provides services without disclosing costs upfront. At least I had an insurance company to review each one and work things out. I was lucky, especially when so many patients lacked proper healthcare insurance and our resources. I knew I shouldn't complain—too much.

Even though Dr. Zeh advised against Proton Therapy, we decided to check it out a little more just in case. On the 21st, we had a video conference with Dr. Jared Sturgeon of the Texas Center for Proton Therapy. Although he was informative, there were a lot of unknowns. UT Southwestern did not have this technology. There was no study we could rely on. Plus, the Texas Center for Proton Therapy didn't appear to have a high volume of pancreatic cancer patients. It seemed to target other types of cancer. It was potentially better, but with a lack of history plus the increased possibility of fibrosis and other unknowns, we decided to keep our radiation therapy at UT Southwestern.

By Wednesday, Lisa felt a little better, though she now suffered from acid reflux, most likely caused by the chemotherapy. She had to sleep sitting up half the night.

We learned that chemo drugs target rapidly dividing cells. The drugs can't distinguish between normal, rapidly dividing cells and cancer cells, so the drugs attack them all. FOLFIRINOX is primarily used to treat gastrointestinal cancers. When cells lining the gastrointestinal tract are damaged, corrosive stomach acid can flow into your esophagus instead of being carefully contained. It's counterintuitive, but in Lisa's case, the acid reflux likely resulted from not having enough stomach acid and/or digestive enzymes to properly digest her food. We believe the lack of stomach acid was caused by her FOLFIRINOX treatments, but it could also be a symptom of a compromised pancreas. It was just another thing Lisa had to suffer through.

We also found out that light-colored or floating stools likely meant the food was not being adequately digested. Thus, she may not have been receiving the proper nutrients. To counter this, she took the enzyme ZENPEP to aid digestion.

By far, the most exciting and promising news was her new CA 19-9 reading. It was 37.9 (the normal range is below 38). This was down from 51.5 and a UT Southwestern high of 71. We were excited to see that and to know that the chemotherapy seemed to be working.

Because she wasn't having oxaliplatin administered, we saved over two hours at UT Southwestern. By 1 p.m., we were home and Lisa was back in bed. After starting a load of laundry, I went to my study to update my notes and do more research. Then I received a call from my good friend Mark Falatovich, with whom I'd been friends since high school. We'd been on the golf team together and had often spent the summer days playing thirty-six holes and enjoying life. Man, that seemed so far away right now.

Mark had gone into IT management and worked for some big companies. Like us, he and his wife, Celeste, had been married for over thirty-five years. When Lisa was diagnosed, Mark reminded me of his mother's story. I'll let him tell it in his own voice…

… Mom was 87 and living in Pittsburgh when she appeared jaundiced. It was mid-April 2016 when my two older sisters took Mom to her primary care physician. After examining her, the doctor sent her for an ultrasound. Then they had her go back to the waiting room with my sisters. The phone rang for the receptionist and she motioned one of my sisters to the counter. "It's for you."

The doctor told her that Mom had pancreatic cancer. As my sister lowered the receiver, her eyes filled with tears. "It's cancer," my mother said. My sister nodded. Incredibly, there was no doctor or personal visit—just a phone call.

Mom went to an oncologist who confirmed the diagnosis through a blood test. He told Mom that given her age and the fact that the tumor encroached on a vein, she wasn't a candidate for surgery. "We could administer radiation and give her some chemo, but it won't change the prognosis. I recommend focusing on her diet to gain weight and increase her appetite." Then he discussed hospice options.

The next week, Mom collapsed at home. They rushed her to the hospital and performed surgery to remove some fluid. They went ahead and installed a port for chemo.

Staring at the end, I returned home and told Mom the derby was coming up. She loved going to the track and casinos and betting on things. "You want to pick a trifecta for the derby?" I asked her. She did, so I bought a racing program and gave it to her. She picked the trifecta and hit it. The two-dollar bet returned over a hundred bucks! It was unbelievable. But that's what I remember about Mom: she just wanted to do what she wanted to do.

Over the next month, Mom continued collapsing due to dehydration. The oncologist reiterated, "If it were my mother, I would focus on making her as comfortable as possible."

She had an appointment for June 17 but died on June 13, just eight weeks after her diagnosis. A week later, my father-in-law needed surgery to remove a large tumor. After the surgery, he never fully recovered and spent his last days in a hospital or hospice. He died three months after my mother. This meant my children had lost two grandparents in a very short time.

Based on my experience with these deaths, I suggest you repeat to the doctor what you just heard because it might not be what he said or meant to say. And to the doctors, I would say phoning a patient in your waiting room and telling them they have pancreatic cancer is not appropriate or professional, maybe even immoral. Finally, I recommend you spend whatever time you can with your loved ones *before* you get that news. Enjoy it so you never have regrets…

***

Mark's story reminded me that on this journey, nothing was guaranteed. I was even more determined to give my wife the best odds of beating this disease.

We did receive some good news about another issue. Before Lisa was diagnosed with pancreatic cancer, she had a faint red spot on her forehead resembling a basal cell carcinoma that was removed from her hand a few years back. After the pancreatic cancer diagnosis and Coronavirus issues, we forgot about it. But last week, that small, almost unnoticeable spot on her forehead became red and angry, growing larger. It concerned us.

A few days later, the mark started disappearing. Dr. Beg's nurse practitioner looked at it and said the spot appeared to be a basal cell carcinoma, and the chemo may have killed it. "A two-for-one!" she declared.

So there's that.

Chapter Thirteen

Lisa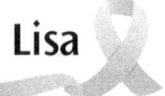

D AY 75 – Tuesday, April 28 – I endured a shortened chemo session yesterday. My CA 19-9 was down to a normal range and the agreement to remove oxaliplatin from my chemo regimen had me feeling better. With a fanny pack of 5-FU strapped around my waist, I took a short walk outside for the first time in months. Though I'd have to return to UT Southwestern tomorrow to have the pump removed and my Neulasta injector attached, today, at least, I breathed some fresh air.

As I walked through the neighborhood, I thought about working at Marsh. I had been planning to retire at the end of 2020. Our first oncologist had said, "I don't recommend patients quit work because they need something to do." I liked hearing that. Then there was that saying, "If you want to make God laugh, tell Him *your* plans for *your* life." So much for working until the end of the year. Cancer changes everything.

It was an easy decision. Robin and I knew I couldn't continue working while fighting this disease and still receive the proper care. I was blessed that losing my salary would not impact us financially. Another reason to retire was Marsh itself. The company had been so good to me that there was no reason to string them along and make them keep my position open. I decided to retire effective May 1, 2020. Still, it was traumatic to face the fact that I would have no job after a lifetime of working. What made it worse was that I wasn't making the decision on my own terms.

Robin helped me get the paperwork started. After twenty-three years, I'd reached the assistant vice president and client representative level and secured two important professional designations—CPCU and ARM. Before my diagnosis, I couldn't remember ever missing a day of work. Because of my tenure, I was eligible for Retired Employee Medical Benefits and able to keep my insurance at a slightly increased rate. That was a valuable and important benefit. I'd been on short-term disability for the last two months and was able to continue my insurance without interruption.

Now that I felt slightly better, it was time for Robin to get out and play golf. He had been so devoted to my care 24/7 that he needed to recharge his batteries. I could tell he was suffering. He needed some social interaction. With the pandemic and my cancer making those connections almost impossible, golf was the perfect antidote. It was outside and people could space themselves six feet or more apart. Unfortunately, we still didn't know how transmissible COVID-19 was by touching objects or other people. This led to the closing of the pro shops. Carts were locked up and unavailable. Flags were secured so the golfers couldn't lift them out, and tiny Styrofoam donuts were placed in the holes, forcing the golf ball back out and stopping golfers from touching the holes. Some players were out on the course, but not many, since you had to walk or pull your bag of clubs, not to mention the ever-present fear of COVID. Still, Robin got out there with a few brave souls and played golf. It wasn't perfect, but at least he had some leisure time.

———————— ◈◈◈◈ ————————

Having a husband take care of me showed me a facet of cancer that's often overlooked: the caregivers. They can run themselves into the ground. Without a chance to relax and recover, they might find themselves sick and depressed, and then they're of little help to their loved ones. Their mental health is as important as the sick person's physical health.

For the past two months, Robin's only human connection had been me. Yet I was mostly in bed, suffering, unable to provide him with any meaningful companionship. It returned me to that unwritten contract that we would experience life together, solve problems, travel, and have fun. Now I wasn't holding up my end of the bargain. There were times I asked him just to leave me alone. I was so sick and tired of suffering. Yet the sun had come out again and I felt a little better. With that, Robin loaded up his clubs and took off for the golf course. I was thrilled for him. If anyone deserved some fun, it was Robin.

Once he'd had some leisure time on the golf course, he was back at the computer. While searching for a cure, Robin checked out some clinical trials that might fit me. PanCAN sent him an email that read:

Pancreatic cancer patients who participate in clinical research have better outcomes. Every treatment available today was approved through a clinical trial.

That led us to a call from our radiation oncologist. During the conversation, Dr. Aguilera discussed a potential clinical trial that might be right for me. It was a "Phase I/II Dose Escalation Trial of Stereotactic Body Radiation Therapy in combination with Radiomodulating Agent GC4419 in Locally Advanced Pancreatic Adenocarcinoma." Definitely a mouthful.

It was a research study to find out if a drug called GC4419 could help prevent side effects commonly seen in radiation therapy that stop patients from being able to receive higher doses of radiation. By now, Robin had learned a lot about clinical trials, and so had I, when I was awake and felt like reading anything. Clinical trials are conducted in phases, each addressing a different research question. The phases, as described by PanCAN, include:

Phase I – Studying the treatment's safety, dose, and side effects

Phase II – Studying the treatment's effect on the cancer

Phase III – Studying if the treatment is more effective than the current standard of care treatment

Phase IV – Studying the long-term safety and side effects after FDA approval

Since I still suffered terribly from chemotherapy, it was hard to be very enthusiastic about signing up for this experimental treatment. And my radiation treatments were a little ways off. Ultimately, we felt it was best to proceed with the current radiation treatment protocol and declined participation in this trial. These are the personal decisions cancer patients have to contend with on a regular basis.

***

DAY 83 – WEDNESDAY, MAY 6, 2020 – I had just endured days three through eight after my fourth chemo session. Without the oxaliplatin, it was better, but not by a lot. I still had waves of nausea and floating stools and was bedridden most of the time.

To brighten me up, professional running back James Conner texted me a personal video of encouragement. He had been diagnosed with Hodgkin's lymphoma, a deadly blood cancer, while playing for the University of Pittsburgh. Doctors found tumors nestled around his heart. When he asked how bad it was, the doctor said, "You have one week to live if you don't get treatment right now."

Not only did he beat cancer, but he played football again and was good enough to be drafted in the third round by the Pittsburgh Steelers. (As of this writing, he plays for the Arizona Cardinals.) Watching him mention my name on the video and tell me to hang in there was uplifting and inspiring. It was a very cool thing for James to do. I recorded a thank you video and sent it back to him. (Thank you so much, James! Also, thanks to Pat Bostick, Chris McFarlane, Athletic Director Heather Lyke, and our other friends at the University of Pittsburgh for setting that up.)

After that excitement, Robin helped me outside to see another inspiring event. The Navy's Blue Angels performed a flyover saluting Dallas's frontline pandemic workers. What those workers endured was extremely tough. It was courageous to treat patients knowing they might contract COVID and possibly die. Sadly, some of the doctors and nurses did die. They took their last breath without family and friends, usually alone with a fellow healthcare provider next to them. They deserved the flyover and so much more.

Later that afternoon, we heard from a Johns Hopkins scheduler, who set up an appointment for the end of June. Their doctors still couldn't telemedicine with us since they had licensing issues operating between Maryland and Texas. The pandemic was causing a lot of issues we never dreamed of. I wasn't sure we'd be able to see them in June, but at least we had an appointment.

Going back to the nausea, it was one of the battles I fought almost every day. We tried everything. Robin searched online and found these little hard candies called Queasy Drops. I ate them like M&Ms and they helped. Another trick that worked was peppermint oil. After dipping some of it into a cotton ball, I smelled the fumes and leaned back in bed, hoping the nausea would disappear. Sometimes it did because it gave me something to concentrate on. I wasn't just lying there feeling sick; my mind was doing something.

I learned that each person deals with nausea differently. Mostly, I just fought through it, though the cumulative effect of chemo made it almost impossible.

The doctors gave me various pills to beat the nausea. One of these was an antipsychotic drug called olanzapine. It spaced me out and made me extremely tired. I remember doing something in the garage and calling Robin to come get me. He practically had to carry me back to bed. It also made me emotional and weepy while doing absolutely nothing for the nausea. When I sobered up, I decided the cure was worse than the disease. After that one pill, I never took another. If you experience nausea, the doctors will keep trying different drugs to see what works. Sadly, none of them ever worked for me.

Last but not least, I was given a prescription for synthetic marijuana. I got the prescription filled and put it in my refrigerator. I started thinking about it and became afraid to take it. A relative in Washington (State) bought some liquid THC, among other authentic marijuana products, and sent it to us. I didn't try the liquid THC but Robin did. He said it relaxed him. A friend's father in Nevada sent us some cannabis-infused gummies. I took half a gummy at night to help me sleep. It calmed me and provided some relief. I never took it during the day, though, as it didn't seem to do much for my nausea. If you haven't taken marijuana products before, be careful of the dosage. Start small and understand it takes some time to kick in.

For anyone going through this, try anything and everything. That's the best way to get through it.

Chapter Fourteen

Robin

DAY 85 – FRIDAY, MAY 8, 2020 – I watched Lisa step on the scale and saw her weight had dropped from 115 to 102. I knew chemo was brutal, but Lisa's side effects were untenable. She had been bedridden or semi-bedridden for the past two months, including two emergency clinic visits to control her nausea. Her inability to process or keep down food was slowly killing her.

As Lisa struggled, we talked about stopping the chemotherapy. We spoke to Dr. Zeh about our options. If she got worse, we could move up the surgery. But that would be a last resort. We all understood the importance of continuing chemo and pushing the boundaries of her endurance.

The uplifting video from James Conner had been a blessing. He said, "Hey Lisa, how you doing? This is James Conner, running back for the Pittsburgh Steelers. I'm here to send you well wishes and tell you to keep going strong. I've been in your shoes before and I know it's getting tough, but just keep fighting through those treatments. It'll be a distant memory soon. I definitely will say a prayer for you. I just want to tell you to keep going strong, Lisa. Keep the faith."

Lisa responded with a video of her own. "Hi James, this is Lisa. Thank you so much for making the video for me. It really meant a lot to hear from you. I see you're having a birthday next week and I hope you have a happy 25th birthday. Chris, thanks for sending this to me. Go Steelers, and go Pitt!"

My friends at Pitt told me no one had ever sent a video back. Apparently, it meant a lot to James.

That video and Adrienne's daily texts helped Lisa inch her way forward each morning. It was tough, but she tried not to look at the big mountain ahead. Instead, she just focused on what was right in front of her.

During a brief window one day, Lisa felt well enough to take a rare short walk. With her 5-FU pump strapped on and me holding her hand, it was good to get some fresh air together. As we walked, I thought about how, just a few months earlier, she hadn't been taking a single pill. So far that day, she had taken Xarelto, dexamethasone (steroid), Pepcid AC, ZENPEP, Compazine, and a Sancuso patch applied that morning. Later in the evening, she would take Ativan, and tomorrow she'd have the Neulasta injector attached. She was a walking pharmacy.

———————————— ◉◉◉◉ ▬————————————

It was easy to be focused on our own issues, but one of my longtime friends reminded me that a lot of folks deal with cancer in one way or another. Michael Donohoe has been a good friend of mine for the past thirty years, and he has his own cancer story, as I'll share here in his words…

…In early 2013, just after New Year's Eve, I became sick with flu-like symptoms. It was bad. A few weeks later, I went on a business trip and felt horrible. When I returned to Dallas, I saw my primary care doctor. He ordered some blood tests and called me when the results came in. "I see something I don't like. It's probably nothing, but I want you to see a hematologist-oncologist."

I went to see this guy and he said, "It's probably nothing, but you've got something going on here that I want to look at. I want to schedule a bone marrow biopsy just to see."

Wow! I thought. *That's serious.* "How bad is it?" I asked.

"Oh, you're going to be fine. Don't worry about it. I just want to do this and see where we are."

I left his office and dragged my feet on getting it done. Ten days later, Saturday—7 a.m., I was upstairs in our house and couldn't sleep, so I decided to get up. As I descended the stairs, I passed out and fell awkwardly to the bottom landing. When I regained consciousness, I found my leg twisted underneath my body. I was a mess.

I dragged myself back into the bedroom and woke my wife, Linda. "I've messed up my leg," I told her. "I feel like crap."

She called a friend of ours who's an orthopedist. He said, "I'm going to be in the neighborhood. I'll come by and take a look."

Around eleven that morning, he arrived and studied my leg. By now, it had swollen up like a balloon. "Well, you've obviously done something really bad there. But that's just carpentry. Something else is wrong because you're pretty sick. You need to go to the hospital and we'll figure out the leg later."

We called the doctor, who wanted to do a bone marrow biopsy. He had privileges at a hospital close to my house, so we drove there and checked in. The ER doctor examined my leg and ran some tests. Then they admitted me to a private room. As I sat in bed, I studied the facility. It was an old building, definitely not modern. That concerned me. I was also on a floor with a whole bunch of other people with all kinds of different illnesses. I heard coughing and screaming. I felt like I was in one of those mental hospitals you see in movies where I was the only sane person.

Sunday, the doctor finally appeared and performed the bone marrow biopsy. On Monday morning, he came into my room and sat in one of the chairs.

"What's the story?" I asked.

He frowned. "Let's just wait until your wife comes in." When she arrived, he announced, "You've got acute myeloid leukemia. AML."

My wife and I looked at each other with puzzled faces. "Okay, what's that? What do we do? How do we fix this?"

The doctor cleared his throat. "It's a blood cancer. I want to start you on chemo right away."

I looked at him and said, "Whoa, whoa, whoa. We need to think about this."

He understood and left. Linda didn't care for the guy, so she spent the next twenty-four hours researching AML. My wife also hated this hospital. She didn't feel comfortable, and neither did I. Back home, she worked the phones and got referrals all over town. We were blessed that we had so many friends.

On Thursday morning, Linda called me at the hospital and said, "I found the guy we need. He's downtown Dallas at Baylor Hospital. I have an ambulance picking you up at nine and taking you there. They're printing out all your records. You're going to take those with you. Be ready."

I was. I'd been in the hospital for almost a week and was on four different antibiotics because I was so infected. And the doctors had determined that I had a torn ACL and PCL in my knee. I was in an awful way and couldn't wait to leave this Soviet Union-style hospital.

When I arrived at Baylor and met the new doctor, I told him the other doctor had used a drill to do the bone marrow biopsy and he had planned to do a spinal tap with the same drill. He inspected the site and freaked out. "Oh my God, that's so out of date. Drilling was something we did a long time ago. But now we've learned if you have cancerous cells in your body, you don't want to open a path into your spinal column to let those cells in, so no one drills anymore. At least, that's what I thought until a second ago."

He explained that spinal taps were now done with needles. "I learn much more from a needle biopsy because I have clean samples."

It didn't take long to see the differences in care from one doctor and hospital to another.

After he checked everything out, he started the chemo a few days later. The chemo was designed to shut down my bone marrow so I wasn't producing anything because leukemia produced the wrong stuff. My bone marrow was kicking out "blasts." It wasn't good for my body, as the white blood cells were overwhelmed. To deal with this, the chemo regimen for AML was a 24/7, seven-day treatment. It was more aggressive than most chemotherapies.

They basically told me, "We're going to try and kill you. If you live, we'll let your body rebuild itself."

It took about twenty-five days, but sure enough, my bone marrow returned and started producing the white blood cells with none of the bad stuff. It worked for me. Between those two different facilities, I was in the hospital for about forty days.

The chemo I received would've been the same mix anywhere. But that wasn't the whole story. The nursing care I received at Baylor was top-notch. And I was also on a blood cancer wing. This floor had patient rooms with positive air pressure to push the air out into the halls, which kept infections and germs from coming into the room. Also, this floor did not have people infected with other diseases. That helped patients like me since my immune system was offline, putting me at a greater risk of infection. Compared to the first hospital, I'd been better off staying at a Holiday Inn with a bushel of COVID victims. I mean, it was better than a third-world hospital, but not by much. For one, they didn't have state-of-the-art equipment.

I thanked my wife since it was because of her that I had received the best care. Based on this experience, I told Robin early on to "Find the right doctor. Find the right place. And find them fast!" I attributed my good outcome to that strategy.

Once out of the hospital, I went through three more rounds of chemo and came out six years later cancer-free with a full release—a clean bill of health. But until you go through it, you don't understand how the health system works…

———— ◉◉◉◉ ————

DAY 85 – FRIDAY, MAY 8, 2020 – Yesterday, we went to UT Southwestern so Lisa could have her CT scan. Today, we had a Zoom call with Dr. Zeh and Lan Vu, his physician assistant.

"The body of Lisa's tumor has measurably shrunk," Dr. Zeh said, sounding very positive. "It's still butting up against, but not encasing, the superior mesenteric artery. When the body of the tumor shrinks, this is common." He emphasized that the chemo was working well and Lisa needed to tough it out for the next month. She would also need three months of chemo after the surgery.

I asked him about our concern for removing oxaliplatin from the regimen and he said there was no real study that showed the remaining cocktail of drugs would not be as effective; it seemed that no one really knew. "But coupled with her CA 19-9 dropping back to normal from 71 to her most recent reading of 37.6, this shrinkage is very exciting."

He also said there was a slight chance Lisa's CA 19-9 might jump back up, but with continued treatments, he hoped that wouldn't happen. Also, the tumor was in a position where he felt even more comfortable performing surgery. Still, the next two chemo treatments were needed to kill any micro-metastases (tiny cancer cells) roaming around the body, as 85 percent of pancreatic cancer patients had these.

I asked him about the surgery and he said it would most likely be a simple distal pancreatectomy. The modified Appleby may not be needed. If this held, it would be less invasive than the modified Appleby. That was the best option Lisa could have. He confirmed the surgery would be done via robot. This would greatly reduce her recovery time. He was still 50 to 70 percent sure that Lisa would need some radiation before surgery, whereas previously, he'd been 100 percent sure. "After the chemo ends," he said, "let's restage in one month and revisit everything."

He closed by talking about Lisa's weight loss. He wasn't concerned—*yet*. He also loved the video from James Conner since Dr. Zeh was from Pittsburgh.

After finishing with him, I got a disc of Lisa's scan and sent it to Johns Hopkins. They looked at it and backed up Dr. Zeh. I had told Dr. Zeh we were consulting with Johns Hopkins and were considering flying up there. He said, "I spent eight years at Johns Hopkins. The top surgeon, the guy who was the head of pancreatic cancer, he's not there anymore. And the other two surgeons there, I trained both of them. So go up there if you feel more comfortable." The way he said it in his cocky-yet-confident manner made me trust him even more. I asked myself why I would load up the fishing boat and cruise an hour across the lake to where the trophy fish were supposed to be when the biggest bass in the lake was right here in my own marina.

By mid-May, we had ended our relationship with Johns Hopkins. They sent me a bill, which I paid. It was nice having them looking over our shoulder, but with the pandemic restricting everything, we had to go with UT Southwestern and hope they knew what they were doing. I was pretty sure they did.

Chapter Fifteen

Lisa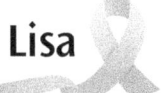

DAY 88 – MONDAY, MAY 11, 2020 – Today, I finished round five of my chemo. With the oxaliplatin gone, it helped a lot to finish much earlier.

Dr. Beg, my oncologist, talked to me before the infusion started. He said my tumor had shrunk about 35 percent. He felt everything had been progressing quite nicely, even though he was unsure how the tumor was reacting to the reduced chemo regimen. "Don't feel bad," he said. "Fifty percent of patients don't complete the full FOLFIRINOX regimen."

We discussed my weight loss. Even though I was taking digestive enzymes to help process food, Dr. Beg said the tumor caused inflammation of the entire pancreas and thus compromised my digestive system. "After surgery, the remaining pancreas usually returns to functioning normally." That was amazing and good to hear.

I slept through most of the infusion session and went outside so Robin could pick me up. He told me that while he'd been waiting in the park, he had befriended an oversized squirrel. I studied the photo of his friendly squirrel and smiled. As soon as I got my seatbelt on, I rolled my head over and fell asleep. I don't remember much after that.

DAY 93 – SATURDAY, MAY 16, 2020 – Robin and I met with a new doctor two days ago, a specialist in palliative care. The sole intent of the meeting was to discuss possible solutions to my ongoing nausea. He suggested a couple of new drugs that might keep the nausea at bay. Unfortunately, he also felt the need to focus on Directives to Physicians (Living Wills), Medical Powers of Attorney, HIPAA, and more. Robin and I thought it was an untimely discussion, especially since we had copies of all that in our medical file. It was like saying, "I just want to make sure you've planned for your death." The way he approached it upset us both.

At my meeting with Dr. Beg, I learned that my CA 19-9 was down to 27.8, well below the upper limit of 38 and down from my last reading of 37.6. That excited me. It also gave me hope the new FOLFIRI regimen was working.

The written explanation from my May 6 CT scan arrived. As we read it, we were stunned to learn that I had growths in my lung. One of the organs pancreatic cancer spreads to is the lungs. Robin panicked, thinking my cancer had metastasized. We checked with our doctors and researched more about these growths. They were called pulmonary nodules. The nodules were never discussed in the February 14 or February 28 reports, which had been completed at our first medical facility before we started at UT Southwestern. We quickly provided these scans to Dr. Beg, Dr. Zeh and our radiation oncologist at UT Southwestern. This reminded me to be sure Dr. Beg and Dr. Zeh received all our past scans and records.

We emailed Dr. Zeh about the pulmonary nodules, who responded immediately on Sunday night. He said most people who grew up in Pittsburgh have them. Even though he may have been half-kidding and we hadn't grown up in a polluted area, we understood his point. They were likely harmless; at least, that's what we believed. It was just another thing to get stressed about in a long line of scary events. However, we would continue monitoring the nodules for any changes in the future.

In the same email exchange, Robin wondered if a PET scan might help see the cancer more accurately. Dr. Zeh replied, "With the exception of a very few narrow indications, PET scans are not helpful in pancreatic cancer."

Sometime later, Robin again pushed the idea of a PET, and Dr. Zeh responded,

> I have never used PET scans for staging or surveillance of pancreatic cancer. I do not believe that there is any evidence that it provides increased sensitivity or specificity in this disease (in fact, there is some evidence that 40 percent of primary pancreatic cancers are not FDG-avid.)

We looked at some notes in the PanCAN.org section regarding PET scans:

- For pancreatic cancer diagnoses, CT scans are more common than PET scans. A PET test is usually used with CT or MRI tests.

- PET scans are more sensitive and useful in some cancers than others. Studies are still looking at the PET scans' usefulness in pancreatic cancer.

- Until it has proven to be the best imaging test for pancreatic cancer, it is important to use PET scans with other imaging tests to build a complete picture of a patient's cancer.

We understood that PET scans would not likely be used in my case. But at least we had raised the question.

————————————— ◉◉◉◉ ▬—————————————

DAY 105 – THURSDAY, MAY 28, 2020 – The last several days have been quite busy. Two days before my final chemo session, I rode around with Robin to the nursery and a golf store. I felt like throwing up a couple of times but didn't. Masks were mandatory, and my interactions were pretty limited. But it felt great to get out.

Around this time, I switched digestive enzymes from ZENPEP to CREON in an attempt to digest food better and take in nutrients. I also experimented with different dosages. I needed to put on weight and still had light-colored floating stools. I soon found that CREON caused me to become even more queasy, so I switched back to ZENPEP.

I found I was also very fidgety and couldn't concentrate. This was a likely side effect of 5-FU. Some might call it chemo brain. Robin was concerned about the long-term effects, and I certainly hoped it would end soon.

On May 26, I endured my sixth and final neoadjuvant chemo session and left with the 5-FU pump attached, but it wasn't easy. I had lost so much weight the nurse couldn't get the fanny pack strap tight enough to keep it over what was left of my hips.

Two days after my chemo session, I returned to UT Southwestern to have my 5-FU fanny pack disconnected and the Neulasta injector attached. Robin was able to come in for the first time during the pandemic. Due to my diarrhea and vomiting, my potassium level was down. So was my weight: 101 pounds.

Thankfully, my level returned to normal after an intravenous potassium treatment. And the big surprise was my CA 19-9 was down to 18.4. It was amazingly positive news!

Dr. Zeh had hoped I would hit 35 but I'd blown past that. He was a believer in the CA 19-9 marker and we hoped the tumor would follow those results. Still, I was worried about my upcoming June 1 CT scan. That date was pretty much right after my final chemo session, where I felt my worst and was highly nauseated. Yet I'd still have to drink plenty of fluids to spread the contrast. I'd just have to concentrate and get the stuff down. Dr. Beg officially confirmed this would be my last chemo session until after surgery. Although I switched from FOLFIRINOX to FOLFIRI for the last three sessions and skipped a week, I made it through every session as planned. I was determined and made it happen. Now it was likely on to some stereotactic radiation.

———————— ⟨❋❋❋⟩ ————————

DAY 108 – SUNDAY, MAY 31, 2020 – During one of the moments when I felt okay, I made my way to the wooden deck at the back of our house. Easing back in a chair, I enjoyed the sun's rays and fresh air. I stared at the sky and saw clouds dancing around the bright ball. Then I said a prayer for God to heal me. As I prayed, I glanced up again and saw that the clouds had formed a smiley face aimed at me. At that moment, I felt like God had heard my prayer and was looking down on me. I was comforted.

Later that day, Robin told me he'd been considering tearing up the deck and redoing it. He also wanted to add a koi pond. I smiled to myself. Robin liked having projects to work on. Then I thought of my dad. He had always been good at building things and remodeling our house. Whenever he fixed up a room or the porch, he'd kid my mother: "I'm just getting the house ready for your next husband." But he was wrong because she went first, and Dad was left in an empty house.

I considered the remodeling project that Robin wanted to start. Then my mind wandered to HGTV and all the remodeling shows. It was funny, but every doctor's office and hospital I'd been in had HGTV on the screens. Really, it made sense. The shows were noncontroversial. There was no dying or death. The most stressful it got was when the paint didn't match or they blew through their deadline. It was just stuff getting built and rebuilt, subjects that work for people trying to recover. And once everything was finished and it was all nice and pretty, everyone felt good about it. There was always a happy ending. They never showed someone accidentally electrocuted or a house collapsing on the workers.

Before my cancer diagnosis, I watched *Investigation Discovery, Forensic Files* and other true crime stories. Now, I didn't want to see anything that had death in it or left me with a downer feeling. All I watched was HGTV, positive shows with maybe a little news. So thank you, HGTV, for keeping it upbeat.

Chapter Sixteen

Robin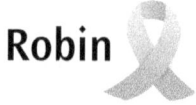

Day 111 – Wednesday, June 3, 2020 – Lisa and I climbed into my car and drove to UT Southwestern. We met with our radiation oncologist, Dr. Aguilera, and discussed the results of Lisa's recent CT scan. It caused us some concern.

"There is encasement of the celiac trifurcation as well as a 1 cm adjacent lymph node," the report said. Dr. Aguilera explained that he believed Lisa's pancreas had atrophied due to her disease and chemo treatments. The initial size of the tumor was 22 mm by 20 mm. Now, it was 12 mm by 10 mm, which was great news. And a 1 cm lymph node was located adjacent to the tumor. Dr. Aguilera said the atrophy had allowed a better view of the new findings on the latest CT scan. Yet he was sure this was not a new development. Regardless, the encasement discussion concerned us. It was a new discovery that could potentially move Lisa back to borderline resectable. Ultimately, though, it was Dr. Zeh's call. I'd found out that everyone interprets CT scans a little differently.

We learned that all our doctors (Zeh, Beg, and Aguilera) would meet tomorrow to discuss a plan going forward. This discussion with Dr. Aguilera differed from our first meeting with Dr. Zeh, when he was cocksure that Lisa was resectable. Dr. Zeh had also told us that it was not uncommon for a radiologist to mistake the tumor for "scar tissue." Lisa had a friend in the same situation. During surgery, the tumor had easily fallen away from the artery because it had become scar tissue. It was another reason Dr. Zeh valued CA 19-9 results.

Dr. Aguilera said the stereotactic radiation protocol for Lisa would be as follows: Week One – two days of radiation; Week Two – two more days of radiation; Week Three – one day of radiation at the beginning of the week. Lisa would need some "gold seeds" implanted as markers for her radiation treatment. After radiation, she'd have four to six weeks of recovery before surgery. However, if any metastasis was found during this period, the surgery could be canceled.

The last thing we heard was that Dr. Aguilera predicted Dr. Zeh would go ahead with the surgery. Due to COVID, this was our first in-person meeting with Dr. Aguilera. We felt comfortable with him, and I hoped this all worked out.

DAY 116 – MONDAY, JUNE 8, 2020 – A stressful day. Lisa was scheduled for another invasive procedure. It was time to have four "gold seeds," or fiducial markers, implanted to ensure accuracy during the radiation delivery. We went to the hospital at 10:30 a.m., and Lisa was put under anesthesia. An endoscope was sent through her mouth and stomach and into the upper part of the intestine. Once the target lesion was identified in the body of the pancreas, four gold seeds, each the size of a grain of rice, were implanted using a special needle. When Lisa came out of it, she didn't have the problems she'd had before. It wasn't a walk in the park, but everything went well—a huge relief.

By 2:30 p.m., we were headed home. It was hard for me not to be with Lisa, but COVID protocols kept me outside. Many cancer patients had their biopsies and other procedures delayed due to the pandemic. Only a few were having these done now, along with critical elective surgeries. We'd been truly blessed that Lisa could have these procedures.

DAY 119 – THURSDAY, JUNE 11, 2020 – Yesterday, Lisa intravenously received a dye called "radiocontrast media" (RCM). She also drank a glass of chalky barium. Dr. Aguilera used those to get a better picture from her CT scan. Then he had two tattoos the size of a freckle added to the middle of her chest and one to her left shin. Those were placed by using a slender needle and a tiny drop of ink. The process wasn't painless, though. Together, the tattoos and gold seeds helped ensure the precision and safety of the radiation treatments. Once that was done, Lisa practiced her breathing. She'd need to hold her breath for thirty seconds while the radiation blasted the tumor. If she moved her chest, healthy tissue could be damaged.

The breathing practice was done by inserting a snorkel into her mouth while she held a control button. She had to press a button to stop the airflow, hold for thirty seconds, and then release the button to breathe. She would have to hold her breath nine times during each session. Dr. Aguilera gave her a score of 99 and was confident she could handle it. I tried holding my breath for thirty seconds and found it challenging, especially doing it nine consecutive times. I hoped Lisa could do it.

But that was all yesterday. Today, I was called upon to drive "Press Three," a vehicle in President Trump's motorcade. After Air Force One landed at Love Field, five White House media reporters with masks climbed in and we took off for Gateway Church in North Dallas. From there, I drove to the home of billionaire Kelcy Warren of Energy Transfer Partners. Then it was back to the airport, and away Air Force One went.

As a tip from one of the media members, I was given a box of M&Ms from Air Force One. All of them were red, my favorite color.

So, how did I land this gig? My good friend Keith "Rosey" Rosenkranz headed the White House advance team. He'd made the local news coverage for his time with Governor Abbott and Lt. Governor Patrick. Rosey also got to meet President Trump as he exited Air Force One. Keith "Rosey" Rosenkranz has a story I'd like to include:

"I served eight years in the Air Force as a T-38 instructor and F-16 fighter pilot. The highlight of my career was flying thirty combat missions in the 1991 Gulf War. During my service in the Air Force, I lost about a dozen friends—classmates, students, fellow instructors, and fellow fighter pilots—to aircraft accidents. As the years passed, I also lost close friends to cancer, including my dad. I've learned that death has a way of showing up when you least expect it.

"Based on everything I've dealt with, I believe that for a patient to have the best chance at success, they need the will to fight the disease. I've seen that in Lisa because she's tough. Also, if they have the support of a loved one like Robin, who can watch over their medication and care, they can get and stay on the path to healing.

"I've watched Robin in action. He's been the lighthouse on the foggy shoreline, guiding Lisa through every step of the journey. I also understand a caregiver's role since my wife has multiple sclerosis. That's why I wanted to be there for Robin and help with encouragement in any way I could. Hopefully, I have."

I truly appreciated Rosey for being there for Lisa and me. I also must mention a book he wrote, *Vipers in the Storm*, which chronicled his experiences as an F-16 fighter pilot during Operation Desert Shield/ Storm. It hits home when discussing the stark realities of war, and I highly recommend it.

Then there was a book by Lou Holtz, the famous football coach. He wrote about how his wife had been suffering from throat cancer, so he decided to put an addition onto his house to take her mind off things. That gave me an idea, especially since Lisa's chemo was over, and she spent so much time watching HGTV that I thought a project would give her some mental relief.

I looked out my back door and focused on our aging deck. It simply had to go. I decided to redo it and add a koi pond along with a waterfall. I called our longtime interior designer, Allison Gimpel, for help and advice.

We'd met Allison roughly sixteen years earlier when I'd read a small article in the *Dallas Morning News*. She and her business partner, Emily Gibson, had just started their business. After seeing them online, I felt they would be a great fit. I called them, and they came over to discuss adding some art to our house. As it turned out, we were pretty much their first client. Over the years, Allison became our main contact. Sixteen years later, she has practically redone our entire house. She likes to say, "I know every nook and cranny in that house."

I set an appointment with Allison and told Lisa about it. She was ready to focus on a project and get back to feeling normal. And since Allison was a former Dallas Cowboys cheerleader, I hoped she could also "cheer" our patient up.

Chapter Seventeen

Lisa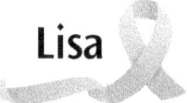

Day 126 – Thursday, June 18, 2020 – Back from his presidential motorcade, Robin drove me to UT Southwestern for my first radiation treatment. The assistants helped me onto the table and raised it so I was about four feet off the floor. Lying flat on my back, I stared up at a wide-diameter cylinder overhead and another large device to my left. I knew the beam came from one of them, but I wasn't sure which one. The device rotated around me as I lay on my back.

The radiation targeted the tumor and the area next to the splenic vein. It also targeted some lymph nodes near the tumor in case the cancer had spread to them. The entire process took about forty minutes. It was like being under an MRI but not fully enclosed, so I didn't feel claustrophobic. The hardest part was holding my breath for thirty seconds nine separate times. After the last one, the doctor said he was happy. I'd performed well.

Back home, I felt no side effects. Dr. Aguilera explained that the main one might be cumulative fatigue as the body worked hard to repair the damaged cells. Nausea might also make another appearance. Been there, done that. Long-term side effects could include calcification of the targeted veins, which could clog up. Ulcers could form in the duodenum— the upper intestine the stomach dumps food into. There were plenty of possibilities, but the doctors decided I needed radiation, so I had to go through with it.

Getting past the first radiation treatment was a huge relief. Truthfully, I'd been really stressed about it. I was fixated on the pressure of holding my breath. I did not want them to start over or risk damage to healthy parts of my body.

Before I went, I weighed myself: 101.4. I had gained a little bit of weight, possibly a half pound. With my pancreas coming back online, I reduced my digestive enzymes. Hopefully, I could eliminate them at some point.

UT Southwestern had assigned me a dietician. She told me which foods my body could digest and would put some weight on me. The plan was working. I hoped to gain ten pounds. I was pretty sure I'd need that extra weight, not only to survive the surgery but also for the final rounds of chemo after surgery. I focused on eating good food whenever I could. It's not often you can say that.

DAY 129 – SUNDAY, JUNE 21, 2020 – James Conner released a book titled *Fear Is a Choice: Tackling Life's Challenges with Dignity, Faith, and Determination*. In it he explained what we already knew—how he'd suffered an injury in 2015 before his junior season and had a lot of fatigue during rehab, so doctors did a chest X-ray and discovered he had Hodgkin's lymphoma. He'd started chemo and finished on May 9, 2016. Incredibly, he got himself into shape over the summer and was ready to play in the season opener against Villanova. During the 2016 season, he managed to run for over 1,000 yards and score twenty touchdowns. He'd even skipped his senior year and was drafted by the Pittsburgh Steelers. It was a miracle.

We bought a copy and started reading it. It seemed more personal after I'd received his video cheering me on. One point I felt differently about was the chemo infusion room. James liked being with other patients and talking to them during his infusions. I preferred a private room so I didn't have to be reminded how bad things could get. Maybe I'd feel the same way as James if I were outgoing like him. Other than that, his book gave me a healthy dose of hope.

DAY 131 – TUESDAY, JUNE 23, 2020 – It was the day after my second radiation treatment. By the afternoon, I finally felt the fatigue Dr. Aguilera had warned me about. At least it wasn't a shock.

I rested in bed and thought about my permanent tattoos. They had put them on me to assist with the accuracy of the radiation beam. Dr. Aguilera tried to distract me with conversation when they applied the tattoos, and I quickly found out why: It hurt like hell. I wasn't bothered, though, that the tattoos were permanent. They were small and looked like freckles. Besides, I had more important things on my mind.

This morning, I met with Dr. Beg. He said my blood work was "spectacular," with my CA 19-9 at 18.9. It was up from 18.4 but within the normal range since it was way below 38.

When we returned home, Robin and I had an appointment with Allison Gimpel, the interior designer we've known for years. Because of the pandemic, no one came to our home, but we made an exception for Allison. That's how special she is to us.

I discussed getting some new bedroom furniture before my surgery. Our old furniture needed an update. I knew I'd be too down after surgery and wouldn't have the strength to deal with it during the final rounds of chemo. Now was the time to get it done, so Allison brought some brochures and her ideas about furniture. Of course, with pandemic-related shipping delays, the furniture wouldn't be delivered until the fall.

Seeing Allison always brightened my day. She was not only a vendor but a really great friend who'd been more helpful to us than she'll ever know. During all this, she took my mind off my situation. Picking out fabrics and other items allowed me to focus on something else, which certainly made me happy.

Another way Allison has been helpful to us was by relating to Robin, my caregiver. She had been a caregiver for her cancer-stricken mother and told us what she'd learned. She also offered great tips on how to navigate the healthcare system. Her story is important for anyone dealing with cancer.

While she was here, we discussed redoing our deck and other changes Robin wanted to make in our backyard. When the meeting was over, I hated to see her leave.

We all know we're going to die one day. Most of us think it's when we're eighty or ninety—way down the road. We always assume we have lots of time. Then, one day, someone comes and says you don't have much time. And your life flashes in front of you.

We just can't know how our life will work out. Only God knows. But while we're here on Earth, there are folks we can learn from. Allison is one of them. We've devoted the entire next chapter to her. It's powerful reading, and I hope you all get something out of it.

Chapter Eighteen

Allison Gimpel

IN 2005, MY BUSINESS PARTNER, Emily Gibson, and I opened Gibson Gimpel Interior Design. Emily had been a classmate in college and was a good friend. We'd been working for a residential designer in Fort Worth, but then we jumped off the cliff and started our business with nothing.

In 2006, Robin and Lisa reached out to us and became our first official client. They had just remodeled their kitchen and wanted to add some art to the space. Because Emily was handling another client, I became the lead on this project. I'm a firm believer that people are brought together for a reason, but in this case, I had no idea what that reason might be. In 2020, I had my answer.

The Stoughs were open with me about Lisa's cancer diagnosis, aware that I had gone through a similar situation with my mom. In 1993, Mom was at a small hospital in Arlington, Texas, when doctors told her she had an advanced stage of colon cancer that had metastasized to her liver. They explained that she wouldn't make it and wanted to do pellet radiation to delay the inevitable. It was a devastatingly grim diagnosis.

At the time, I was working for a company with a board of directors, one of whom I knew was also on the board of the Baylor Medical System. I called him at 10 p.m. and he got Mom transferred to Baylor that same night, where she was reassessed. They found that although she had advanced cancer, it had *not* metastasized to her liver. They successfully operated and followed it up with radiation and chemo. Mom survived and continued living a happy life. Had I not questioned what that small hospital wanted to do, she would've died.

Just as we caught our breath from this experience, in 1996, my mother-in-law in Amarillo, Texas, was diagnosed with breast cancer. It was not very aggressive. The doctors told her she needed a radical mastectomy, chemo, and radiation. And they hadn't even performed a biopsy!

My husband and I said, "Hang on!" and brought her to Dallas, checking her into Baylor Hospital. They performed a battery of tests, including a biopsy, and decided that all she needed was a lumpectomy. She, too, went through chemo and radiation and continued living her life.

So, I've learned that doctors don't always have the right answers. They aren't all educated on the latest discoveries and techniques. They're also human, so they can misdiagnose. Fortunately, my mother-in-law lived another fifteen years. She passed away in 2011.

But just as I was mourning my mother-in-law, Mom came down with breast cancer, and it was very aggressive.

She had a left breast mastectomy, and on the door of her hospital room, doctors posted a sign that warned, *No IV Sticks In Left Arm*. They explained that any needle stick in her left arm could affect her lymphatic system and cause her to swell up. I was sitting in a chair on Mom's first day of recovery when a nurse came in and began preparing an IV for her left arm. I jumped up and said, "Did you not read the sign on the door?!" She glanced at it and said, "Oh, sorry." If I hadn't been there, that nurse would've put that IV in her left arm, and Mom would've swelled up. You must be there to protect your loved one from mistakes and incompetence. It's sad but true.

Mom's breast cancer was inflammatory, relatively rare in older people and usually seen in younger women. The cancer gets more into the skin tissue and advances quickly. Very aggressive radiation treatment was prescribed. By the sixth or seventh radiation treatment, her skin was so raw that it looked like third-degree burns on her chest. She had to be hospitalized to deal with it. I was upset that we were not informed it would get that bad.

In the first two days in the hospital, we saw her palliative care doctor. By the third day, we still had not seen her radiation oncologist. I'd been there the entire time and knew this for a fact. I called his office and learned he was not on vacation and had been at his office for the past three days. I asked the nurse if the doctor was going to see her. She asked, "Is there something wrong?" I said, "Well, she's hospitalized because of the radiation, so I would say, yeah. I think since he's the one doing the dosing, he would want to know about her situation." Instead of saying they'd be right over, they were flippant. That offended me.

On the fourth day, I asked Mom if she wanted to go for a little walk, and she nodded. I got her into a wheelchair and pushed her across the parking lot to his office. I walked up without an appointment and demanded to see the doctor. This shocked them. But they found a way for Mom to slip back into an examining room. When the doctor entered, I asked him why he had not come to see my mother in the hospital when his therapy was the reason she'd been hospitalized. "If this was your mother, is that the treatment you would want her to receive?"

He was stunned and quickly apologized.

"This is a human being," I reminded him. "She's dying. I think you would want to give better care than that."

He teared up as I reminded him that he was treating human beings, not numbers, not files, and not charts. I encouraged him to think a little about his patients beyond just what radiation dose he decides to give.

Did all this make a difference in his future behavior? I don't know, but I hope it made him think. As I wheeled Mom back to her hospital room, she patted my hand and smiled. She felt loved and supported because she knew I had her back.

Mom had always been a strong advocate for us as kids. She had to be because my dad committed suicide when I was thirteen. In terms of her ability to fight for what's right, she was a warrior. But Mom was not a very strong person in terms of her emotional health. At times, this led her to become a victim. She'd had a tough life, enduring an abusive father and more.

I've never been a mother, so I don't know what having children is like. I'd never had to take care of anything other than my cats. But as Mom got sick and her health started to decline due to the radiation treatments, my husband told her, "You'll move in and live with us." I don't think I realized what we were taking on when we did that. I didn't understand the day-to-day grind because I was working full-time and caring for Mom full-time. It's a tough job, and it *is* a job. It's emotionally demanding beyond anything I think most of us will ever experience.

Fortunately, there's a community of caregivers online. I learned a lot from them, like the importance of taking some time for yourself and doing self-care. If that means getting away from whatever, then do it. My sister would come over and stay at our house for a week to give me a break. She bathed Mom every night, washed her hair, fixed her meals, everything. Thank goodness for my sister.

If you can find someone to help you with that, it's wonderful. I know it isn't easy because some people don't have financial or family resources. Still, there are a lot of very loving, helpful people out there. You just have to look for them.

As for my health, I knew I couldn't care for someone else if I wasn't well myself. Sure, I felt guilty when I took some time for self-care. It reminded me of when I was a kid and had asthma. I was pretty sick, yet Mom had to go to work to pay for our food and housing. I was sick on the sofa, and she said, "I'm so sorry that I have to go and can't be here with you." On days I had to leave Mom at home to go to work, I understood that feeling because our roles were now reversed. But my husband worked from home, so we were very fortunate that Mom usually had someone with her.

Still, there were times he had to travel. When I left the house and Mom was alone, I felt terrible. We were also going through marital problems at the time and I was seeing a counselor who continually brought up self-care during our sessions. I think that things happen the way they do for a reason. Had I not experienced that counseling while Mom was sick, it would have been even more difficult because I don't think I would have taken care of myself.

Right before Mom's breast surgery, she was supposed to attend a class that would tell her what to expect from the surgery. My mother couldn't go that morning because she felt sick, so I went instead and met two fabulous nurses. They asked me why Mom wasn't there, and I told them she'd had colon cancer and explained her problems to them. They said, "Oh, you need Dr. Levy. He's a palliative care doctor."

"Palliative care? Isn't that end-of-life care?"

"Oh, no! That's what people think. But sometimes it's for people with chronic problems and pain."

After hearing such an optimistic point of view and some great things about Dr. Levy, we went to see him. Sure enough, he was truly my mother's savior. Those last three years of her life, Dr. Levy was it. He was compassionate. He listened to her. He validated the pain she felt. He was never dismissive. He never made light of something. He sat with Mom face-to-face, usually a couple feet from her, looking directly into her eyes, sometimes even touching her knee. It was compassionate care, just what Mom needed.

It was no surprise that I noticed a change in her attitude once she started seeing him. She felt understood. Because my mother had high anxiety, doctors sometimes dismissed her as dramatic or exaggerating. Now she felt validated and understood, and I firmly believe people need this kind of acceptance and peace to recover properly.

As Mom deteriorated, I wanted Dr. Levy to oversee her end of life, but he couldn't do it. He had to transfer Mom to a hospice doctor. But he was there till the very end. In fact, I talked to him the night before she died. He was the exact opposite of that radiation oncologist.

People who face a chronic illness like cancer or any painful disease would gain so much from a relationship with a palliative care doctor. This really matters. Fortunately, we hit the jackpot with Dr. Levy.

When Mom finally entered hospice, I learned that being in hospice doesn't always mean you will die tomorrow. It just means that you're not expected to live more than six months. If you thrive, they take you out of hospice. But there's a lot of value in hospice. I know that spiritual and religious beliefs make some people hesitant to seek out hospice, as they feel they're helping the patient die. "It should be God's will," they'll say. We ran into that a few times and had to explain that Mom was enduring a painful death and hospice was helping her body deal with the pain by using morphine. It's a myth that morphine enables you to die faster.

Caring for my mother and watching her pass away was a blessing but also a little bit of a curse, at least initially. So many emotions hung around for a while. But it did change who I am as a person, a woman, a friend, and a wife. Being there at the end for the person who brought you to life was an unforgettable experience. The most challenging aspect was accepting that she was no longer caring for me; I was caring for her and had to embrace that.

She always told me, "I'm so sorry you have to do this."

"Don't be sorry," I'd reply. "It's an honor to be able to do it." And I really meant it.

I also told her the truth—there were times that it was a burden and it was hard. I was very open and upfront with her. But I also explained that I carried tremendous joy and satisfaction. "You raised me and got me through some pretty tough times." She knew I had endured a rough childhood with a mentally ill father, and she was a great mom. I said, "It's my turn to return the favor."

I was with Mom when she passed, and so were two caregivers from hospice. They were there twenty-four hours a day and those people were unbelievable. But it wasn't a smooth passing. Some people say, "Oh, they gave her morphine, she closed her eyes, and went to sleep. That was it." Neither my mother-in-law nor my mother passed that way. For both of them, it was very dramatic and, I imagine, painful.

They say sometimes death has to do with people's personalities. If they're not ready to go, they cling and hold on to life. My mom was not ready to go. When a patient hits the point where they know they're actively dying, it's usually three days. Mom lost consciousness, and it took her two weeks to die, which is very unusual. It was hard to watch her struggle so much.

Once she was unconscious, I sat with her and said, "Just let go, Mom. It's time. You've fought as hard as possible and it's time to let go."

I found the process of death brings out different reactions in people. Some of my relatives didn't face it well, while others were prepared. Regardless of who was ready or not, Mom finally passed on November 1, 2015.

With all this knowledge and experience, I listened to Lisa's story and watched her deal with pancreatic cancer. Unlike my situation, Robin was caring for someone who was getting better. For me, I knew there wasn't going to be a happy ending, so I expended a different kind of energy.

I did see Robin struggling, however. Men tend to want to fix things, to make things right. They're problem-solvers. I know that feeling of being out of control. You're at the mercy of the illness and whatever treatment is prescribed. It was heartbreaking because, as a woman, I had girlfriends and a sister to cry with. We could show empathy. I could tell Robin, as a man, didn't feel that comfortable having those relationships. I tried to encourage him to find a support group but was pretty sure he wouldn't do that.

Instead, I let him tell me what he was feeling, the frustration and uncertainty. Then, one day, he asked me, "What did you do with your mom? How did you handle that?"

I told Robin all about it, including how my husband had helped. He had been phenomenal. I couldn't have asked for a better partner. I knew that because I saw how he was with his mom, and he was stellar. Even though we'd considered getting a divorce, my mother's health issues had nothing to do with our marital issues. Today, we say that my mother's illness saved our marriage because it made us take the focus off us enough to care for her.

As for Lisa, she's a very strong lady. I saw her body change from all the chemo and radiation. The weight evaporated off her. Each time I rang their doorbell, I never knew what I would see because she could've lost ten pounds in one week. I watched as frailty set in. But Lisa's mind was sharp. There were days I could tell her body was tired and she didn't feel like working on a project, so I adjusted to her situation.

After the first chemo phase, I watched Lisa regain some weight. It made me appreciate the human body. It's a pretty remarkable thing. It can be pushed so far to the edge and still manage to heal itself, with the help of doctors and modern medicine, of course.

What I found through all this is that people are either comfortable talking about the ugliness of cancer and illness or they're not. There's not much space in between.

We tend to judge people on outward appearances. If someone's tall and muscular, they must be strong in all ways. Yet Lisa is this tiny little person, fragile and quiet. But she's probably one of the strongest women I've met. The way she's faced this has been phenomenal. I was totally inspired, and one thing I know for sure—Lisa has the inner strength to make it.

Chapter Nineteen

Robin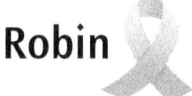

Day 139 – Wednesday, July 1, 2020 – Visiting all these cancer treatment centers and clinics was heart-wrenching. It made everything real. That's why it was an incredible relief when Lisa completed her fifth and final radiation treatment this morning. She has now endured three months of chemo and three weeks of radiation treatments. It was a deeply stressful and difficult time.

When Lisa finished her last radiation treatment, the staff asked her to "ring the bells." It's a tradition for patients once they complete radiation treatments. The bells are long tubes mounted on the wall, similar to a vertical xylophone. Lisa took the mallet and happily did her duty. Then she received a certificate of completion. I grabbed my phone and snapped a photo of her in a mask, oversized glasses, and a baseball cap. Wearing this getup, she could've robbed a bank.

We drove home and I sat her in a comfy chair and then vacuumed the hardwood floors, which I did frequently. By now, I was used to seeing clumps of hair everywhere. I noticed Lisa's flaky scalp and thin, brittle hair, mostly gray and white. Her natural red color was long gone. She had mentioned that after her last radiation treatment, she would check out some wigs. This made me think back to my friend Michael Donohoe, who'd been treated for acute myeloid leukemia. He'd lost his hair in the hospital. One morning, the doctor came in, studied the scene, and said, "It looks like Chewbacca slept on your pillow." I told Lisa that and she laughed—a little bit.

I know hair loss for men can be distressing, but it's somewhat expected, cancer or no cancer. For women, hair is an important part of their identity and is not expected to fall out. Lisa was devastated by the hair loss and color change. It was also a daily reminder of how sick she was and the treatments she was living through. Up to this point, she had resisted shaving her head, but today, she finally gave in and let me buzz it all off. It was freeing, at least for me.

Michael also told me to stop sending so many emails and sign up for CaringBridge instead. This excellent site allowed me to create a section for Lisa and upload photos and a journal of events. As our friends and relatives logged in, they would see these posts. The great thing about CaringBridge was not only the time it saved but also that it allowed everyone to support Lisa. I thought the comments would be uplifting for her, and they're open for everyone to see. Anyone going through something like this should consider signing up at CaringBridge.org.

With Lisa's treatments over, it was time for Dr. Zeh to formally enter the picture. After our interactions with him over these past three months, we had tremendous confidence. And his resumé was impressive. It was time to watch the rubber meet the road.

———————— ❖❖❖❖ ————————

DAY 147 – Saturday, July 18, 2020 – Lisa carried her new buzzed look well, with confidence and beauty. However, she experienced fatigue, indigestion, and some nausea after her final radiation treatment. Last night, she felt full and couldn't eat dinner even though she had eaten nothing all day. We were told radiation symptoms like these could continue to appear for a few weeks after the final treatment but had forgotten about that possibility, not to mention the latent chemo effects.

This morning, I asked how she felt, and she replied, "About seventy-five to eighty percent." Other than last night, her appetite had been good. This allowed her to concentrate on eating the right foods to gain weight and strength over the coming weeks leading up to her surgery. It's vital to get her body as healthy and strong as possible.

This morning we received confirmation of a surgery date: August 3, 2020. The clock was now ticking. We just needed to make it to surgery with no more problems.

We weighed Lisa and found she was up to 106; significant progress from her low of 98 pounds but still off the 115 she weighed a couple of weeks before her diagnosis. She'd been walking each morning and working with light weights. I loved to see her doing both of those.

She still took the pancreatic enzyme ZENPEP to aid digestion. Our oncologist recommended continuing ZENPEP, even if the enzymes may not be needed. We believed she would be fine without the enzymes but continued the small dosage to ensure proper digestion.

There's an informational website for pancreatic cancer called LetsWinPC.org. Our oncologist, Dr. Beg, and our dietician, Shelli Hardy, were interviewed for an article on it, "Pancreatic Enzymes Explained." It was very informative and gave us a sense of confidence in both Shelli and Dr. Beg.

Lisa has also been taking Xarelto 20 mg (one tablet) daily to protect against any blood clots. So far, we have not been aware of any clots other than the ones that materialized at the onset of her chemo treatments.

At the direction of our radiation oncologist, Dr. Aguilera, Lisa took pantoprazole SOD DR 40 mg (one tablet) daily and a sucralfate 1 mg tablet four times daily. Pantoprazole would be continued for six months to minimize the risk of developing ulcers due to radiation. This risk existed with or without surgery. Sucralfate was being continued until the end of July.

Finally, to close out the day, we learned about the vaccines Lisa would receive on July 31. This was necessary because her surgery would include a splenectomy. With her spleen being removed, her immune system would take a hit. People without spleens are more vulnerable to infections, which was the reason for these vaccines. She was scheduled to receive shots for:

- Prevnar 13
- Menactra (meningococcal conjugate, groups A, C, Y, and W)
- Bexsero (meningococcal group B)
- PedvaxHIB (Haemophilus Influenza B)

Then, eight weeks from the initial immunization date, she would receive:

- Menactra (meningococcal conjugate, groups A, C, Y, and W) second shot
- Bexsero (meningococcal group B) second shot (plus every two to three years for life)
- Pneumovax 23

Five years after the initial immunization date, she would receive:

- Menactra (meningococcal conjugate, groups A, C, Y, and W) third shot plus one dose every five years for life
- Pneumovax 23, second shot and one every five years for life

When I studied this immunization schedule, I rubbed my arm, thinking about all those needles. It wouldn't be fun, but it was nothing compared to everything she'd already been through.

⁂

I leaned back in my chair and took a deep breath. I thought of all my friends who had encouraged me. Paul Crane was a friend I played golf with at the Four Seasons. He had suffered from prostate cancer and chose a high-intensity focused ultrasound to pinpoint and heat up the cancer cells, effectively killing them. It was a noninvasive outpatient procedure that let him keep his prostate. Paul called me at least once a week, checking in to see how I was doing. It was great therapy to speak with him and very much appreciated.

By now, I'd learned that the caretakers of sick people endured a considerable burden. Having someone to chat with was extremely helpful. It gave me a way to vent without bothering Lisa. Paul took the updates I provided and passed them on to our other playing partners. This saved me from calling everyone with regular reports.

My friend and longtime personal trainer, Erin Cooper-Epperson, was always there to listen and provided much-needed positive support. Other friends called, too. I heard from Joe Kienast, Bruce Palumbo, and others. My CPA, Ralph Neal, called regularly. He was with us at our estate planning meeting and was among the first to know of Lisa's diagnosis. Ralph had known us for thirty-five years after meeting me at Hackberry Creek Country Club. His wife, Sandy, had undergone quadruple bypass heart surgery, so he'd had some experience with health issues.

Then there was Jack Zimmermann. Lisa and I had known Jack for over thirty years. We had played a lot of golf together. From day one, Jack had been very encouraging to us. He'd also had some cancer experience when his father, Chris, had suffered from cholangiocarcinoma, or bile duct cancer. Only one in 1.2 million people get this form of cancer.

Chris was 65 when he received the diagnosis. He needed surgery right away but only three places in the world would do it: Sloan Kettering in New York, Johns Hopkins in Baltimore, and some hospital in France. Jack took his father to New York and had Dr. Blumgart perform the surgery, which clipped off part of the liver. It was a hazardous procedure.

Dr. Blumgart cut a Mercedes-Benz emblem on Chris's chest and dove right in while Jack, his sister, and his mother waited. When the surgeon came out to talk to them, he said, "Your father is too far gone to do the procedure. He has a tumor the size of a walnut encroaching on a portal vein. He'll die if we remove the tumor."

"What now?" Jack had asked.

"We'll see if he survives this surgery, then discuss the options."

Jack and his family were devastated. They understood that Chris would not live to see his next birthday.

Chris recovered from the surgery and returned home to Ashville, North Carolina. One of Chris's golf partners there was a general surgeon. He had been researching this disease and recommended an experimental drug that Duke University was trying. "They have an excellent cancer center," the surgeon told Chris.

Chris landed an appointment at Duke with Dr. Lee. Jack wanted to be there, so he flew in. At the hospital, Jack and his parents waited for Dr. Lee to appear. Assuming he was of Asian descent, they were stunned when the door opened and revealed a Joan Lunden lookalike. And she had an incredible bedside manner. Chris fell in love with her immediately.

Dr. Lee explained that Chris was not a good candidate for the experimental drug. "You know what?" Dr. Lee said. "Sloan Kettering has a different philosophy than I do. They like to cut it out first, and I like to try to shrink it with chemo and radiation first. Let's try my way and see how it goes. What do you think?" Jack's father would've followed her to Mars.

Chris endured the chemo and radiation. There wasn't much to get excited about until one day, Dr. Lee said, "Hey, your tumor is actually shrinking!"

After four months, the treatments ended. Chris began enjoying a good quality of life. He kept in touch with Erika, a young teenager he'd met at the hospital who had brain cancer, and her family. Chris and his wife saw her during his appointments and prayed for the young girl daily. Apparently, she was doing great the last time they checked in.

Chris lived almost five good years after his initial diagnosis. Just when it had looked grim to Chris, a path forward appeared and extended his life. I could only hope the same thing would happen to my wife.

I told Lisa that story as we sat down and watched TV. With the lights on, we looked at her hair and saw a little fuzz starting to emerge. Life had found a way.

Chapter Twenty

Lisa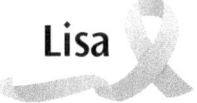

D AY 157 – Sunday, July 19, 2020 – My hair thinned quickly, then turned gray practically overnight after my second chemo treatment. I had a few gray hairs before my chemotherapy, but now it was completely gray. Every morning, there were clumps of hair on my pillow. When I showered, it came out in my hands as I washed it. When I turned the water off, the drain was clogged with hair. Robin urged me to shave it off but I wasn't ready. Then, after my last radiation treatment, I reached a point of no return. Patches of hair dotted my scalp; anything left was long, scraggly, and brittle. I had taken to wearing a baseball cap, so it wasn't like I needed the hair there. "I'm going to shave it off," I finally declared.

Robin had purchased clippers to cut his own hair since the pandemic had made it almost impossible to have someone else do it. We grabbed those, went out on the back deck, and he shaved my head. I cried. It felt like another hard step down into the dungeon of this disease. But after a few days of getting used to it, it was kind of liberating. Suddenly, I didn't have to worry about what my hair looked like or how I would fix it. I rid myself of another thing to worry about while giving the birds some material to pad their nests. It felt right.

I was so grateful Robin had learned about CaringBridge. I read every post and comment. They meant a lot to me; it was an easy way to keep people updated. I didn't have to keep repeating the same stories over and over again. I wasn't up to contributing to the site myself while I was going through chemo, of course. The last thing I wanted to do was sit in front of a computer and tell people how awful I felt. Thank God for Robin and his excellent writing.

Every morning, if the weather was decent, I went for a walk. During one recent stroll, I looked down and saw a postcard on the ground near a neighbor's house. I picked it up and read the words, "I'm praying for you." Before my diagnosis, I ignored stuff like this. Not now. I should've put it in the mailbox but kept it instead. When I got home, I read the entire note.

> "God has placed it on my heart to pray for you today! I pray that God will bless you in everything that concerns you. I pray the Lord will guide and lead you in every decision and in each situation you encounter. I pray that our Father will bless you and your family in ways that you have not considered and cannot be measured. I ask that our great God increase your health and renew your strength. I pray that the love God has for you will make you smile and bring real joy, now and always! I pray this prayer in Jesus's name, Amen.

It was from the pastor of a local church. I stuck it to my bathroom mirror so I could see it every morning, and it's been there ever since.

I finally received the schedule for my August 3 surgery. It was drawing near. The instructions said I needed to arrive at 5 a.m., with surgery scheduled for 7 a.m.

My cancer had been staged as "AJCC Stage 3 locally advanced, T4 by stage grouping." The cancer was growing outside the pancreas and into nearby major blood vessels. It may or may not have spread to nearby lymph nodes.

The tumor was in the body/tail region of my pancreas. As we neared surgery and they reviewed my scans, Dr. Zeh offered these thoughts. The surgery would likely be the modified Appleby procedure (distal pancreatectomy with celiac artery resection). However, if the chemo and radiation had moved the tumor away from the artery, the operation would be a simple distal pancreatectomy. During surgery, Dr. Zeh would take additional biopsies, including removing some of the surrounding lymph nodes.

Approximately 60 to 70 percent of my pancreas would be removed. My spleen, attached to the tail of the pancreas and sharing its blood supply, would also be removed. Dr. Zeh had explained that CT scans couldn't always distinguish between the tumor and scar tissue. Because of this, the absolute need for resection of the celiac axis (cutting out a vital artery) couldn't be determined until the time of the operation. Dr. Zeh would only operate if he could achieve an r0 resection (clean margins all around the tumor). So this could all be for nothing.

The procedure would take roughly three hours. I'd be in the hospital for about five days with a recovery time of six weeks. The most common complication after a distal pancreatectomy was leakage of pancreatic juices, more commonly called a "pancreatic leak" or "pancreatic fistula." This would be addressed with a drainage tube.

Delayed gastric emptying or other gastrointestinal issues, such as diarrhea, could also appear, but most of these issues should be resolved in a few weeks. The surgery should not cause me to be on insulin or change my diet in any meaningful way. My long-term need for pancreatic enzymes would be evaluated after surgery.

The surgery was a two-person operation and would be performed robotically. Dr. Zeh would be assisted by Dr. Patricio Polanco. Dr. Polanco completed a postdoctoral research fellowship and a general surgery residency at the University of Pittsburgh. He later completed a complex surgical oncology fellowship. During their time at UPMC, we understood Dr. Zeh provided robotic training to Dr. Polanco and now they were working together again at UT Southwestern.

Because this surgery put the body in a catabolic state, I would lose fat, muscle, and overall mass. I would need to get back on my feet as quickly as possible and build lean body mass with exercise and increased protein intake. Hopefully, this would quicken my recovery.

My dietician, Shelli Hardy, recommended an immunonutrition drink called Impact Advanced Recovery. There was some research to support this drink reducing the length of the hospital stay as it supported the body's immune system after surgery. I needed to drink three of these special beverages daily, starting five days before surgery and five days after.

Shelli also emphasized carbohydrate loading before surgery. This has been shown to decrease insulin resistance and hyperglycemia, minimize protein losses, and improve comfort, well-being, and postoperative muscle function. To achieve this, she recommended (and Dr. Zeh approved) a carbohydrate drink called Ensure Pre-Surgery (100 grams of carbohydrates). I needed to consume two of these drinks the evening before surgery and one more on the morning of surgery up to two hours prior. So far, Shelli Hardy's diet and other suggestions had been spot-on. I was grateful to have her.

If I survived the surgery, I'd face more chemo eight to twelve weeks later. Not much of a reward, and something I didn't want to think about.

DAY 166 – TUESDAY, JULY 28, 2020 – Today, I weighed 113.8 pounds with clothes and shoes on. That was up from 98 pounds with clothes and shoes just two short months ago. I looked better and my hair was growing. Yet I still felt some occasional indigestion. I was unsure if this was the result of chemotherapy, medication side effects, radiation therapy, pancreatic enzyme deficiency, or cancer.

My lab work was fantastic, with the CA 19-9 at an all-time low of 12.7. This was well below the upper limit of the normal range of 38 and way down from the high of 78.1.

As planned, I received several immunizations. Since my spleen would be removed, I could be more susceptible to infection, so these vaccines were the first line of defense. The shots weren't fun and those meningitis shots hurt like hell. I mean, they really hurt! But what could I do? I had to have them.

DAY 169 – FRIDAY, JULY 31, 2020 – We met for almost two hours with Dr. Zeh, his physician assistant, Lan Vu, and his nurse, Jacqueline Davis. The CT scan showed the lesion to be "similar to decreased in size" from June 1, when it was 1.2 x 1.0 cm. "Similar appearance of adjacent soft tissue density surrounding the celiac axis and an adjacent 1 cm node." Essentially, this meant there was no change or a slight decrease in the tumor size. But the best news was that the scan showed no evidence of metastasis.

Dr. Zeh mentioned a 7 mm liver lesion and a couple of 2–3 mm nodules in my lungs that were seen on scans from February 14, 2020, the first scans I'd had on this journey. These were thought to be benign, and today, Dr. Zeh and Lan Vu confirmed that opinion—more good news.

Dr. Zeh's confident attitude was infectious (no pun intended). He told us significant positive indicators were my feeling well and gaining weight. And he loved seeing the low CA 19-9.

He told us he'd proceed with the surgery using a modified Appleby procedure. He'd done 1,000 to 1,500 pancreatic surgeries, although only 50 to 60 had been modified Applebys. However, he told us his Appleby total might be the most anyone in the world had performed. It was definitely a surgery that required special expertise. He had gone back and forth on whether it was necessary but ultimately decided it needed to be the modified Appleby. We were so thankful we'd found him. I also was reassured that 98 percent of his surgeries involved the pancreas.

He reiterated that symptoms tended to appear much later when the tumor was located in the body/tail region of the pancreas. "You did a great thing moving quickly on your moderate pain."

I knew only 20 percent of pancreatic cancer patients overall were eligible for surgery. (Unfortunately, I learned that up to half of those patients were told they were ineligible.) If their tumor is in the body/tail region, the number eligible for surgery is even lower, and you also may need a doctor who's heard of the modified Appleby procedure. Those are pretty low odds. The late presentation of symptoms for cancer in the body/tail and slow reaction to them is one reason fewer modified Applebys and distal pancreatectomies were performed. Also, how many surgeons are capable of a modified Appleby? The Whipple procedure was the most common operation and removed cancer in the head of the pancreas. It was the most common because symptoms usually manifested sooner when cancer was located in the head of the pancreas. In other words, it was not too late. Hopefully, this book will educate patients by introducing them to the modified Appleby procedure.

We asked Dr. Zeh (again) if surgery was the only curative alternative. He told us there was a 95 percent chance chemotherapy and radiation did not entirely kill the tumor. "So, yes, you still need the surgery." He also told us that some patients felt chemo was more brutal than surgery. I hoped he was right because the chemo had been extremely harsh.

Finally, I learned that my last dinner would be on Saturday evening. After that, I'd be on clear fluids until surgery.

Now that I was barely three days away from a very serious and complex surgery, my mind raced. Even though I had the best surgeon around, that was no guarantee of success. As I watched the minutes and hours tick by, I could feel the weight of the moment coming. Early one morning, I sat on the backyard deck thinking about the risks of this surgery and how I might not have a positive outcome.

I flashed back to my childhood and growing up in Irwin, Pennsylvania. I had lived my entire childhood in a friendly middle-class neighborhood with many wonderful neighbors. I always had kids to play with. I could still see their faces. My parents did an excellent job providing for me and my two younger brothers, Paul and Dan. As I've recounted, Mom died in 1987 of brain cancer, but Dad, 87, was still around, though suffering from heart disease and other health issues. His body was breaking down. I prayed that he would not have to attend my funeral.

As I ran through memories of meeting Robin, getting married, moving around the country, and now this, I realized one thing: Gosh, my life sure had gone by fast. Now, it moved so fast I couldn't slam on the brakes to slow it down.

Robin and I had never really talked about what would happen if I died. We'd been so focused on solving the problem and seeking the best care that those conversations never took place.

Before I was diagnosed, we sometimes talked about finances and money for retirement. We were determined not to outlive our money. Robin always said, "We need to make sure there's money for you." And I would reply, "That doesn't mean you'll go first." He would say, "Statistics show that it's probably going to be me first."

Now, the possibility that I might go first turned all that upside down. He might be a widower. For the past 169 days, I'd thought about that often and wanted to tell him to get married again if he so desired. After all, he could live another twenty years. And since we had no kids, there would be no stepchildren issues.

Up to this point, I'd always felt I had a long runway ahead. Recently, I learned it's not so long. I just felt like I would miss out on the rest of his life, making Robin happy and doing things with him. I remembered what Bill Edwards, Robin's brother-in-law, had told me. He had prostate cancer, and we'd been emailing each other. I told him how scared I was of dying, and he emailed me with, "I'm not afraid of dying. I'm afraid of what I'm going to miss out on." That's how I felt. I was going to miss out on growing old with Robin. I was going to miss out on my family and friends. Cancer makes you think like this.

Everyone knows they're going to die. But when you believe you only have so much time left, you wonder what the end will be like.

Will I be in a lot of pain?

Will I go to sleep one night and not wake up?

I feared dying in bed with Robin next to me. I didn't want him to wake up and find me dead. That would be horrible for him to have to live with. Now, all I could do was pray my surgeon knew what he was doing and that God would get me out of this mess.

Chapter Twenty-One

Robin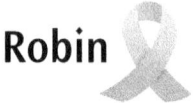

D AY 171 – Sunday, August 2, 2020 – I could feel the anxiety of
Lisa's impending surgery tomorrow. On the one hand, we'd been
praying and pushing for this date to get here. On the other hand, I knew
it was serious, and the news could be bad when it was over. To push past
the fear, I focused on getting things done and working on my checklist.

Before the operation, our surgeon recommended Lisa shower with
Hibiclens or a similar product. Hibiclens was an antiseptic skin cleanser
that killed germs for twenty-four hours after using it and helped lower the
risk of infection after surgery. I double-checked with Lisa. Even in this
time of great stress, as I expected, she was on top of it. Since we were due
at the hospital at 5 a.m., she showered that evening.

I went to the study and looked at my notes. The surgery would be
performed at UT Southwestern, specifically the William P. Clements,
Jr. University Hospital. It was northwest of downtown, in the hospital
district. For the fourth consecutive year, U.S. News had ranked this
hospital number one in Dallas and Ft. Worth and number two in Texas.
I liked seeing that.

I continued reading my notes from all the meetings with Dr. Zeh. He
said there would be five incisions, the largest in the lower left abdomen at
two inches long. Three circular incisions would be made mid-abdomen,
about the size of the end of a thumb. The last incision would also be a
circular cut but only the size of a pencil point. I was happy the surgery
was being done robotically.

Right before the surgery, Lisa would have a urinary catheter inserted.
This would remain in place for about twenty-four hours.

During the surgery, approximately ten to fifteen lymph nodes would
be collected from the resected section of Lisa's pancreas and nearby

tissue. These samples would provide vital information about the cancer and its possible spread, although, according to Dr. Zeh, the data from the lymph nodes may not be as telling as the CA 19-9 readings.

Lisa would also receive a shot of Duramorph. It would be injected through a needle into her lower back. About 15 percent of patients undergoing this surgery develop diabetes, and approximately 30 percent need pancreatic enzymes for the short- or long-term. Immediately after surgery, Dr. Zeh might know better if Lisa would develop diabetes.

In addition to all this, Lisa may receive an injection of Lovenox (blood thinner) for two days after surgery. There was also a chance she would have one or two JP drains for a few days after surgery. This would allow any pancreatic "juice" to leave the body. Usually, the drainage is resolved before the patient goes home.

I stared at the screen and finally closed the file before turning off my computer. There was nothing more to do. I trudged to bed and found Lisa already there, trying to sleep. The more rest she got, the better. The alarm was set for 3 a.m.

I was still a ball of nerves but tried to calm myself down. Then I put my pajamas on and climbed into bed. I'd need my brain fully functioning to make sure she arrived on time and was ready for the surgery, so I turned out the lights and tried to get some sleep.

DAY 172 – Monday, August 3, 2020 – It was 4:45 a.m. We were fifteen minutes ahead of our scheduled 5 a.m. arrival time. As the only two people in the waiting room at this early hour, we nervously waited until Lisa was called back at 5:30 a.m. With tears in my eyes, I kissed her as she walked through the door to her prep room. Due to the pandemic, I couldn't accompany her past this point.

Around 6:30 a.m., Lisa called me on her cell phone and said she was hooked up to an IV. She sounded good but had to end the call quickly as her nurses and doctors were coming in. I told her I loved her. I knew it would be our last conversation before her surgery. As I disconnected the call, I felt limp and helpless. Still, I tried to stay strong.

At 7:05 a.m., Dr. Zeh found me in the lobby. He said everything was going fine and Lisa was just given Duramorph. It would be an hour or so before they began. He turned and went back to the operating room. I sat in the waiting room, watching him disappear. Now, my long wait began.

––––––––––––––––◈◈◈◈■––––––––––––––––

I tried to keep my mind distracted, but it was impossible. At 8:10 a.m., I received a call from a woman who said she was calling from the operating room. Before I went into shock, she said the procedure had just begun and everything was going fine. It was a quick call and one I appreciated.

Then, around 10 a.m., another woman called from the operating room. She was also very quick to talk, eliminating my shock and stress. She told me everything was going fine. They had just finished removing Lisa's spleen and were now working on her pancreas. I thanked her and waited for the next update.

It was a Monday, and the waiting room was now about half full, the other men and women looking as edgy as I felt. COVID-19 likely eliminated some surgeries. I was not much of a coffee drinker and didn't need it, but it looked like a lot of folks were overcaffeinated. I just found a lonely corner and sat there thinking about things.

I was two-and-a-half years older than Lisa and a man, so I had assumed I'd go first. It's natural to think that. I'd even expressed that belief to her during our estate planning sessions. And then there was my lifestyle. Even though I'd changed a lot, there had been a lot of drinking during my hard-charging business years. In my eyes, I drank too much, though in reality, it probably wasn't more than my peers. But I completely stopped drinking after she was diagnosed, to help her through this trauma.

Even though I never smoked, the aggressive business life of late dinners, travel, company politics, making a profit, and managing people had taken a toll. Like Lisa, I was in the commercial insurance business. After leaving AIG in the early 1980s, I became a wholesale broker and managing general agent. Over the years, I served as the president of multiple companies. At the end of my career I started two companies from scratch with our personal funds. After selling my second company in November 2014, I retired. With all the stress I'd been under creating, running, and selling my businesses, I knew I would probably receive the bill later in life. I expected it.

Then there was Lisa. She rarely had more than one drink when we were out to dinner and often had no alcohol. When she did, it was wine. I'd never seen her drink hard liquor. And she was a low-key person, rarely upset or out of control. Nothing bothered her. She simply did not put stress on her body. Yet now, she faced this harsh disease while I was completely healthy.

I leaned my head back and closed my eyes. I recalled Dr. Betam, our initial surgeon. He told us Lisa had only six months to two years, which had slammed me right in the face. When I heard him say those words, I told myself we could find a way to beat this. I'd always come through before and would surely do it this time.

When Lisa heard that her life was ending, I reminded her we hadn't failed yet. "We're going to figure this out," I'd assured her. Too often in business I'd been told, "It's impossible" or "You can't do that." But I'd always busted down the doors of "impossible" and "you can't do that." Now I could do the same for Lisa. I owed it to her.

I glanced at the double doors. My wife was a few hundred feet away in some operating room in another man's hands, and there wasn't anything I could do. Despite putting on a brave face, I was scared. I didn't want to face life without her. I tried not to think about what I'd do if she died. Where would I live? What would my life be like?

Once, Lisa told me, "I want you to marry again. I want you to be happy and have someone to talk to and care for you."

I shut that talk down fast. "Look, don't even bring that up because A, that's the last thing on my mind. And B, I can take care of myself. And C, I don't even know if I'd want to do something like that." I let that sink in before continuing. "That's crazy! Don't ever bring that up again." She never did.

My mind switched to everything she had endured—her port redo, blood clots, anti-nausea medicine, steroids, high-powered antihistamines, biopsies, gold seeds, and chemo drugs. I thought back to the nurse who'd always come in holding a bag and scanned the barcode to make sure it was correct. Then she said aloud the contents of the bag and called in another person to check it. Only after two people had signed off on it did Lisa receive fluids. I liked that.

Then there was the radiation. The tattoos. The CT scans. The scanxiety. We had lived a lifetime in five-and-a-half months. Now, as we approached the six-month mark, Dr. Betam's words bounced around in my head: "Six months to two years." What if Lisa died during surgery? People did. It could be a blood clot, or the anesthesia, or weakened blood vessel walls from the chemo. So many things could go wrong I didn't want to think about it. We had found the best, and like a football game, you had to trust your players to get the job done—one way or another.

I got up and paced around. After waiting, I ripped through several water bottles and even decided to have a coffee. Trips to the bathroom were a nice diversion. It took my mind off this whole experience for a few minutes. Occasionally, I checked my phone for headlines. They had several televisions playing on different channels. I couldn't focus on any of it. I just wanted my Lisa back safe and sound.

Around noon, the nurse let me know they were wrapping up the surgery. "The doctor will be right out to talk to you," she said. *What does that mean? Was it successful?*

I was summoned to a small conference room, where I waited for what felt like an eternity. I felt my entire life pass before me. Finally, the door opened and Dr. Zeh stood there with a serious look on his face. My stomach dropped. This was it. I was about to find out how long I'd have my precious wife with me.

Chapter Twenty-Two

Robin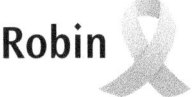

D R. ZEH WALKED INTO THE SMALL WINDOWLESS ROOM and pulled out a chair. After sitting down, he got straight to it. "The surgery went according to plan."

I heaved a deep sigh of relief.

"We did the modified Appleby procedure as we predetermined, and there were no surprises." He continued. "We took her spleen and about 70 percent of her pancreas, achieving an r0 resection. No other cancer was seen; the growth on her liver was just a cyst. We'll have a full pathology report in about seven days."

My eyes filled with tears as I felt my body relax, the stress draining out of me. "When can I see her?"

"She's not in ICU so they'll take her to a room shortly. I believe it's room 1158. She has a urinary catheter and we put in a drain tube, which will be there for maybe three days."

I asked Dr. Zeh a few questions about her prognosis. He told me we would know more once the pathology report came in. After he left, I collected my things, which included my heart and stomach. They had dropped to the floor. I knew it would be a little while before Lisa was moved to her room, so I grabbed a quick lunch. Suddenly, I was hungry.

After eating a sandwich, I headed to room 1158. Sure enough, I caught them wheeling Lisa in. Perfect timing. She was extremely groggy and didn't recognize me. As they set up her bed and connected everything, I stepped to the side and checked my watch. It was 1:30 p.m. This had to have been the longest day of my life. Nothing else was close.

Over the next several hours, Lisa slowly recovered from the anesthesia. She slept for a while and woke, a little delirious at times. When I asked about the pain, she mumbled that she felt very little unless she moved her body. The nurse returned and I asked her about Lisa's pain.

"Over the next few days, she'll feel the worst as the Duramorph wears off. However, pain varies a lot among patients. You can never predict who will feel more of it and who will feel less."

The nurse checked the urine bag to ensure Lisa's catheter was working. Then she inspected the pancreatic drain tube and was happy with it. Before she left, she inspected the oxygen tube in Lisa's mouth and made some notes on the computer.

"Once we remove the oxygen tube," the nurse said, "I'll come in and have her use the spirometer." Lisa had been practicing with one at home before her surgery. "We need her working on breathing exercises as soon as possible."

"Is she doing okay?" I asked.

"Yes, her vitals are good," the nurse said.

I watched her leave and continued feeling the stress. It was a helpless feeling and left me wishing I could do more. I walked over to the window and looked at the new cancer center under construction. The workers hurried along, unaware my wife was up here in bed trying to beat pancreatic cancer. I guess that's life. I never thought about pancreatic cancer until my wife got it.

Dr. Zeh arrived and inspected his patient. "How's she doing?" he asked me.

"She seems okay," I replied. "The nurse checked everything out and was satisfied."

Dr. Zeh read the computer records and examined Lisa. He walked over to the window and gazed out. "I promised you a room with a nice view of downtown Dallas. Want me to move you to another one?"

I considered his question and appreciated him remembering the offer. We weren't on vacation, so the view was the least of my worries. The recovery seemed to be going well and I didn't want to change a thing. "No, we're good right here."

"Okay," he said. "Let me know if you change your mind."

I wasn't going to change my mind. Instead, I took a seat on the couch. It converted into a bed for overnight visitors. The room was well-equipped and the nurses had already set me up with blankets and a pillow. They were on top of things.

As I watched Lisa in bed with a urinary catheter and drain tubes, I wished I could do more to help. I tried talking to her but she was still pretty much out of it. After communicating the best I could, I went out to discuss with the nurses and other attendants the idea of me going home for a few hours of sleep. It was after midnight. Everything seemed to be going well so the nurses were comfortable with me leaving for a while. It was only a twenty-minute drive home and I planned to return before dawn to be sure I saw the doctors on their morning rounds. It was a stressful decision at a stressful time, but I left the hospital.

⬛————◎◎◎◎————⬛

DAY 173 – TUESDAY, AUGUST 4, 2020 – I was back in Lisa's room before dawn. The nurses said she was doing well. Throughout the night, they monitored and checked her vital signs. They also sat just outside her room, watching their patient through a window. I was impressed and reassured by the setup. Thankfully, no issues or complications arose. Lisa was still out of it, so I rested on my "bed" until the morning rounds began.

It was still early when the nurse ran a glucose test. The results showed 99, which was normal, an excellent early sign regarding the potential for diabetes. Her vitals were good, too, except for a 99.8 temperature. Infection was always a risk when going through an operation of this magnitude, but a low-grade fever was typical.

The nurse also injected heparin, a blood thinner, into Lisa's abdomen at three locations. It wasn't fun to watch. These injections would happen once every twenty-four hours. They had talked about Lovenox, but heparin it was.

Speaking of her abdomen, it remained swollen and bloated from the carbon dioxide gas pumped in during surgery. The gas inflated the abdominal cavity so the surgeon could better see the organs and have plenty of room to operate. Even though the surgical team tried to suck out the gas right before they closed her up, they couldn't get it all. Sometimes, the gas migrated to her shoulders, looking for a way out. Unfortunately, there was no way out, so it caused pain until the body dissolved and eliminated it. The pain was temporary, but it did hurt.

Today was busy with plenty of visitors. Dr. Zeh returned and said everything was progressing according to plan. "No red flags. And the fluid in her drain shows no pancreatic leak. If that holds, the drain can be removed earlier." Lisa loved hearing that.

Dr. Zeh explained he had already performed a Whipple on another patient that morning. He said he does one surgery a week on average, less than in Pittsburgh. So far this week, he'd done two, so he was ahead of his average.

Dr. Polanco, the assistant on Lisa's surgery, sent three residents, two nurses, his physician assistant, and a "vitals tech" to check out Lisa. It was comforting to see her getting so much attention.

Another visitor this morning was a physical therapist. I turned to Lisa and said, "The physical therapist is here. This is going to be hard, but getting up and moving will help your rehabilitation." Lisa had no response. The nurse removed her urinary catheter. Then, the physical therapist slid her out of bed and positioned a walker for her to grab onto. Slowly and carefully, the pair moved about seventy-five feet down the hall and back before putting Lisa in a chair. During the walk, Lisa felt pain and nausea. She sat for thirty minutes before being moved back to bed. Watching all this, it was clear her recovery would be a long process.

Lisa's drain bag was continually checked. Thankfully, it was mostly empty and any fluid in it was clear—more good news.

Lisa's liver was functioning properly with the new artery supporting it. A big test down the road would be eating solid foods and the reaction of her digestive system. She was still on a clear, liquid diet. We ordered some juice and Jell-O from room service, though she had a minimal appetite.

At 3 p.m., Lisa awoke and felt real pain. She told the nurse it was a four to five out of ten on the pain scale. It was tolerable when lying down but when moving around it hurt. The nurse gave her half of a hydrocodone, which soon worked. The next time she felt pain, Lisa told me she'd ask for a full dose.

Without a catheter, Lisa had to get in and out of bed to go to the bathroom but needed help. But that movement was part of the healing process, even though it caused pain. Each time she did it, she got a little faster.

I urged her to practice breathing into the spirometer as much as possible. The medical staff explained that the bottom half of the lungs are "asleep" during this surgery and need to be "awakened" afterward. Lisa worked at it some, but of course, it was slow going.

More blood tests were run. Aside from low hemoglobin, her blood work was good. No one seemed concerned about her lungs because her oxygen level was good. The low hemoglobin pushed her to practice breathing more.

Lisa still wore a yellow gown and had an alarm on her bed. The goal was to graduate to a blue gown with no alarm or nurse assistance required.

I watched everything that went on and asked questions. I didn't want them to give her the incorrect medicine or do something wrong. It was also important to know what to expect when she came home. It appeared the medical staff had it completely handled, which was a huge relief.

DAY 174 – WEDNESDAY, AUGUST 5, 2020 – Lisa's pain level rose during the night, starting at 8 p.m. yesterday evening and continuing until this morning. "It's a six when I'm lying down and a ten while moving around," she told the nurse. The nurse left the room and returned, holding a clear bag.

"I'm going to give you hydrocodone intravenously. It starts working faster and is more effective than the pills."

She was right. But there was no rest for the weary. Lisa was encouraged to move and walk as much as possible. It was her best therapy, though difficult to execute due to the intense pain.

Earlier, her glucose reading was 137, which was elevated. This could be due to the intravenous fluids. That was being evaluated.

Lisa's swollen limbs and bloated body led to weight gain. Her gaggle of doctors, nurses, and physician assistants said they would've been surprised if she wasn't bloated and gained weight. They were happy to see no evidence of internal bleeding and slowed down Lisa's IV fluid intake.

So far, there was no fistula or pancreatic leak, although it was still possible one could appear. Lisa's liver and hemoglobin readings were fine now.

She had no appetite, but the staff encouraged her to eat. She was still on a clear liquid diet, although we hoped to get approval for a milkshake and some light foods. They just kept pushing her to get up and move around.

Around 9 p.m., things quieted down. With Lisa asleep, I leaned back on my couch/bed for a while, feeling optimistic. There were no red flags and it looked like her discharge would be on time. I hoped and prayed her progress continued.

Chapter Twenty-Three

Lisa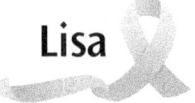

D AY 174 – WEDNESDAY, AUGUST 5, 2020 – Even though my oxygen tubes were removed shortly after surgery, I lay in bed with an IV, being closely monitored. The machines beeped constantly. It was very disorienting.

Last night, around 8, the pain hit me. Since then, I've received intravenous hydrocodone to dull the pain caused by moving around. I especially needed it today when my pain level was a 10. That was really tough.

I glanced over at Robin and saw his eyes closed. What a job he'd done to get me to this point. All the time he'd spent researching every aspect of this disease, finding the doctors, scrutinizing my treatment, and questioning everything. I couldn't imagine what this would look like without him.

Of course, I couldn't forget about God. I was raised Catholic but hadn't attended church in years since we'd been married. Regardless, I'd been praying every morning and every night since all this started. It got me talking to God and asking for help, which was good since He can do it.

The early days in the hospital were a blur. I slept a lot and the drugs kept me loopy. The fatigue was unlike anything I'd ever experienced. Before I got sick, whenever I took a nap or slept well at night, I awoke refreshed. Not now. No matter how much sleep I got, I always felt tired.

Earlier in the day, a physical therapist helped me out of bed. It was almost impossible. My legs felt so heavy whenever I was in bed; I could hardly move them. No matter what I did, I couldn't get comfortable. I just closed my eyes and did the best I could to sleep.

DAY 175 – Thursday, August 6, 2020 – There was a drain in my left side—a short tube leading to a clear plastic ball hanging off my stomach. It looked like a Christmas tree ornament and I was the Douglas fir. Every two hours, a nurse emptied the ball into a container. From there, the contents were measured and studied. Then they snapped the ball back into place and waited for the next cycle. This prevented me from sleeping on my left side, which added to my misery.

It had been three days since the surgery when Dr. Zeh came in and stood at the foot of the bed. He had another doctor and a resident assistant with him, and they watched everything. They were part of a group of young doctors, RAs, nurses, and a PA who had been looking after me.

As he had before, Dr. Zeh moved to the side of the bed and checked my five incisions. The scene was a war zone with a bloated abdomen and ugly-looking scars surrounded by serious bruising. Add in the spots where three heparin shots were administered every twenty-four hours, plus the hole for the drain, and I wouldn't be modeling on a runway anytime soon.

Dr. Zeh pressed my abdomen and studied the landscape, something he had done from the moment I'd arrived in my room. I guess he wanted to make sure the incisions weren't opening up or leaking.

His normal procedure was to check everything and then wiggle my toes on his way out of the room. But this time, he moved back to the foot of the bed and allowed a young doctor and resident assistant to check me out. I started to close my eyes and wait for them to finish. Then I heard Dr. Zeh telling me something and saw him gesturing with his hands. I watched him, confused for a few seconds, until I felt something inside my body being pulled out. It seemed a mile long, and the pain was intense, the worst I'd felt so far. And that was saying a lot, especially since I was on painkillers. Before I knew it, the plastic tubing and clear ball were being handed to a nurse. Dr. Zeh applied some skin glue to my wound and covered it with a bandage. My JP drain was gone.

"Sorry about that," he said. "It was my job to distract you."

I breathed in heavily, which was something I needed to work on. Finally, Dr. Zeh wiggled my toes and left with his entourage. It sure hurt, but seeing that contraption gone was a huge relief.

Later that day, they took me off IV fluids and I was approved for soft foods, a diet that led to immediate diarrhea after eating. I was concerned this indicated a long-term need for enzymes, but it was too early to really know. My body and whatever pancreas I had left would have to adapt to a new normal.

By now, the remaining gas from the surgery was gone. Initially, it had worked its way up to my shoulders, causing some pain. Still, it was more of a nuisance compared to the pain from the surgery.

As for Robin, he never did stay overnight, not even that first night. I didn't want him to. I wanted him to go home and sleep in our bed. After my first night, his routine was to leave the hospital around 9 or 10 p.m. I hated this since it was always dark when he drove home. I told him not to rush up here, but he ignored me and showed up every morning between 6 and 7 a.m. He wanted to catch Dr. Zeh and his staff making their rounds.

Robin always had questions. One day, Dr. Zeh didn't come in early. As the lunch hour neared, Robin wanted to get something to eat at the cafeteria, so he wrote out his list of questions for Dr. Zeh. Sure enough, he'd been gone for only a few minutes when Dr. Zeh appeared. "Okay," Dr. Zeh said, clapping his hands, "what are his questions?" He was always a good sport.

While Robin was gone, I ruminated about the surgery. He had done so much research on my surgery that I knew everything about it. Many pancreatic cancer patients have tumors in the head of the pancreas. This can actually be somewhat of an advantage as it often sends signs of pancreatic distress earlier. A patient can get jaundiced, have stool problems, and generally show symptoms earlier. If they immediately go to a doctor, they could be eligible for a Whipple procedure. This surgery removed the head of the pancreas (where the tumor is), the gallbladder, the bile duct, and the first part of the small intestine.

My tumor was on the body, near the tail of the pancreas. Surgery to remove the left side (body and tail) of the pancreas is called a distal pancreatectomy. However, tumors in this part of the pancreas can be more troublesome, as symptoms often appear later, sometimes too late. It was one reason patients with cancer in the body and tail of the pancreas are less often eligible for surgery. They don't develop symptoms until it's too late.

My tumor abutted the left ventral aspect of the SMA and regional splenic vein. This invasion necessitated a celiac axis resection. The surgery required was a robotic distal pancreatectomy and celiac axis resection, commonly known as a modified Appleby procedure.

In the 1950s, a doctor named Lyon Henry Appleby developed a procedure for gastrointestinal cancer. Dr. Appleby died in 1970, but his procedure lives on. In fact, it was modified for pancreatic cancer. The surgeon now removes the body and tail of the pancreas and the entire spleen and resects the celiac axis. The pancreas then relies on collateral arterial circulation to "feed" the liver. This modified Appleby was a complex and delicate operation, but with robots to help with precision, pancreatic cancer patients like me have a chance to live. I couldn't be thankful enough for the robotic experience and expertise of Dr. Zeh and Dr. Polanco. Finding doctors with the knowledge to diagnose and perform a modified Appleby procedure was crucial in my case.

DAY 176 – Friday, August 7, 2020 – Dr. Zeh studied my incisions and abdomen. He checked the records and saw that my low-grade fever had resolved and the pain was much lower. I was still on painkillers but hoped to soon be on Tylenol since the opioids could produce constipation. We needed to get my digestive tract back to work.

Given all this, Dr. Zeh announced he was issuing a discharge. I was surprised, but I didn't question it since I was eager to be back home in my bed. As I prepared to go, I realized the huge benefit of having a physical therapist. She'd gotten me moving pretty fast after surgery, pushing me to get out of bed and walk so I didn't feel I was leaving too early. The nurses had been great, too. My only complaint was the 2 a.m. wake-up to take my blood pressure and check my vitals. I just wanted to sleep and didn't like being jolted awake. Still, it was essential to do that, and I respected them.

A patient transporter helped me into a wheelchair. I took one last look at the spacious hospital room. It was almost like a hotel suite; really, the place was that nice.

The transporter pushed me through the halls to the elevator. Before I knew it, I saw Robin waiting with our car in front of the hospital. The transporter belted me in and we headed for home. I was both excited and a little scared.

How will I do at home? Will I have any complications? When will I be healed enough for the next round of chemo?

I didn't need to hear the answer to that last question—at least not yet.

Chapter Twenty-Four

Robin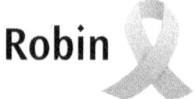

D AY 179 – MONDAY, AUGUST 10, 2020 – It was great to have Lisa home after such a serious surgery. Even though her return was three days ago, we'd still been on pins and needles waiting for the pathology report. *Did Dr. Zeh get clean margins? Is the growth on her liver really benign? Has the cancer spread to the lymph nodes?* This report would tell us much about Lisa's chances of survival.

As we waited for the results, I worked hard to ensure her recovery would go smoothly. One worry was diabetes. I constantly checked her glucose levels. In the hospital, it had been checked every four hours. Now, it was up to me to do it.

I kept track of the readings on a spreadsheet. They bounced around, some normal and others in the 130–150 range. But the last two days had been in the normal range between 86 and 91. Dr. Zeh felt things would work themselves out and told me it wasn't necessary to monitor her, but I insisted. At one point, Lisa mentioned my continued testing to Dr. Zeh, and he shot back, "You should be allowed to prick his finger if he continues."

Lisa's digestive system was another area we worked on. She experienced diarrhea shortly after eating, even with pancreatic enzymes. Since surgery, all her bowel movements have been diarrhea with lots of cramping. We worked with her dietician/nutritionist to experiment with different foods and levels of enzymes while hoping the enzymes wouldn't be needed long-term.

Pain continued to be another issue for Lisa as it ebbed and flowed, depending on her movements. Her pain seemed to increase as the day wore on. We had hydrocodone if needed, but she controlled her pain during the day with extra-strength Tylenol. Last night, she woke up in pain and needed a tramadol to sleep.

The fatigue was very hard on her. "It's like nothing I've ever had before," she told me. "It's like you're tired, so you take a nap, and when you wake up, you usually feel better. It's the same thing when going to bed at night. In the morning, you feel better. With this fatigue, though, sleep doesn't help. I'm so tired I can barely get out of bed. And my legs feel so heavy. If I'm lying in bed, I can hardly move them when I roll over. It's hard getting comfortable in bed and having a solid or restful sleep."

I watched her struggle to get out of bed, walk to the living room, and sit in a chair. She didn't feel like doing anything. It was even hard for her to get to the bathroom and brush her teeth. But she walked more and more around a loop we set up in the house. I liked seeing her do that, even though, the past few days, she spent two-thirds of the time in bed. Today was the first time she spent only a quarter of the day in bed. She even walked up and down our stairs with a long break in between trips. It was great news, although this would definitely be a long recovery.

Finally, the pathology report came back. A Zoom meeting was set up between us and Dr. Zeh. Whatever the results, our lives were about to change. As I got Lisa in to place in front of the computer screen, I thought back to how nerve-racking the waiting had been for each new test. The pathology report was like a jury verdict in a criminal case. Lisa and I were about to find out if it was life or death.

"Okay, Dr. Zeh," I said, staring at him. "We're here."

"Ready," Lisa added, grabbing my hand.

There was a maddening silence as Dr. Zeh looked down at the report. "I have the pathology report here and there's no other way to say it other than that it's very positive."

Lisa and I exhaled. We'd just aged ten years in five seconds.

"We achieved an r0 resection. The distance of invasive carcinoma from the surgical margin was 0.7 cm, and chemo achieved a nearly complete destruction of the tumor."

From my research and conversations, I knew this didn't always happen in pancreatic cancer. He continued.

"A total of 76 lymph nodes were biopsied: abdomen 1, spleen 3, pancreas 72. All were negative for metastatic adenocarcinoma—meaning they were all cancer-free. That's a lot of lymph nodes!"

Based on my research and our expectations, it may have been a lymph node world record. I was thrilled by their thoroughness. Again, more exhaling as Dr. Zeh continued.

"And there was no perineural invasion."

Before surgery, we knew Lisa had *vascular* invasion—her tumor abutted the left ventral aspect of the superior mesenteric artery (SMA) and regional splenic vein. Dr. Zeh said a very high percentage of his patients had this presentation: "It's the way pancreatic cancer is." Perineural invasion means cancer cells are taking another route to spread through the body—by invading nerves—and Lisa's test was negative. More good news.

"Lisa's remaining tumor was measured at 0.5 cm by 0.2 cm by 0.1 cm," Dr. Zeh said. "Also present were single cells or rare small groups of cells and a near complete response score of 1. It's the best report possible without the complete destruction of the tumor." We heard the happiness in his voice. He was genuinely thrilled to give us this good news.

According to Dr. Zeh, three of the most critical indicators after surgery for a patient's survival are (1) CA 19-9 readings, (2) how much of the tumor was destroyed by chemo, and (3) negative lymph nodes. Lisa hit the ball out of the park on all three—so far.

We discussed the report in depth. Theoretically, if the chemo had worked well on the tumor, it should have the same effect on any micrometastases floating around in the bloodstream. With Lisa's low CA 19-9 and this piece of excellent news, there was hope for her to fully recover and remain cancer-free. Still, we weren't naïve about the future.

At one point, we asked Dr. Zeh about her prognosis. He told us, "With this pathology report, she has a 60 percent chance over five years of this not recurring and a 40 percent chance that it could come back. If it does come back, it's often in the first two years. We'll discuss everything in more detail during our next telehealth visit on Friday."

After ending the Zoom meeting, we felt relief and hope. Her pathology report was just about as good as you could get.

As we came down from this high, the next iceberg was heading our way: adjuvant chemotherapy—three months of it. This disease had taught us not to think too far ahead. *Just focus on what's in front of us.*

Step by step. Brick by brick. I knew we could do it together.

Chapter Twenty-Five

Lisa

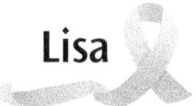

D AY 186 – Monday, August 17, 2020 – Two full weeks from surgery, I was still dealing with pain, mostly at night. When I sleep on my right side, I'm good. If I shift to my back, the pain is immense. This makes it hard to get comfortable. I didn't like the prospect of taking painkillers, but I needed them.

The biggest issue has been cramping after eating. Everything I eat causes me intestinal distress, along with some nausea. The diarrhea is always there and I'm concerned about constipation from the tramadol. I have a cornucopia of conditions to manage.

I learned about a test called "fecal elastase," which could determine if the diarrhea is caused by enzyme deficiency or simply inflammation from surgery. As the stomach is situated next to the pancreas, it takes some time to settle down after surgery. Dr. Zeh said I could take a muscle relaxer to help with cramping, but he voted against doing so, as well as taking the fecal elastase test, at least for now. He didn't even want me taking Imodium because I had too much going on inside me and we couldn't be sure what was causing what. Again, time was the main prescription.

Against all this was my weight, which had dropped to 103 pounds. This was not good, especially with the next round of chemo rapidly approaching. If I didn't gain enough weight, I might miss the final rounds of chemo. The main goal of adjuvant chemotherapy is to lower the chance the cancer will return. In no way could I afford to miss those sessions. I needed to gain weight now!

———

DAY 190 – Friday, August 21, 2020 – Eighteen days after surgery, I felt like I hadn't improved much, especially in the last few days. I still spent at least 60 percent of the day in bed. My appetite was minimal because of nausea and a gag reflex while eating. If I could manage to get something down, I felt pain from the surgery and cramping. These symptoms came and went, with at least one usually present. I was tired and weak, barely able to walk from the bed to a chair.

Pantoprazole, an antacid, is another issue that has popped up. I'm taking it to reduce my chances of an ulcer after radiation, but antacids can reduce the effectiveness of pancreatic enzymes, which could be causing some of my problems. Managing the interaction of these medications was an art form. Our dietician, Shelli Hardy, suggested I try the drug simethicone found in Gas-X and other over-the-counter medications. Seemed like a bit of a stretch, but I was willing to try almost anything to be able to eat food.

I kept a log of my reactions to different foods. On an experimental basis, I only used pancreatic enzymes with fatty food. To ease the cramping, Robin bought a heating pad for me. It helped a little. Then I received a shock. My tramadol prescription wouldn't be renewed. It was an opioid and they wanted me to start using extra-strength Tylenol, along with a wooden stick to bite on. Okay, I made up that last part. The reasoning was twofold: Tramadol can cause constipation and could be responsible for the cramping. Or the cramping could be due to my surgery, adjusting to a new digestive process, inflammation, or healing. No one knew for sure. I counted my pills and had eight tramadols left. I planned on making each one count.

On the plus side, I had my first "normal" bowel movement with no diarrhea. Who would've thought seven months ago that this would be something to celebrate?

———————◄ ❂❂❂❂ ►———————

DAY 195 – WEDNESDAY, AUGUST 26, 2020 – The nausea simply wouldn't go away. Eating a small piece of white bread even made me sick. This would be followed by several bouts of dry heaves and gagging. I couldn't seem to eat or drink without feeling nauseous.

The anti-nausea remedies were the same ones from my chemo days. I was taking Ativan before bed, which put me to sleep. During the day, I alternated between Zofran and Compazine (different drug groups). These offered little relief. I was reluctant to take Phenergan, which pretty much put me out. Other anti-nausea drugs I still had at my disposal included Marinol (synthetic marijuana), Tigan, and a few others. We also discussed the steroid dexamethasone. During chemo, my desperation led me to try anything. A number of these drugs work by changing the actions of chemicals in the brain and I experienced some concerning side effects from a drug called olanzapine. I would never try that one again.

As before, I experimented with pressure point bands, ginger gum, ginger tea, and ginger ale. One thing that helped a little, just like before, was sniffing pure extract peppermint oil. With access to all these drugs, it became a question of how strongly I wanted to treat myself.

Robin and I called the physician assistant and dietitian with our concerns. After discussing it with Dr. Zeh, they asked me to come in for lab work, so we drove to UT Southwestern. They couldn't draw blood from my veins and had to use the port, which probably should have been used initially. But the vein issue showed I was a little dehydrated. My lab results were available in forty-five minutes and didn't reveal severe dehydration or any other problems. That was a relief, especially since I didn't want to spend a few hours there receiving fluids.

When we got back home, I was depressed about constantly feeling horrible. I just wanted it to end. Having 70 percent of your pancreas removed was not for the faint of heart. It continuously caused me digestive chaos.

I quickly discovered that protein drinks, which I'd wanted to drink to gain some weight, for some reason triggered cramping. I was also told the acid-reducer pantoprazole was not causing the cramping, nor was it causing an enzyme dilution problem. Then there was the tramadol. Ever since I'd stopped taking it, I'd been out of bed and walking more—a positive step. Robin was 90 percent certain that the opioid caused constipation and contributed to my bowel/stomach pain and cramping. We both felt it added to my nausea as well.

All the professionals believed my digestive system and remaining pancreas would ultimately recover and reach a positive, fully functioning new normal. Still, it was not going to be quick or easy.

The pending chemo date was always on my mind. Yet I wasn't gaining weight, and likely below 100 pounds again. Right now, I was burning through weeks and going backward. I knew I had to start moving forward. I needed to stop the nausea and gain weight fast.

Chapter Twenty-Six

Robin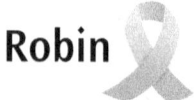

DAY 196 – THURSDAY, AUGUST 27, 2020 – Lisa's weight was going in the opposite direction. Seeing this, I worried she couldn't start or complete the next six rounds of chemo, so I read papers published in various medical journals discussing this matter. Dr. Zeh, a prolific writer, was the author of one of them. Apparently, a high percentage of pancreatic cancer surgery patients never recovered fully enough to receive adjuvant chemotherapy. The question I had was: Does Lisa still need adjuvant chemo?

I talked with Dr. Zeh about this. He had recently coauthored a paper that concluded patients whose CA 19-9 normalized after a decrease of more than 50 percent might not benefit from adjuvant chemotherapy. When I brought up this paper, he suggested he wasn't "brave enough" to recommend against adjuvant chemotherapy in Lisa's situation. "More evaluation is needed." Thus, Lisa was still scheduled for adjuvant chemotherapy. He wanted me to focus on getting her better and gaining weight.

DAY 197 – FRIDAY, AUGUST 28, 2020 – Due to Lisa's ongoing nausea and our continued concern, Dr. Zeh scheduled a CT scan this morning before our meeting. The results came back immediately and did not show any major concerns. Dr. Zeh did note a hematoma surrounding Lisa's largest incision, which was still swollen and noticeably bruised. He said sometimes these situations needed assistance, but he didn't feel any attention was warranted in this case. Otherwise, the scan and the lab work Lisa completed a few days ago checked out fine.

The surgery resected veins and arteries to her liver (and stomach and more). Now, the body had to figure out how to reroute the blood supply. Without this "natural rerouting," a condition called "ischemia" could occur. This basically meant a lack of blood supply. According to Dr. Zeh, Lisa was not suffering from ischemia.

We asked about her nausea. Dr. Zeh believed she had an exacerbated sensitivity to nausea because she was somehow wired that way. The sensors in her brain triggered it more than other patients. This surgery caused nausea in many patients; it's just been worse for Lisa.

Dr. Zeh also noted her extreme nausea during chemotherapy. We also discussed Lisa previously being diagnosed with Mal de débarquement syndrome (MdDS)—a rare but temporary disorder experienced after traveling (especially by boat) that makes you feel like you're moving when you're not. After returning from a cruise, Lisa suffered for months and it was a real ordeal.

During our meeting, she became nauseous, so Dr. Zeh saw it firsthand. His favorite expression was a "tincture of time." Time should resolve the nausea and diarrhea.

Lisa weighed in at 100.8 pounds with clothes and shoes. Dr. Zeh looked at the weight issue and wanted protein in her diet. It was not easy because of how she felt. He also wanted her to keep taking pancreatic enzymes, maybe for a year.

One thing I liked about Dr. Zeh (among many things) was that he was unafraid of questions. He looked at it like a challenge—could he measure up? So I always came loaded with questions whenever we met with him. Looking down at my pad, I saw another question and asked Dr. Zeh if the pathology report's definition of "lymphovascular invasion" meant cancer had entered Lisa's bloodstream. He told me lymphovascular invasion was not defined as cancer entering the bloodstream. "No one knows if cancer entered Lisa's bloodstream." He stated again that the two most important prognostic indicators after surgery were CA 19-9 and tumor destruction after chemotherapy.

With Lisa's permission, I again asked Dr. Zeh straight up, "Now that Lisa has finished surgery and we have the pathology report, what is your prognosis for her?"

It was so quiet I could hear a hair follicle hitting the floor. Lisa and I both held our breath. Finally, he said, "You are in the very highest prognostic category. Still, I can't promise anything, but the statistics you read about pancreatic cancer are not you."

We exhaled.

As I drove her home, I considered how bad Lisa felt and how we might not make the adjuvant chemo starting window of eight to twelve weeks after surgery. Somehow, we had to get her well so she could take the chemo and get sick all over again. One day in the future, I was sure doctors would look back at this logic and laugh. But today, I wasn't laughing.

Chapter Twenty-Seven

Lisa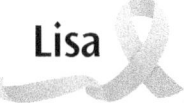

DAY 200 – MONDAY, AUGUST 31, 2020 – This morning, Robin drove me to UT Southwestern for my scheduled meeting with my oncology nurse practitioner, Leticia Khosama. I had to admit I was somewhat nervous. The last meeting like this was in March, before I started chemo. At that time, I had no idea what I was in for. Now I did.

I could only handle three FOLFIRINOX sessions before we cut out oxaliplatin. This left me with FOLFIRI, which was somewhat more tolerable. But first, I had to go through projectile vomiting for days on end, two emergency trips to the clinic to address nausea, blood clots, and more. I wasn't looking forward to going through that again.

As Dr. Zeh had told us, the purpose of this meeting was to start evaluating my readiness for chemotherapy. Since my recent lab work had checked out fine, this was just a discussion and a chance for the oncology team to get a firsthand look at me. Aside from my continued nausea, I seemed to be on a normal course of recovery.

"How is your nausea now?" Leticia asked.

"It's improved," I replied, "but I still have it every day. I can't shake it."

She reiterated the standard line that adjuvant chemotherapy needed to begin eight to twelve weeks after surgery. If I waited past twelve weeks, the benefit would become questionable.

"Your response to chemotherapy was very good, even rare," Leticia told me. "The oncology group believes you should continue with FOL-FIRI for three months, even though pancreatic cancer can develop an immunity to chemotherapy drugs. That treatment was very effective for you. We still have gemcitabine as a second-line chemotherapy regimen."

She told me I'd have more lab work and meet with our oncologist, Dr. Beg, on September 29. Depending on how I was doing then, I could start on Monday, October 5, 2020. After chemotherapy ended, I would be scheduled for lab work and a CT scan every three months for the first two years. Then, in year three, it would shift to every six months. That point seemed like a distant island in the Pacific Ocean—so far away I couldn't even see it.

We left the meeting with a feeling of determination. I just needed to get better fast, put on weight, and eliminate the nausea so I could start the chemo on time. Not starting at all was too depressing to think about.

In the car, Robin said, "No one knows if your good response to chemo was mostly due to your three sessions with FOLFIRINOX or continuing with the FOLFIRI. This UT Southwestern team follows all the newest published and established protocols. I bet if you talk to other people about this, you'll be shocked to find out how many other institutions don't follow a six-month regimen of chemotherapy. Maybe they don't even know about it."

He made a good point. I was blessed to be at UT Southwestern.

DAY 203 – Thursday, September 3, 2020 – Despite the decreased cramping, constipation, and pain, I wasn't pleased. The nausea and gagging continued to wear me down, setting back my recovery. I could not get past it.

Earlier this evening, I gagged on a single ZENPEP capsule and threw up. Robin was in touch with my medical team at UT Southwestern more than once today. We were desperate for relief. My dietician, Dr. Zeh, and his physician assistant were all involved. My dietician, Shelli, told me petite females seem to disproportionately experience ongoing nausea. Lucky me.

During this call, we discussed a Sancuso seven-day anti-nausea patch, which I had worn during my first round of chemotherapy. Carafate was another option. This liquid coated the lining of the GI tract and might help soothe and heal my esophagus. Next up was marijuana—medical or otherwise—and Marinol, a synthetic marijuana. Finally, there was the old standby of steroids. These could tamp down any inflammation while giving me more energy. Steroids were what Dr. Zeh and the team wanted me to take. It would be a low-dose steroid: Decadron 4 mg once a day for five days. Dr. Zeh wanted me to try that and see how things went.

———————— ◉◉◉◉ ▮————————

DAY 210 – Thursday, September 10, 2020 – Surprisingly, the steroid began relieving the nausea. For a few days, I was nausea-free. But then a day came along when I felt extreme nausea and stayed in bed all day. The steroid did give me a boost of energy, allowing me to walk outside past four or five houses before turning around. Yet, six weeks after surgery, I didn't feel like I had made much progress.

Yesterday, I tried the drug Reglan (Metoclopramide). They used it to treat the symptoms of slow stomach emptying (gastroparesis), a side effect of pancreatic cancer surgery. This condition was a possible cause of my nausea. Reglan worked by affecting different receptors in the gastrointestinal (GI) tract, including a dopamine receptor that had a relaxing effect on the gut.

About ninety minutes after taking this drug, I became so weak that Robin had to help me get into bed. I lost all my energy and then became extremely emotional. It scared Robin. As if that wasn't enough, my diarrhea quickly reappeared. The whole experience was a total disaster, so that drug was gone.

Dr. Zeh and his team decided against me trying liquid Carafate. They were worried it would make me more nauseous. Right now I was trying Tums and Maalox—a "lite" version of Carafate.

One thought regarding my nausea was that chemotherapy (FOL-FIRINOX) damaged healthy cells in the stomach's and digestive tract's lining. Radiation could also be a culprit, although no ulcer was indicated. Coupled with the trauma of surgery, these prior treatments could be part of the problem. Once again, all I heard was, "Time is the best cure." But how long?

In four days, I was scheduled to meet with a palliative care doctor to hopefully get other ideas for my nausea. I was at 97 pounds, my lowest weight, including chemotherapy and going backward. I needed some help big time.

On the pain front, I still experienced surgical pain. For some reason, it seemed more frequent. Maybe it was a healing pain? I managed it with extra-strength Tylenol. Regardless, I still felt lousy and uncomfortable. And I napped at least one-third of every day.

I still couldn't have a bowel movement without a laxative or other drug-induced assistance (see the Reglan experience above!). Even though we experimented, I continued to experience cramping after eating certain foods. And I stayed with ZENPEP, my pancreatic enzyme of choice, hoping it would kick in.

My medical team continually assured me that these issues would slowly resolve. All it would take was_____. I think by now, you can fill in that blank.

In preparation for seeing a new palliative care doctor, I spoke to Allison Gimpel, our interior designer and good friend. She reminded me about her experiences with palliative care and told me that her husband, Dewayne Gimpel, had a lot to say on the subject. So I thought it would be good to give him the next chapter. I hope you find the information valuable.

Chapter Twenty-Eight

Dewayne Gimpel

ALLIE TALKED ABOUT SOME OF THIS A FEW CHAPTERS BACK, but I want to add some additional information I feel you will find helpful. First, my mother's name was Reita. She was diagnosed in 1997 with breast cancer. Because I was the oldest and we'd been through a lot together, she turned to me for emotional support.

Mom called and said the doctor had palpated her breasts and decided on a full mastectomy without a biopsy. We knew that wasn't right, so we had her come to Dallas for a second opinion.

In 1997, the internet was just starting to catch on. Mom didn't have a lot of faith in doing her own research, and she was kind of in shock with the diagnosis. Our role was to help do a lot of homework for her. We assembled a thick binder of information with helpful articles for Mom. It felt like the more we equipped her with facts and information, the less fear she had of the unknown, which lowered her anxiety.

Allie used her contacts at Baylor and Mom was reassessed. Her oncologist, Dr. O'Shaughnessy, was and is an amazing lady. She really impressed Mom and let her know that yes, it's something we need to take care of, and it's going to change your life, but it's not a death sentence. "We can get you there because you're in good hands," the doctor had said. "Trust us. We're going to take care of you."

Early on, Dr. O'Shaughnessy was an advocate for Mom, an enthusiastic ball of fire. When it came time, she recommended a good surgeon. So, for me and Allie, our first job was to help Mom through the shock of that first diagnosis and navigate the healthcare waters to find the best treatment, then plan for the aftereffects.

Allie and I agreed to have Mom live with us. As the tests were completed, the doctors agreed they only needed to do a lumpectomy of the affected breast. It was still difficult for Mom to handle since it was life-changing but much less traumatic than a full mastectomy.

Once Mom recovered, she underwent chemotherapy and radiation. She was with us for six months before heading back to Amarillo.

For the next ten years, Mom regularly returned to Dallas for checkups. They ran blood work and checked her CA 27-29 markers. She did well. Allie and I learned plenty more about the medical and the clinical side of it than a lot of family members do. Thankfully, Mom's annual checkups did not find any spread or metastasis.

At the ten-year mark, Mom's breast cancer returned. Additional treatments kept her alive for four more years until she passed in 2011.

So what lessons did I learn?

The first was how important it was to be an advocate for someone who's sick. Mom leaned on me to be her spokesperson with the doctors. She leaned on me to help interpret the clinical information. She leaned on me to help take notes during sessions with the doctors because she was often emotionally upset.

There was a point where I finally had to tell Mom, "Look, I love you, and I want to be there for you, but you need a counselor for some of the issues you're going through—a professionally trained therapist. You need the space and privacy to be more open with that person than you can be with me, to express your concerns and fears about your life and maybe about the past."

It was difficult to set that boundary and even harder for her to hear it. So I'd tell someone who's about to go through this the following:

> Go easy on yourself and realize that you can't fill every role the patient will need. You can be emotionally supportive. You can help them with some of the clinical, technical, and factual side of it. You can be an advocate for them with the doctors. But you can't be everything for them. Work on getting them some professional help; that's the other side of the emotional support they really need.

Mom did connect with a wonderful therapist who worked with her for the remainder of her time with us. It was super helpful for her to have some closure and emotional peace that she would've never found without it.

When Mom's time drew near, we offered to have her come live with us in Dallas, but she didn't want to. Her grandkids and her friends were there in Amarillo. My younger brother and his family were there, too. She had a great support system full of loving people. The only ones who weren't there were Allie and me.

Mom stayed in her home for a long time, even when she became really sick. That part was hard because we wanted to arrange either home-care for her or placement in a nursing home. Looking back, I don't know if we could have afforded it, but we wanted to.

Mom was 64 and ineligible for financial assistance or aid from the government. We helped financially, but our funds were limited, and it wouldn't have been sustainable. All the same, part of the reason we put off getting her into a nursing home for so long was because she was stubborn and willful and independent. The research we found suggested this was common; as people give in to a debilitating disease, they struggle for control and hold on to their routines like feeding and bathing themselves. But it wasn't easy for her. She lived alone and was on significant amounts of morphine for pain associated with the bone metastasis.

One of the most comforting aspects of this experience was that Allie and I were on the same exact page as to how hard to push Mom and how much to let things be her decision. I tried to be persuasive while also respecting Mom's ability to choose for herself. One example was her driving. She was on Vicodin and morphine and still wanted to drive. One day, she said to me, "I've got to go the store. It's just there and back."

I said, "Mom, I have no issue with you being able to get there and back. I know you can probably do that just fine. But if a child walks across the street and your reaction time has been dulled by the medication, you could kill that child. If that happened, you couldn't live with yourself, much less deal with the pain the child's family would have to go through." I made my point, and she got it.

Another piece of advice I have is to be compassionate and empathetic. You may go through something like that one day and want somebody to empathize with you. But at the same time, step up and be as thoroughly persuasive as you can because just like Mom wouldn't have been able to live with herself, I wouldn't be able to live with myself if I hadn't argued as effectively as I could to stop her from driving. The way I was raised, it was always going to be her decision unless she was incapacitated. But I needed to try everything I could to get through to her in a loving, respectful way.

There were a few times I had to scare Mom to get her to see things my way. As the disease progressed, her arm was so brittle that she broke her humerus just opening the closet. She also broke her ribs frequently since they were brittle, too. Even though it was all so painful for her, she maintained that it was worth it if she could stay at home instead of going into a nursing home.

At one point, I knew I had to get through to her by playing on her fears and pushing her buttons. I said, "Mom, if something were to happen and you fell and hurt yourself, how would you get to a phone?"

"I'd push my Life Alert," she insisted.

"If you fell on your Life Alert and couldn't get to it, how does that look? Or your arms are broken and you can't press the button, then what? It might be twelve hours or longer before someone checks on you. I don't want you bleeding on the floor, in severe pain, hoping somebody might come. Do you want to pass away like that? Is that the way you want to go out?"

I was about to leave but I must have finally made sense to her because before I reached the door, she said, "I get it. You're right. I'm ready to make arrangements to go to a home."

We placed her in a nursing home, which was much better for her. She finally passed on June 4, 2011.

Right after this, Allie's mother, Barbara, a colon cancer survivor, was diagnosed with breast cancer herself. Because of what we'd been through with my mother, we knew the journey Barbara was about to go on.

We insisted that she move in with us. She was hesitant at first. This seemed to be a recurring theme, so for people about to go through this, I would say, be aware that the patient's thought process is going to be overwhelmed at first. There might be times when they need you to see things clearly and help make important decisions for them. We found that as long as our hearts were in the right place, motivated from a place of love, respect, loyalty, and kindness, our heads would catch up. If we later found that we made a mistake, at least it was a mistake made out of love.

As the body becomes incontinent, it gets tougher on the patient. Your mom may not think about it beforehand, but what happens when you, her son, have to clean her up? What if you are the son-in-law? This loss of independence weighs heavily on the patient; the mental and emotional indignity of losing those freedoms can't be overstated. That's why a nursing home and hospice care are so vital for helping a sick person maintain their dignity. People like my mom and Allie's mother don't usually think about all of this.

Of course, I would tell anyone to get their affairs in order way before they need to. Sign a living will, a power of attorney for health care, and anything else needed. Do it now so everyone can have peace of mind. As the caregiver, you don't want to be making those decisions at the end because you're not in the best state of mind to make informed decisions, and neither are they.

If you have been entrusted with the medical power of attorney, be aware there may come a time when you must make decisions that other loved ones might question. Make sure your heart is in the right place, then give yourself permission to make those difficult decisions. You won't have to look back and second-guess yourself if you've done it with love, and you're much more likely to find consensus among siblings or other family members. If you're coming from a place of kindness and compassion, then it's kind of hard for anyone to argue with that.

Both our mothers were involved with hospice. At the very end, Barbara lived in our home and died in her bed. My mother was in a nursing home receiving hospice care. I was with both at the end and watched them pass away. Allie was there for her mom and nearby with my mom. Allie had needed a good night's sleep and just happened not to be there, but she was the first call I made.

Let me say to anyone about to go through this that hospice is a godsend. But there are some things you need to know. First, in choosing and taking advantage of hospice, educate yourself about it. For Allie and me, we found that being more informed helped us get rid of fear and anxiety. The information allowed us to be prepared to make better decisions. Not all caregivers feel that way, but it's worked for us.

Hospice has a very specific function for the end of life. It can be tough for a caregiver to get to that point emotionally because you need to admit the end is near and it's time to surrender the care to someone else. If you've been so involved in their care, it's hard to let go of the process.

Make sure you communicate openly and frankly with the hospice provider. Get answers to every question you have in the initial hospice interview. Once they're hired, take care of the nurses because they're going to show up and be there in the last hours. They are angels and deserving of our respect. Not only are they there to help the patient, but also the caregiver.

Right after my mother-in-law's death, I visited an endocrinologist for my thyroid condition. He took regular blood work and always tested my PSA. One day, I received a letter from my doctor that read, *Thyroid's fine. But your PSA is elevated. I've scheduled an appointment for you with this Baylor urologist.* I thought about this. I had smoked for twenty-eight years but finally stopped. Could I have cancer?

I went to see Dr. Matthew Shuford at Baylor and had a digital rectal exam. He didn't feel anything out of order. He repeated the PSA blood work and determined that I needed a biopsy. From the biopsy, prostate cancer was confirmed. The Gleason score was low, so the cancer was slow-growing. He recommended "active surveillance." This meant periodically having both blood work and biopsies to catch the cancer before it grew too much. "We're going to watch it closely," he said. "We may never have to treat it, or we may have to treat it in a year. We don't know. But we do know it's there and it's not growing. As long as we keep an eye on it, we can catch it."

The doctor shared with me the literature and the findings. It explained how active surveillance was a better approach, less invasive, and good for long-term health. "If you were much older, well, we wouldn't even worry about it," he said. "You'd be more likely to die of old age before you die of this."

A year later, the cancer turned bad. Following a biopsy, he said, "It started to spread, so unfortunately, we've crossed the threshold from active surveillance to recommending treatment. There are a couple of options available. Let's talk about radiation or prostatectomy."

I learned all I could and opted for the prostatectomy. That was the ultimate recommendation based on the medicine at the time. However, I was due for a colonoscopy. Dr. Shuford said, "Let's go ahead and do the colonoscopy now, just in case they find something."

Sure enough, they found a mass at the elbow of my colon where my appendix was situated. I soon learned our colons have three parts:

ascending, transverse, and descending. They needed to remove my ascending colon, reconnect it, and rewire the plumbing. However, the prostate cancer was growing inside me. What to do?

My doctors agreed the confirmed cancer trumped the mass, which could be benign. So I had a prostatectomy first. Dr. Shuford used the Da Vinci machine and robotically removed my prostate. I recovered from that in about three weeks. Then I was back at the hospital having a right hemicolectomy. This put me on sick leave for another ten weeks as I recovered from the two surgeries.

Both my doctors were good at providing information and talking through it with me. But based on everything I went through with our mothers and now this, I think it's probably useful for any doctors reading this to hear the patient's perspective:

> This may be the 700th time you've had to deal with this disease or condition, but it's the first time I'm dealing with it. Please have some empathy. In my profession, I must treat every client with personal attention as though I have no other clients. It's what professionalism demands. And I think it's the same with healthcare. The fact that you have a great pedigree and extensive experience gives me intellectual confidence in you. But for me to have *emotional* confidence, I need to know you're human, too. I don't want condescension or minimizing any of my questions. I want you to be patient not just with me, but with my wife, who's been through this with her mom and my mom and is as anxious about this as I am.
>
> As for the administrative staff, you're an extension of the primary doctor. Your competence, your follow-up, your sense of urgency in returning calls, and your ability to handle the administrative stuff well can inspire confidence in the competency of the doctor and the office. If you're a day late, or I call you for results and you say, "The doctor has gone on vacation," or whatever it may be, that can diminish my confidence in the competency of my doctor. The administrative side is just as critical to the

patient's emotional well-being as the doctor's bedside manner. We talk to the doctor only when we absolutely have to. Yet we talk more frequently to you, the administrative staff. You're our lifeline.

If I put myself in your administrative shoes, it probably feels like busywork. A lot of the time, you're filling out forms and making sure the i's are dotted and the t's are crossed. I want you to know that to me, your work is really important. You're helping me feel better and more confident about the process. You're also helping me feel confident in my recovery. So the attitude you take on the phone, the follow-up, the sense of urgency, and making sure you get the details right are all critical to me. Just ask yourself, how would you want her treated if this was your mom? How would you want to be treated if you were on this side of the phone?

The hospice end of things is extremely difficult. It's very hard to lose somebody and hold their hand as they pass away.

As laypeople, we're not familiar with the routines of death. We don't know how the body and the mind start to let go. I had no idea until we went through it with hospice that there are stages of dying, including when they become "active." This phase is generally 24 to 72 hours out. There are ways hospice nurses can tell where the patient is in the process. As laypeople, most of us don't know what to expect. I really appreciated learning from the hospice nurses what we should expect.

Near the end, patients can lose the ability to clear their throat or swallow. This causes fluid to build up, which makes a wet rattling sound as they breathe. It's not painful for them, but it sounds terrible. If you choose to be close during those final hours, you should prepare yourself not to be distracted by the signs of death. Prepare yourself to be able to be present and know what's coming so that you're able to be there for them and not be taken by surprise. For me, it was helpful to make those final moments fully about the patient and about being there with people you love.

Make good use of the hospice folks. Have them educate you about the process. Get as much information as possible to be knowledgeable and prepared. It's still going to hurt. It's still going to break your heart. At least you'll know what to expect, and you won't freak out at what you're seeing and hearing because you'll understand what's normal.

With any cancer—prostate, breast, colon—the more you know going in, the better outcome you will have. Don't scare yourself or worry over worst-case scenarios. Just arm yourself to turn on the light in a dark room so you are less afraid.

You may never experience some of the things other people have gone through, but at least you'll be prepared if they happen. If you benefit from something somebody else has shared, you'll be more willing to share it when it comes time to help someone else with their journey.

Chapter Twenty-Nine

Robin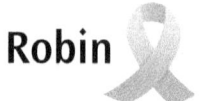

DAY 212 – SATURDAY, SEPTEMBER 12, 2020 – Lisa and I met yesterday with Dr. Zeh and his PA, Lan Vu. He reconfirmed there were no red flags regarding her surgery. Lisa's incisions were healing well, and her recovery was going as expected.

Dr. Zeh said there was something magic about the eight-week mark after surgery: he expected her to feel better then. That would be Day 228 or Tuesday, September 29, 2020, only sixteen days away. But he did tell us that Lisa's weight wouldn't increase while her body still expended most of its energy on recovery. That wasn't encouraging.

As we anticipated, they still had no real answers about Lisa's nausea. The doctor said he saw about one patient a year with this problem. Lucky us.

Lisa had a pretty good day yesterday, and things started out well. But this afternoon, she was in bed again for her nausea. Dr. Zeh said marijuana could be a real answer and would prescribe it if he could, as some of his other patients had benefited from it. But sadly, in Texas, we didn't have legal marijuana—medical or otherwise.

In two days, Lisa would have a CA 19-9 test. Dr. Zeh had deemed other lab work unnecessary since her other blood work had been fine a couple of weeks ago. We also had a telemeeting coming up with a new palliative care doctor specializing in anti-nausea drugs. I created a long list of anti-nausea drug suggestions from a local doctor friend, which would be part of that discussion.

Although it was still a problem, Lisa's nausea had become less frequent, which again led me to an uncomfortable truth: none of Lisa's suffering and pain were directly related to her cancer. Her only cancer symptom had been pain in her side and her back. Between chemotherapy, radiation, surgery, biopsies, blood clots, harmful drugs, and nausea, all her agony had been caused by the treatments.

We understood the treatments were and are very much needed. After all, where would we be without them? But I suspect they'll be considered barbaric a hundred years from now.

DAY 215 – TUESDAY, SEPTEMBER 15, 2020 – Lisa went in for her CA 19-9 test and met with our new palliative care specialist, Dr. Hana Yu. Lisa didn't like our previous palliative care doctor because he made her cry. He kept saying how horrible it was she had this disease and he didn't seem to understand where she was in the process. He thought she needed end-of-life treatment so he wanted to help her with the pain. We kept trying to get him to understand that we didn't need help with the pain; we needed help with her nausea. Basically, he had nothing for Lisa, so we fired his ass. Hopefully, this provided him more time to understand the needs of his other patients or be retrained for another profession.

We met with Dr. Yu and discussed anti-nausea drugs, including marijuana. These doctors were all for trying marijuana, so I quickly learned a lot about THC, CBD, and blends and the best way to administer them. I wanted to have it available for Lisa when she needed it.

Over the past couple of days, Lisa's nausea had continued to improve. For the first day in a long time, she was nausea-free. What an enormous relief! As Dr. Zeh said, "Just give it time." We were hopeful the nausea was under control and starting to disappear permanently. Maybe now we could work on Lisa's other digestive and bowel movement issues.

Although every doctor's visit gave us a little more information, we didn't get many new ideas from Dr. Yu. We were meeting with her again in four weeks, if not sooner. But we really needed an updated nausea plan for the coming adjuvant chemotherapy.

The best news was Lisa's CA 19-9 result, which came in at 11.9. Her reading before surgery was 12.7, with a normal range below 38. Everyone has their own "normal" number under 38, and we were not looking for a "0." But this was an impressive number and perfectly in line with her recovery. By the way, yesterday marked exactly six weeks since Lisa's surgery.

DAY 225 – FRIDAY, SEPTEMBER 25, 2020 – Earlier this week, Lisa experienced some "come and go" nausea. At least she could brush her teeth without gagging, so that was good news. Yesterday was her best day in a long time, and so far today she's felt well.

Her bowel movements have been approaching normal and she still took ZENPEP, the pancreatic enzyme to help digestion, but there hasn't been a specific medication to account for her general improvement. Just time.

Once again, Lisa and I met with Dr. Zeh and his PA, Lan Vu, this morning. She had made the 7½-week mark since surgery and Dr. Zeh continued to call this point "magic." His prediction was starting to look accurate.

Lisa still had difficulty lying on her left side because of the pain it caused. She had general surgery pain, which seemed to come and go. Dr. Zeh believed this was normal, and she could still experience intermittent pain for up to six more months.

He checked her incisions and found the glue still hadn't dissolved. The hematoma on her lower left abdomen near her largest incision was improving. Then, something pretty incredible: Dr. Zeh felt she was healed enough to resume normal activities. Up to this point, she had certain limitations. It was a very positive visit, and he said everything had gone very well and according to plan.

We discussed the protocol Lisa has endured: diagnosis on February 14, chemotherapy for three months, radiation for three weeks, and surgery with an eight-week recovery. Now, Lisa faced another three months of chemotherapy. If Lisa had been treated at Johns Hopkins, MD Anderson, or UPMC, the basic protocol would've been the same. (MD Anderson and UT Southwestern are both part of the UT system and share a lot of information.) If you're treated outside a major medical center that doesn't have pancreatic cancer experience, there is no telling what protocol you'll be under.

Of course, a protocol rarely holds to form. Three major "calls" outside of protocol were eliminating oxaliplatin after it became so toxic that Lisa couldn't tolerate the FOLFIRINOX and was switched to a new regimen called FOLFIRI. And then there were the radiation treatments. No one could say if we had treated cancer cells or scar tissue. Finally, she had a modified Appleby procedure instead of a distal pancreatectomy. Sometimes, the pilot needs to deviate around the storm clouds, and Dr. Zeh had done that for us.

It was not easy getting through this, but we hired experienced doctors who specialized in pancreatic cancer and believed we'd done everything right to this point. I had always told myself bad decisions had consequences, so we tried hard to make good ones.

Lisa was tentatively scheduled to start adjuvant chemotherapy on October 5. In our hearts, we knew that wasn't doable, but I felt October 12 (the ten-week mark) was a possible start date. We had a scheduled meeting with Dr. Beg, our oncologist, for next Tuesday, so we'd see how that went.

Today, Lisa weighed 97.4 pounds. Even though her weight was barely stable, Dr. Zeh believed she was well enough to begin chemo, so he turned us over to Dr. Beg and the oncology department. They all had offices on the same floor and met weekly, which comforted us. We were not scheduled to meet with Dr. Zeh until after chemo. We'd miss his direct involvement and advice, but we knew how to find him.

Chapter Thirty

Lisa

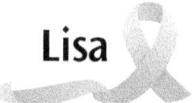

D AY 229 – TUESDAY, SEPTEMBER 29, 2020 – This morning, I had a video conference with my oncologist, Dr. Beg, and detailed my off-and-on nausea. It was worse in the evening as I tired out, but it didn't seem to correlate with eating. Before the call, I weighed myself and saw 96.5 displayed on the scale. That was without clothes.

I told him my bowel movements were almost regular, which was one thing to celebrate. It appeared I'd be taking pancreatic enzymes for quite some time, definitely after chemotherapy began.

Dr. Beg subscribed to Dr. Zeh's philosophy of time being the great healer, especially for my nausea. He believed my lingering nausea was an accumulation of everything I'd been through, citing my cancer, chemotherapy, radiation, and surgical changes. He was not overly surprised I still had nausea. Then he dropped the news. "I want you to begin chemotherapy on October 5."

Silence.

I finally spoke up. "This coming Monday?"

Silence.

I felt my stomach drop three stories. I had hoped for more time. "But I still feel sick," I pleaded.

Dr. Beg didn't budge. "I don't consider your lingering nausea a reason not to start, and your weight has stabilized. There's a lot of value in starting now."

Stabilized? My weight has been dropping. "Is there any chance I could start next week? I'll be more ready then."

Dr. Beg studied a calendar. "So that's October 12. That's ten weeks from your surgery." He rubbed his jaw. "Okay, I can live with that. But no longer than October 12. We need to get this going to maximize the benefit."

I sighed. Robin had been ready to jump in but let me handle it. "Is that all we need to talk about?" I asked.

"No," Dr. Beg said. "I believe the original FOLFIRINOX treatment will have the most value, but I think you should start with FOLFIRI. Every two weeks you'll receive a treatment, a total of six—twelve weeks total. I want the last three treatments to be FOLFIRINOX. It's not perfect to administer FOLFIRINOX after FOLFIRI, but if you can tolerate it, I think that's the best course of action." He paused for a moment. "But I understand how harsh FOLFIRINOX is for you, so just keep an open mind for now."

An open mind? I almost lost my mind last time. I'm not sure I could ever be open to FOLFIRINOX. "I'll try," I replied grudgingly.

Dr. Beg congratulated me on the pathology report. He said pancreatic cancer was notorious for a reason, but the pathology report was as good as we could expect. Both Dr. Beg and Dr. Zeh were cautious but very optimistic, yet none of us were naïve. We were well-versed in recurrence statistics.

Before we ended the meeting, Dr. Beg said that immunotherapy wasn't better for treating pancreatic cancer than chemotherapy unless I had certain genetic predispositions. I already knew that, but I was glad we'd brought it up again.

Robin and I ended the call and looked at each other. Now I just had to get my mind right and be ready for one last chemo dance.

DAY 237 – WEDNESDAY, OCTOBER 7, 2020 – Today, Robin and I met with our radiologist, Dr. Aguilera. We hadn't seen him since the end of June. He was part of our three-legged stool: Dr. Zeh, Dr. Beg, and Dr. Aguilera. Since they met regularly, Dr. Aguilera was fully aware of my situation.

My vitals were taken and my incisions examined. "I'm feeling better in tiny increments," I told him. "My symptoms seem less frequent and not as long-lasting or severe. Unfortunately, I've had very few days without nausea, surgical pain, or cramping."

Dr. Aguilera took mental notes as I continued. "My surgical pain still comes and goes and is controlled by Extra Strength Tylenol. I can't lay on my left side without discomfort. My bowel movements are still problematic. And my abdominal cramping starts up after my meals. Any protein drink causes serious cramping."

"Are you seeing any progress?" he asked.

"Yes, but the cramping and bowel movements are an issue since I need to be able to eat more normally to gain weight. It's hard to figure out which foods cause cramping and what dose of pancreatic enzyme to take. My system is still adjusting to the new normal."

Although there wasn't much he could do, Dr. Aguilera empathized and said he understood my situation. He then confirmed I should continue the ulcer-preventative drug Protonix for six months post-surgery.

"Unlike a few weeks ago," I told him, "I can deal better with these issues now since I'm out of bed all day. I've even gone for some short drives in my car. Then, this morning, I weighed 95.4, my lowest since all this began. I have barely turned the corner, yet here comes adjuvant chemotherapy in five days, knocking at the door."

Dr. Aguilera nodded. Sticking up for his profession, he believed radiation had helped me. He also commented on how effective the chemotherapy had been: "A very small percentage of patients achieve that result." He also told me some patients still feel poorly one year after surgery, while others have permanent issues. Then he told us he wouldn't be surprised to either see me make it one chemo treatment or the full three months. "After everything you've endured, we're not sure how your body will respond."

Between meeting separately with Dr. Aguilera's nurse, PA, and Dr. Aguilera himself, we were there for about an hour and a half. Dr. Aguilera and Dr. Zeh were willing to sit and answer questions until we exhausted ourselves, which was great because Robin usually had plenty of them.

Dr. Aguilera said lymphovascular invasion was a pathology concern (which we knew about at the onset of my diagnosis). He said *if* the cancer recurs, it could return to the "localized" area where the tumor started. "If that happens, it could possibly be treated with radiation."

Robin and I didn't hold back. We pinned these guys down and asked for opinions on everything. Our doctors were pretty matter-of-fact with their responses, but the good thing was that they were all very optimistic about my long-term prognosis.

Dr. Aguilera's advice regarding adjuvant chemotherapy: Don't fret about it. Do the best you can.

DAY 242 – Monday, October 12, 2020 – The dreaded day finally arrived, ten weeks since my surgery and eight months since I began this journey fighting pancreatic cancer. Truthfully, I was not physically or mentally ready to begin adjuvant chemotherapy. But I knew it was crucial. So, at 7 a.m., I had lab work done, which was good. Dr. Beg reviewed everything and approved the start of chemo. And away we went.

First up was a cocktail of symptom-reducing drugs administered through my port. For nausea: aprepitant (CINVANTI), palonosetron (ALOXI), prochlorperazine, and the steroid Dexamethasone. For diarrhea: atropine. For twitching, itching, and that antsy feeling: Benadryl.

I also received follow-up immunization shots in the arm for pneumococcal, 23-Valent, meningococcal conjugate, and meningococcal B. Due to the removal of my spleen, I was scheduled for another round of immunizations in six months.

Next up was FOLFIRI. It consisted of three drugs: Fluorouracil (formerly called Adrucil or, more commonly, 5-FU), irinotecan, and leucovorin. This took 105 minutes to administer.

Before I could leave, the nurse hooked up my 5-FU fanny pack pump. Like before, the drug Fluorouracil would continue to be slowly released into my port over the next forty-six hours. It still had a faint but annoying clicking sound we could clearly hear in the dead of night. All this was the same routine as my neoadjuvant chemo, and I didn't have any good memories to rely on.

My treatments were scheduled for three months, and the cumulative effect was real. If all went well, my last treatment would begin on December 21. I couldn't wait!

DAY 244 – Wednesday, October 14, 2020 – Robin and I visited the infusion clinic this morning at 8 a.m. I was scheduled to remove my

5-FU pump later that morning, but I wanted to take advantage of every resource, so I arrived early for fluids along with an intravenous anti-nausea drug called Zofran. The fluids were mainly saline and offered hydration and a little energy boost. Having Zofran administered intravenously worked much better for me than the pill form.

Since this appointment was impromptu, I was put in the community room. Due to the coronavirus, Robin could only come to the private room, but that wasn't available, so I was on my own.

It was tough to watch all these cancer patients push themselves to the brink of death to survive another day. It honestly looked like something out of a horror movie. I felt so sorry for those folks and prayed they made it.

While I was there, the nurse disconnected my 5-FU pump and, like before, attached the Neulasta injector to my abdomen. Twenty-seven hours later, the device would automatically inject a drug to keep my white blood cell count up. Robin and I would remove it after the injection.

Before we left, we picked up a prescription for a Sancuso patch, an anti-nausea drug taped to my arm for seven days. We had an array of other anti-nausea drugs as well.

When all was done, it was 10:30 in the morning.

Back at home, I was worn out and had some off-and-on nausea. I was in bed most of the afternoon and evening. At the moment, everything was manageable. Still, I was sure I'd spend much time napping over the next few months. Hopefully, I could keep under control the nausea and whatever other symptoms appeared.

Hopefully.

Chapter Thirty-One

Robin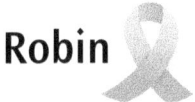

DAY 260 – FRIDAY, OCTOBER 30, 2020 – Lisa started her second adjuvant chemotherapy treatment last Monday, the 26th, and it quickly became too much for her to handle. The cumulative effect of Lisa's treatments caused her to fall last night around 12:30 a.m. She was returning to bed from the bathroom and fainted, hit her head on a wall, and was semi-conscious for thirty seconds or more. It was terrifying. I was very close to calling 911.

I checked her blood pressure, which was good—110/74. (Throughout this ordeal, her blood pressure was always good.) We kept the lights on and I observed her for an hour or so. It took that long for her to fully recover. Aside from a bruise and some swelling on her forehead, she seemed fine in the morning. Still, I quickly contacted our doctors, who gave me a list of other things to look out for. We also discussed how hard the chemo was hitting her. Everyone was concerned about her hydration, so that was a focal point.

Lisa had her pump disconnected two days ago after the second chemo session and has remained in bed since then. Even though she received additional fluids and anti-nausea medication during that visit, it didn't do much for her. She also suffers from extreme fatigue, along with the strange combination of being very antsy.

The cumulative effects of her treatment continued to overwhelm her. After her collapse in the bathroom, I was very concerned. I could see it would be an extreme challenge for her to make all the scheduled treatments.

DAY 264 – Tuesday, November 3, 2020 – We weighed Lisa this morning and it showed a shocking 89.8, by far her lowest. This was very concerning. She barely managed to get up and eat very small meals and take bathroom breaks. Almost all her time has been spent in bed, although she did manage to sit in a chair for about an hour today. She threw up a couple of times and had some gagging episodes. The extreme fatigue has not disappeared.

She was very concerned about taking the third treatment of FOLFIRI in six days. I didn't feel like she could handle the treatment. Nor did I think it was wise. It was clear she couldn't continue on this path.

After taking my concerns to Dr. Beg, he agreed to give her one more week to recover. He and his team began discussing how best to proceed. We scheduled a meeting with them in about ten days to evaluate how Lisa was doing and further discuss a plan going forward.

Regarding Lisa's fall, our doctors decided it would be best to get a CT scan of her head for a better evaluation. She had experienced severe fatigue before her fall, and now, everything seemed okay, but the imaging was still a good idea. To be honest, it probably should have been done a couple of days ago, but hopefully, we can get it done tomorrow.

DAY 265 – Wednesday, November 4, 2020 – Lisa completed a head CT scan this morning to ensure there was no damage from her fall. We received the results two hours later, and everything checked out perfectly, as we felt it would, but it was good to have this confirmation. It was a very concerning incident, probably best described as a collapse.

It was a no-brainer for Lisa to skip her next scheduled chemo treatment. It had been an extremely difficult week for her. She needed the week off and had to focus on getting well and gaining weight. Having chemotherapy when you haven't fully recovered from surgery was an awful lot to endure. At least we dodged injury from her fall. That was something to be thankful for.

DAY 273 – Thursday, November 12, 2020 – This morning, Lisa and I met with Leticia Khosama, Dr. Beg's nurse practitioner. Based on instructions from Dr. Beg, Lisa would not have a chemotherapy treatment this coming Monday, which was in four days. We had already skipped a week, so this news came as a shock.

"The cure cannot be worse than the disease," Dr. Beg explained. Usually, they asked for Lisa's thoughts. But this time they didn't. They knew she was in a bad way. With some pushback, Lisa finally agreed with the decision.

She would be "off" until we met with Dr. Beg for further discussion and instruction on November 24. Lisa had been receiving the "full strength" FOLFIRI. Most likely, she would continue with a scaled-down version of that regimen. It was also possible she could get a different version of the regimen or even just the drug 5-FU. That would be further discussed on the 24th.

Lisa weighed in at 92.8 this morning. This is up from 89.8 pounds a couple of weeks earlier. She needed a longer break to gain more weight. They wanted her to feel much better and her weight to be 100 pounds.

Lisa's last few bowel movements were very light in color. This had also happened during her first round of chemotherapy. Since it happened after she'd had a proper stool color, they asked her to go in for full blood work this afternoon, including bilirubin. A blockage of the bile duct could cause light-colored stools. That would be a concern since a recurrence of cancer or scar tissue could cause that blockage. It could also be caused by inflammation, liver damage, breakdown of red blood cells, tumors in the liver or pancreas, general side effects from chemotherapy, or Lisa's "new digestive tract." We didn't believe the cancer had returned but appreciated the full diligence of the oncology team. Hopefully, this was just something that needed to calm down during the chemotherapy break.

Four days ago, on Sunday, Lisa was having a bad day, nauseous for most of the afternoon and evening. Then she developed severe diarrhea. We think it was from eating an avocado on half of a turkey sandwich. Protein drinks, iced tea, and avocado triggered her nausea. Some of this was hard to figure out.

Her hair started to become brittle again. More and more, I saw hair on the floor. It didn't fall out. Instead, it became brittle and broke off. It was the same pattern as her initial chemo treatment. Back then, Lisa's hair had returned. It was very curly and gray. Yet her new hair roots seem more of a red color. Between treatments, the beginnings of normalcy appeared. That stopped as she moved forward. That's what life was like with chemotherapy.

And if all this weren't enough, Alec Trebek just died of pancreatic cancer—twenty months after diagnosis. From what I could tell, he'd been unable to initially have surgery on his tumor. Near the end, he did have surgery, but it was three weeks before his death. At least he lived to be 80. A lot of us would take 80 right now if we could.

Chapter Thirty-Two

Lisa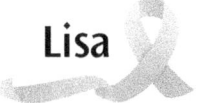

D AY 283 – Sunday, November 22, 2020 – Since stopping my chemo after only two sessions, I was doing better, even getting my weight up to 94.5 pounds, yet nowhere near the 100 pounds my doctors wanted. Still fatigued, I had digestive issues like heartburn and minor nausea after some of my meals.

We were scheduled to meet with Dr. Beg in two days to discuss resuming chemo. So far, I'd enjoyed this "holiday" and the ability to eat more. And I had a lot to be thankful for. That's why it was such a terrible blow to get a call from my brother Paul that Dad had passed away. Gordie O'Dell was 87 and would have celebrated his 88th birthday in January. He had been admitted to a skilled care nursing home, Transitions Healthcare, in Irwin, Pennsylvania, two days earlier after spending about ten days in a local hospital. Dad's health had been deteriorating, so it wasn't a total surprise, but I still felt the shock.

Dad had undergone heart bypass surgery in the 1990s and suffered a mild heart attack a few years ago. He had been previously diagnosed with congestive heart failure and suffered from Lewy body dementia. Although his health had declined, until his recent hospitalization he lived with and cared for my stepmother, Dorothy, who had Alzheimer's.

Basically, Dad's body just shut down, although the official cause of death would probably be listed as complications from congestive heart failure. With Mom dying in 1987 from complications of brain cancer, now I had lost both my parents. It was surreal.

Robin spent time on the phone dealing with the funeral. Even with small funerals being allowed in Pennsylvania under the pandemic rules, we wouldn't be returning to Pittsburgh. I was not well enough to make the trip, not to mention the risk of COVID-19 exposure. It was just bad on top of worse in what had been an extremely difficult year.

––––––––––––––––◆◆◆◆■––––––––––––––

DAY 285 – TUESDAY, NOVEMBER 24, 2020 – Losing my father knocked me back, but I had to keep going, trying to get better so I could beat this terrible cancer. Dad's funeral was scheduled for December 1, in seven days. I wouldn't be there but it would be broadcast over the internet. At least I could watch it.

I felt good that the funeral home suggested donations to the Pancreatic Cancer Action Network at PanCAN.org instead of flowers. That was a nice touch, set up by my sister-in-law, Janet.

With Dad's death hanging over my head, I met with Dr. Beg this morning. He said I would resume chemotherapy next week, probably Monday, the day before Dad's funeral. I'd stay on FOLFIRI but reduced to a 60 percent dose. If I tolerated that, the dose would gradually increase for future treatments.

We discussed gemcitabine again, which would have its own side effects. Dr. Beg was not hung up on keeping gemcitabine as a second-line treatment; he just felt in this situation I should continue with the reduced FOLFIRI regimen. Of course, I would continue treatment since I needed to maximize what my body could withstand with no regrets. However, I did regret not being able to tolerate the full dose of FOLFIRI or, better yet, FOLFIRINOX.

This morning, my weight was 93.6 pounds. Much like Dr. Zeh, Dr. Beg said gaining weight after surgery would be a marathon, and any weight gain would take a while to kick in.

I still suffered some intestinal cramping and a full feeling after eating. I was also fatigued very easily. But even with these side effects, in general, I was improving. The time off from chemotherapy had definitely helped.

My bowel movements and stool color were getting close to normal. That was probably more of a chemo side effect that would change when I started back up.

My diet was only restricted based on food tolerance, but I still took pancreatic enzymes with every meal. Dr. Beg gave me a few ideas on how to increase calories.

He said I would have a CT scan after finishing chemo, which was now scheduled for mid-January. He would only test me earlier if my CA 19-9 was really elevated, like approaching 100. Dr. Beg was definitely not as strong a believer in CA 19-9 testing and reliability as Dr. Zeh. He did say the same thing as Dr. Zeh: "If your CA 19-9 is under 38, you can't get more normal than normal."

Hopefully, my chemotherapy would be more tolerable as I grieved my father's death.

———————————◈◈◈◈▮———————————

DAY 292 – Tuesday, December 1, 2020 – Dad's funeral was held at the Immaculate Conception Church in Irwin, Pennsylvania. It was broadcast on the internet but I couldn't watch it. The chemo I had endured the day before had knocked me down. I was in bed feeling really bad. The last thing I wanted to do was watch a funeral, even if it was Dad's. I just needed to shut down and take care of myself. Dad would've understood. He'd been a survivor, too.

Chapter Thirty-Three

Robin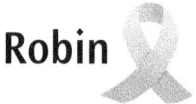

D AY 300 – WEDNESDAY, DECEMBER 9, 2020 – Gordie's death seventeen days ago was another hurdle Lisa had to overcome. And believe me, she was in no shape to jump over anything.

There was really no way we could go to the funeral. Lisa was still very weak and suffering from the lingering effects of her surgery and ongoing chemotherapy. She was certainly in no shape to travel. Having her spleen removed wasn't going to help her immune response either. Being as sick and immunocompromised as she was made it an easy decision. Even though doubts ran through the country about how harmful this virus was, we couldn't risk it.

Lisa's brothers and immediate family went to the funeral. Despite the many precautions in place, many still came down with COVID. After hearing that, it reconfirmed how disastrous the trip could have been for us. Lisa might not have recovered as quickly as her family members. In fact, I truly believe she could have died. The bottom line was that Gordie's death and missing the funeral did not help Lisa get well. Unfortunately, death is often very inconvenient.

After all that, Lisa received the 60 percent FOLFIRI dose on November 30. Then, yesterday, we met with Nurse Practitioner Khosama. There was no lab draw; it was just a meeting to evaluate Lisa's chemotherapy treatments. Although Lisa was not without side effects, the dose reduction to 60 percent had made a very measurable impact. It was decided Lisa would continue with the same regimen, but the dose would increase to 70 percent of "normal" at the next treatment. We'd continue to evaluate how this new strength worked and look for any chance to increase it.

We also talked about her CA 19-9 results. The normal range was under 38, and her numbers have been:

11.9 on September 14

13.0 on October 12

16.3 on October 26

16.4 on November 12

17.2 on November 30

We worried about this steady increase but were told by Dr. Zeh, Dr. Beg, and various nurses that it was not a cause for concern. The comments were, "The difference is not clinically significant," or "The normal range is normal range," or "This doesn't define a trend," or "You're placing too much faith in the accuracy of CA 19-9 results."

Lisa's next CA 19-9 test will be taken during her December 28 infusion visit. Larger and continued increases outside the normal range would definitely be a concern.

————————— ◈◈◈◈ ◼—————————

DAY 313 – Tuesday, December 22, 2020 – Eight days ago, Lisa had her fourth adjuvant chemo infusion, this one with a 70 percent FOLFIRI dose. She was feeling better before the treatment, but after this 70 percent dose, she really felt it again. The oncology team used the term "stacking" rather than "cumulative effect" to describe this effect on patients. Lisa's treatments were approaching one year, so it was not hard to understand how stacking had worn her down. It was really indescribable what she had endured, both physically and mentally.

The fourth infusion was completed without any complications. Again, she survived the forty-six-hour 5-FU pump and the Neulasta device. She continued with the Sancuso patch, wearing it for seven days. Everything else was the same as her previous treatment.

Lisa's hair finally bothered her enough that she cut it short, and what remained on her head was thin and dry. She dressed every day but got increasingly tired as the day progressed. She had some nausea and threw up once, although her most significant issue was now fatigue. Her surgical side effects have been much better lately, though.

This morning, we met again with Khosama, our oncology nurse practitioner. Lisa's vitals were taken and her incisions checked. Those looked good. No lab work was done. She was weighed with clothes on and the results were 92.6 pounds. I couldn't see her gaining any weight until chemo was over. We discussed the final two treatments and decided to stay at 70 percent.

We also learned that Lisa's present designation was officially called "No Evidence of Disease" (NED). She had no physical evidence of disease on examination, lab work, or imaging tests. This was obviously very positive and meant her treatment was effective. The term "remission" is not normally used these days for solid tumors, and UT Southwestern preferred never to use it, as they believed the term suggested an inevitable recurrence. I get it. I liked NED better. In fact, NED could stay awhile—like forever.

DAY 319 – Monday, December 28, 2020 – Lisa received her fifth and second-to-last adjuvant chemotherapy treatment this morning, a 70 percent dose of FOLFIRI. Everything went according to plan.

Lisa's fasting glucose number was high at 128. We were surprised to see that number, as her fasting readings over the past couple of months were in the 90s range. None of our medical team were overly concerned, though, and, as they kept reminding us, one reading was not a trend. We just had to continue monitoring it and hope it was an outlier.

One aspect of chemo that bothered me was the attire of our infusion nurses. They wore chemo gowns that looked like a HAZMAT suit. Due to the toxicity of the drugs, it was too dangerous not to wear them. That pretty much told us all we needed to know about chemo.

We expected Lisa to feel reasonably well until her pump was removed on Wednesday, two days from now. For nausea, she had to take Compazine and wear the Sancuso patch. She'd also take the steroid Dexamethasone for two days. After that, she was in for a rough ride for several days. Then she should slowly recover until her last scheduled infusion treatment on January 11. It was almost here!

Chapter Thirty-Four

Lisa

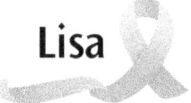

DAY 329 – THURSDAY, JANUARY 7, 2021 – New Year's Eve came and went without a whimper. I stayed in bed and tried to keep from throwing up. While I was lying there, I thought about our last New Year's Eve celebration, which had rung in 2020. Robin and I had enjoyed dinner at Perry's Steakhouse in Grapevine. The dinner was great, and afterward, we brought in the New Year together at home. At the time, I couldn't have ever imagined what my next New Year's Eve would be like—trying to defeat pancreatic cancer. Life could change so fast.

It seemed like yesterday when I first noticed the pain in my back, and suddenly, I was on FOLFIRINOX. I was so weak from the chemo that I could barely make it to the bathroom. During video conferences with my doctors, I worked hard to stay awake and alert. Then I gagged from brushing my teeth. I had switched to a child's toothbrush, which helped a lot, but I still gagged until I was too sick even to brush my teeth. I was nauseous every day until they removed the NOX and gave me FOLFIRI, which helped a little. What a horrendous ride it had been, and what a difference one year could make.

My most recent and fifth chemo treatment was on December 28. Now, ten days later, I felt a little better. I had some nausea and gagging but kept improving as I aimed for my final chemo session in four days.

***

DAY 333 – MONDAY, JANUARY 11, 2021 – Once again and for the last time (at least for a while), I went to UT Southwestern and had lab work done. It looked good, with a fasting glucose level of 95 and a CA 19-9 of 14.3. All the other test results were in line.

I weighed 91.8 with clothes on. Then I took the last dose of chemo and other fluids through my port and had the 5-FU pump attached. Throughout the infusion, I just kept telling myself, "It's almost over. It's almost over." I was pretty sure the anti-nausea drugs would keep me sleeping for the next twenty-four hours.

It was difficult for me to eat well as I had a tiny appetite. I still took ZENPEP, the pancreatic enzyme that helped digestion. I also took Protonix daily to prevent ulcers from the radiation treatments. I would probably continue taking the blood thinner Xarelto until my port was removed, hopefully in a year or so. At least I was not experiencing any noticeable side effects from the surgery.

My treatments would officially end two weeks from today (January 25). On that day, I would complete more lab work, a CT of my abdomen and pelvis, and another chest CT... but no more chemo! We'll then meet with our oncologist, Dr. Beg, on January 26, the radiation oncologist, Dr. Aguilera, on January 27, and Dr. Zeh, our surgeon, on January 28. Assuming the lab work, CT scans, and our meetings all went well, we anticipate I'll be asked to report back every three months for lab work and CTs. That routine will go on for at least a year. On February 14, 2021, I will have spent one full year dealing with this disease. I could only pray it didn't return.

⬥⬥⬥⬥

DAY 350 – THURSDAY, JANUARY 28, 2021 – Four days after my last and final chemo session on January 11, it really hit me. I'd had the chemo on Monday, and by Thursday, I was bedridden. I also stayed put all day Friday but got up a little bit on Saturday. Fatigue was super difficult, probably due to the stacking effect from a full year of treatments. I was just thankful we'd switched to FOLFIRI and then 70 percent of the full dose. I couldn't have made it at full strength.

I still experienced nausea to go with the fatigue. It was a wicked little double shot of misery. I definitely needed some physical and mental relief. I was doubtful I would have been able to finish another round if it had been necessary. Instead, I was done. Just done.

Chemotherapy had affected my mind. Doctors used the term "chemo brain." The last couple of rounds made me very antsy. I had difficulty concentrating and my mind felt like it was cloaked in a haze. Plus, the mental stress of going through the treatments while trying to stay alive was incredibly taxing. I was actually glad I hadn't known what I was in for. Sometimes, it's better to jump out of the plane and feel the panic when you pull the rip cord than to do it a second time and remember the panic from the first jump.

And chemo also affected my body. Look no further than the weight loss. No telling what these chemicals had done to my overall health. But right now, I don't have any other choice. This was it.

Four days ago, Monday, I had lab work and CT scans. Of course, I was nervous and apprehensive. After my three doctors' visits, I learned that NED was still in the house. The CT scans and lab work showed No Evidence of Disease (NED). NED was going to be my new best friend. Because of this, I was not scheduled to be back at UT Southwestern until the end of April—in three months, which was fantastic news. It felt like the last day of school before summer vacation. And I felt like I'd just won a boxing match. I took everything they threw at me and made it to the bell.

My last weigh-in was 90.6 pounds. I'd been communicating with my dietician, Shelli Hardy, regarding my diet and possibly hiring a personal trainer. Diet and exercise were extremely important for me going forward for a number of reasons. I'd need to recover from chemo before implementing anything, but gaining weight and adding muscle mass would be job one.

Of course, I still had ups and downs, with the occasional nausea and fatigue. I was usually ready for bed after dinner. All our doctors agreed it would take me some time to recover and gain weight. They weren't sure I'd ever get back to my pre-cancer weight. We'd just have to see.

There were a few things that concerned us this week. My CT abdomen scan showed a 7 mm lymph node (slightly enlarged). This same lymph node, while maintaining the same size, had appeared on a number of my CT scans over the past year. Dr. Zeh unequivocally stated it was not a concern, so we decided to go with that for now.

Additionally, much to our surprise, my scan showed a superior endplate compression fracture at the L1 with approximately 25 percent loss of vertebral height. This was new compared to my most recent scan on August 28. Dr. Zeh assured us the compression fracture had nothing to do with my cancer, but I was still worried. (Maybe it isn't typical for pancreatic cancer, but cancer can invade and weaken bones.) We believe this spinal compression fracture happened during my bathroom fall (better described as a collapse) at the end of October. At least I felt no pain from it. At some point in the future, Dr. Zeh recommended I get a bone density test to check for osteoporosis. I understand that 30 to 50 percent of all women will have at least one spinal compression fracture before age 80. Many go undiagnosed and can cause back pain.

My CA 19-9 came in at 12.9, which was a great reading and well under the normal of 38. Dr. Zeh advised us that continually elevated CA 19-9 readings would likely indicate a recurrence before it showed up on a CT scan, so this would remain an important diagnostic marker.

Dr. Aguilera stopped the antacid called Protonix. I had been taking it for the past six months to prevent ulcers from radiation. One less pill was a welcome thing.

Both Dr. Zeh and Dr. Beg told me I could discontinue the blood thinner Xarelto in six months. But they wanted to keep my port in for a year.

Dr. Zeh and Dr. Aguilera only wanted to see me every six months. Dr. Zeh had even said there was no clinical evidence that visiting every three months was helpful. Dr. Beg asked us if we preferred three or six months. The main downside of the three-month trips would be "scanxiety." This happened when I had scans and blood work and then had to wait a few days before meeting with the doctor. During that time, my mind wandered and it was hard to focus on other things. *Did they find something? Has it come back? Am I going to die in six months?* Scanxiety was real and debilitating.

Robin and I talked about it and decided we would endure the scanxiety in exchange for getting a jump on any recurrence. I understood that, ultimately, it might not make a difference, but I felt better going in every three months.

Regarding my treatment and chemo regimen, no research showed that switching my chemotherapy regimen to gemcitabine versus continuing with diluted FOLFIRI would have been any better. However, no one knew for sure. In talking about it, Robin and I were reminded how much research was needed for pancreatic cancer. Compared to other cancers, doctors admitted it was poorly funded.

Some of the best advice Dr. Zeh gave me was, "Live life as robustly as you can." Robin and I plan on doing just that.

Again, we asked Dr. Zeh for his prognosis. He had previously directed us to several papers he was involved with, so his answer was not surprising. He told us patients with my pathology report, CA 19-9 history, surgery, chemotherapy results, etc., have an 80 percent favorable prognosis after two years and 60 percent after five years. Dr. Aguilera and Dr. Zeh emphasized that I had a lot going for me, and I recognized that statistics could be interpreted in several ways. Yet, I was a statistic of one. I know the word "cure" is not often used with cancer, but cuddling up with NED is an incredible blessing. Robin, NED, and I plan to be a nice little family and live happily ever after.

I can dream, can't I?

Speaking of dreams, I received an inspiring message from Elvira Bond, a former coworker, to start my recovery off right. She wrote:

> Praying for you for strength and always looking up to God for reassurance. I had the most beautiful dream... I was at the front desk at Coppell High School and out of the blue you came over to me, smiling and looking great! I was just so happy to see you and my heart was smiling. You said the pain was gone and you were elated! The doctors said this was a miracle. You left and I was still smiling ear to ear as I was just happy to see you happy. I still have that smile while I'm writing this to you... Miracles do happen, and I will continue to pray for you.

It was a much-needed boost of encouragement at the right time. I hoped and prayed Elvira's dream was true. Now it was time to roll up my sleeves and get this recovery going.

Robin and Lisa

Thank you for reading this book and following Lisa's progress. We sincerely hope it helps you or someone you love. But don't stop now. Please read the next section, which is from doctors who treated Lisa. You will find valuable information straight from their mouths.

Next, and perhaps the most important part of this book, is the Survivors' Stories section. Each story is different, riveting, and full of hope. Again, these survivors provide plenty of critical advice from pancreatic cancer patients on the front lines.

Finally, we have an Epilogue. It's there that we have updated Lisa's story from the end of her final chemo session. We highly recommend you read that, as not only will you see how fast she recovered, but you'll learn about her participation in a clinical trial. If you decide to do that, the Epilogue will lay out what Lisa went through so you can have some understanding of what clinical trials are all about. The Epilogue also details the recurrence scares Lisa endured. Future updates to Lisa will be at the end of the Epilogue.

After the Epilogue is a photo section. Hopefully, it helps you connect with us and everything we went through.

And don't forget Dr. Zeh's words: "Live life as robustly as you can." Wise advice to us all.

God bless you
    Lisa and Robin Stough

Comments from Medical Professionals

Dr. Phillip M. Aronoff
Doctor of Internal Medicine

Background: *Raised in Dallas, Texas, Dr. Aronoff attended the University of Michigan at Ann Arbor, where he majored in biology and was a Phi Beta Kappa. He attended UT Southwestern Medical School in Dallas and performed his residency in Internal Medicine at Presbyterian Hospital of Dallas. He started his practice in 1986 and continues to be a highly respected primary care physician.*

Practice: My patient priority is preventive medicine, which includes physicals and checkups as well as routine issues such as colds and blood pressure problems. As a primary physician, I'm often the first point of contact before referring a patient to other medical specialists.

Pancreatic Cancer Diagnosis: Having pain is something everyone experiences. If the pain lasts for four weeks and it's in your knee or elbow, that's not an uncommon experience. However, Lisa had pain in her abdomen for four weeks. That's a big red flag that must be evaluated. And she had pain on the left side of her abdomen. There are a few organs on that side: a kidney, the spleen, the colon, the heart, and the stomach. On the right side is the liver, gallbladder, appendix, kidney... lots of things that can cause pain. And the pancreas goes from the right to the left side across the very back of the abdomen.

   Her symptoms were left-sided abdominal pain, which would tend to move into the left side of her back when she laid down on the left side. She had some indigestion symptoms, too. It wasn't clear what was causing her pain, but to be hurting for four weeks was certainly not normal. So, rather than trying to treat her for different issues, I recommended getting a CT scan. I also recommended Advil because if it's muscular, that might help. But if it's gastritis or a stomach issue, Advil might make it worse. The idea was to see the response and then try Prilosec for a few days. But the CT scan found the abnormality and made those other treatments unnecessary.

Each year, I diagnose six or seven patients with cancer. Three of those will have a serious cancer like colon, kidney, and pancreatic. If their eyes turn yellow, the cancer is blocking the bile ducts. This blockage blocks the flow of bile from the liver. It's a form of painless jaundice. It usually means cancer of the pancreas or bile duct and that the cancer has been caught too late.

It's tough to catch pancreatic cancer early because once it's causing pain, it has usually invaded another area to cause that pain. Once pancreatic cancer spreads beyond its original confines and gets to the surrounding tissue, removing it does not usually cure the patient. It's already spread microscopically, and chemotherapy is often very ineffective for it. Yet that's the only way we have to treat it. Unfortunately, pancreatic cancer cannot be caught with a blood test. At least, not currently.

Are Body Scans a Good Idea? People constantly come to me asking, "Well, what do you think about me getting a whole-body scan?" Those body scans can be MRIs, which are relatively expensive, or CT scans with a lot of radiation. When you do those scans, you invariably find something abnormal, which you call "incidental findings." You don't know their disease process. All you know is you see something abnormal. Then the hard part comes.

Many times, when you delve further, what you find is of no concern. An example of this is that almost ten percent of people will have a tumor—a nodule—on their adrenal glands. It's not cancerous. It's not anything that you would've ever known about or would ever come to know about in the future if you hadn't done this test. But now that we see this, do we ignore it? Or do we pursue it? If you pursue it, there may be expensive tests and scans to do, and if biopsies are done, then there's risk involved. If you don't pursue it, will you worry about it? Lose sleep? Stress about it?

Another common issue is to see nodules in the lungs, especially here in Texas. This happens because when people inhale fungus spores, granulomas in the lungs develop. They're benign nodules. So my wife had a whole-body MRI, and they said, "You've got nodules in your lungs *and* you used to smoke years ago." So, they did a CT scan every three months for two years, making sure the nodules didn't change. After two years of no change, they said, "Oh, it was nothing." Well, it wasn't *nothing*. She went through the expense and radiation of eight CT scans. That's not insignificant. So, when you look for things or scan the body, sometimes you have to take what you find with a grain of salt and not go overboard.

You may also hear about a person who had a routine scan and, lo and behold, they found pancreatic cancer. The scan saved their life. You're going to hear about those events. But there's also the opposite that can occur where you find things that were absolutely nothing to be concerned about, and you end up going through further procedures to evaluate it, which can both be somewhat risky or costly. So, it's a very tough situation to manage these abnormal findings when a person does not have symptoms.

There are some recent studies I've seen about a new blood test that's out now. It's supposed to detect fifty different cancers based on the tumor's DNA, which it releases into the bloodstream. This is what the future may be, that we'll be able to screen this way. But again, it may lead us down the road of false positives. You may put a person through a lot of testing to find nothing. So, it's a tricky area, especially when people have no symptoms.

I heard about a doctor who had a whole-body scan and they told him he had a tumor on his kidney. They saw the tumor and removed his kidney. But his kidney was fine. So, it's really hard. You don't want to hurt people in the process of doing these things. So, whenever anybody asks about these scans, I tell them what I know. It's of very little concern when an abnormality isn't causing any symptoms and may have been there a very long time. If you could do these scans and understand that you don't have to pursue everything or that there's a risk to pursuing it, you could just monitor the abnormality. It's not unreasonable to do it this way because there's always that rare individual in which something bad is found.

Another commonly done test is getting calcium scores of the coronary arteries. Sometimes, you find very high calcium levels in patients' coronary arteries. In many cases, when you go looking for blockages in the arteries, the answer is no, there's no significant blockage. You've got a lot of calcification. That's usually not a high-risk problem and doctors will do stress tests and further imaging to go looking around. But if you have to put them through a heart catheterization, that's a potentially risky procedure. So, it's a tough area. It really is.

Dealing with Bad News: The absolute worst thing in the world for a doctor is to tell somebody they've got cancer. It's just the worst. It's incredibly awful if it's something you think there's little hope of being able to fight or cure. So, how does a doctor mentally deal with it?

First, you didn't give them the disease. It was there, and you will do everything you can to help them through it. As a physician, it's gratifying to help them, even though it's very stressful to have to tell a person something like that. I just always think to myself, *I didn't cause this problem, but I'm going to do everything I can to help them.* If they have a good outcome, then I did a good job. If they have a terrible outcome, it doesn't necessarily mean I didn't do a good job; it's just that they had a bad outcome, and we did the best we could.

Many of my patients have been with me for thirty years. The patient is like a family member and so it's horrible to have to watch them do poorly if they don't respond to treatment. But they're always so appreciative. It's quite uncommon for patients to want to take it out on me or ask how we could have missed it. If you show them that you're going to be there and try to do everything to help them through it, they're hugely grateful. It's a very rewarding part of the job, but it's a horribly stressful thing to deal with because of the stress it causes the patient.

Minimizing the Risk of Cancer: Obviously, not smoking is the biggest one, but it's so tough to know about other causes of cancer. I hate restricting people's lifestyles unnecessarily unless there's a known reason for it. I'm all for people trying to follow a good diet and exercise, but diseases happen anyway. I think the smart choice is focusing on good screening and attention to your body, looking for things that are different, and not ignoring anything that goes on, something that's staying with you for a couple of weeks and should be checked out and not ignored. But as for prevention, it's a tough deal. You eat right, exercise, avoid alcohol in excess: that is your best chance. Smoking is probably the biggest one, I'd say, to avoid.

Maximizing the Chances of Surviving Cancer: It depends on the cancer. If you go to a surgeon, they may want to cut it out. That's often an essential part of the treatment, but sometimes it's not. I think a medical oncologist is generally the first step because they coordinate treatment and are up-to-date on all the latest available treatments.

If you have cancer, getting in with an excellent medical oncologist is the first step. And then they have to decide: do we need to operate, do we need radiation, do we need chemo, or do we need a combination, and if so, in what order will we use those treatments?

The field of oncology is changing so rapidly with the work from the Human Genome Project and all the different genes that we can link to the tumors—normal and abnormal. They're making antibodies to attack only the tumor and not the rest of the body, which is what chemo does. Chemotherapy is aimed at destroying all rapidly dividing cells in the body. So, it can cause a lot of side effects. But that's one of the best parts of what's going on right now: all the new cancer treatments coming out. Sure, they're very expensive, but eventually they'll be more affordable and not break the system.

All these drugs you hear about on TV are hugely expensive. But I have a patient who came to me three years ago. She was about 60 years old and had pain in her chest and shortness of breath. It turned out she had breast cancer that had spread to her lungs and ribs. She was not an American citizen and didn't have insurance. They did the biopsy and found that it was all breast cancer, and she had specific genes that responded to a drug called Ibrance. It's a pill that you take once a day. The pill doesn't make you sick. It doesn't make you lose your hair. It's what they call a "biological," an antibody that's directed against cancer cells. The tumor cells have abnormal proteins that are part of the cancer and don't exist in the other cells. You can make antibodies against those proteins so they will attack only those cells and not the other cells.

You take the drug for three weeks, then you're off for a week. That's twenty-one pills a month at $1,000 per tablet, which equals $21,000 a month or $240,000 a year. The one thing about pharmaceutical companies is that they may charge a lot, but they often offer patient assistance to indigent people. Pfizer has given her a year's supply of this for three years now, and she has been in remission the entire time. She's had no recurrence. It just knocked it out completely. She has been asymptomatic; she has led a normal life—no shortness of breath, no pains until recently when it started to come back. Nonetheless, it gave her three years of a very high-quality life. So, to me, that's a fantastic drug.

The $1,000-a-pill is a game played by the insurance companies. A big insurance company might negotiate a 70 percent discount off the drug manufacturer's listed price, so the final cost to the patient is $300, which is still a lot of money. If you're indigent, you're going to get it for free. If you're a billionaire, you don't care what it costs. The people who suffer are the ones who have some money but don't have health insurance. They won't be able to afford the pill, and they won't get it for free. So, either be really poor, super-rich, or have good insurance.

I had another person with melanoma. For six years, she came in and refused mammograms. Now, she had a big lump in her armpit and thought it was breast cancer. We did a mammogram, which was normal. We biopsied the lump, and it was six centimeters across. It was melanoma, and it had spread to the lymph nodes in her armpit from an unknown primary source. We didn't know where the source was, but she had it, and it had already spread. Yet there was a new drug out called Opdivo. It was one of the newer ones, so she got on that and the lump went away. The medicine just ate up the melanoma. The surgeon went in to operate and removed everything from that area. Incredibly, there was not one tumor cell they could find. That was about six years ago, and she's still cancer-free.

Some amazing drugs are coming out for cancer. Although these things are hugely expensive because they're brand new, they have the potential to give quality of life where people would've died quickly from some of these cancers. It's promising, and I'm hopeful that we'll start seeing more of those treatments become available.

PET scans are one of the better tests for certain cancers but they're tough to get insurance approval for because they're so expensive. For example, you have a person who comes in and says they've lost thirty pounds over the last year. You can get a CT scan done from the neck to the pelvis, looking for cancers. A PET scan would be a better test, yet you can't get insurance to pay for it. Thus, they're generally used only in people who already have a cancer diagnosis.

Once you've been diagnosed with cancer, you may do a PET scan so it can map the location of cancer throughout the body. This will provide a baseline for when you start treatment. With this baseline, you can redo the PET scan and see if the medicine is shrinking the cancer or if new areas are springing up. It can also pinpoint the area for a biopsy if needed.

A PET scan is more involved than a regular CT scan. It involves injecting the patient with a radioactive tracer (usually glucose) and doing a CT scan. It will then pick up the rapidly dividing cells because of glucose metabolism. It could show up in other potential conditions, too, like an area of infection where there are many rapidly dividing cells. That makes PET scans a great tool for detecting certain cancers and measuring treatment progress.

Advice for Caregivers: I think that most caregivers, like doctors, get a lot of reward from what they're doing, but it's painful to see the person you love going through this. Sometimes the caregiver needs a little counseling or some external support.

I know that seeing the person you love dying and ill and going through horrible treatments is just the pits. There's no easy answer to this and I don't have any great advice to offer. Sometimes counseling is necessary to ensure they're sleeping, eating properly, and taking care of themselves so they can be there for the person they're caring for.

I would say to look for help; find someone to come in and give them breaks. There are websites like Care.com and there are people who will do this kind of work on a short-term or an hourly basis. There are agencies, as well, that do all this. But the problem with agencies that I've found is that the agency keeps about half and gives the rest to the employee. So, a $20-an-hour employee is getting $10 an hour. You may not get great quality or experienced care for that rate.

However, agencies carry insurance, so you can be a little more trusting of them. If you're just looking for someone to sit there for four hours, that's probably fine. But if you're looking for somebody on a longer term, I encourage people to ask around and not go through agencies if they don't have to.

If you're using long-term care insurance, you must go through agencies because the long-term care insurance often won't cover it if you hire the caregiver on your own. The insurance companies are afraid people will hire their daughter or a relative to come and live with them and get a twenty-four-hour-a-day fee that could be abused. Nonetheless, when you use an agency and get a $20-an-hour person, the agency will not let that person help you with medications because they don't want the liability. They want a nurse to do that, and nurses will bill at $100 an hour.

I always try to look around for people seeking that type of work and keep a few names so that when I have a patient who needs it, I can let them check these folks out and see if it could work for them. It's a big help to have somebody give you a few hours or even a whole day off because it's very tough being there all the time and having to take on the burden of the illness of your loved one.

Primary Care Surprises: Like in Lisa's case, once I diagnose a person with cancer, I sometimes don't see them as often because the surgeon and oncologist take over their care. There's just nothing more for me to do. But fourteen months later, I picked up a chart and walked into an exam room to see Lisa. She had made it! She had survived. I was like, "Oh my gosh, you're alive!" That was such a thrill because I had worried she would have a terrible outcome. This was one of the most rewarding things I could ever get from my work.

Dr. Herbert Zeh III, M.D.
Surgery and Surgical Oncology

Background: *Dr. Zeh was born and raised in Western Pennsylvania. He attended the University of Notre Dame, receiving his bachelor of science in biology and philosophy. He then went to the University of Pittsburgh School of Medicine. This was followed by a residency in General Surgery, Advanced Hepatobiliary, and Surgical Oncology at the Johns Hopkins Hospital. After this, he returned to the University of Pittsburgh and served on the faculty there for eighteen years before coming to UT Southwestern Medical Center to be the Chair of Surgery.*

During his training at Johns Hopkins, Dr. Zeh was exposed to the leading experts in pancreatic surgery and cancer research. It was during this formative time that he took a serious interest in cancer. When he looked at the tallest mountain to climb—pancreatic surgery—he decided to dive right in. And, as the firstborn of six children, it just fit his personality—tackle the toughest job.

Dr. Zeh has published extensively about his experiences with robotic pancreatic surgery at the University of Pittsburgh. There is probably no one with more time behind a robotic machine while performing pancreatic surgery.

Expertscape.com is a website that provides experts in all sorts of medical fields and where pancreatic cancer patients can find the top experts in their geographical area. Currently, Dr. Zeh is shown in the top 0.047 percent in terms of published authors on pancreatic cancer.

There are also other physician-ranking services online, such as PanCAN. org, which is another great site for getting dialed into top surgeons and oncologists. PanCAN has a PALS, or Patient and Liaison Services program, where they can help patients navigate all this and find experts in their area. Then they provide a list of questions to ask the experts. Dr. Zeh is listed on this site too.

Modified Appleby: It's important to understand the medical terms here. Modified Appleby, otherwise known as a Distal Pancreatectomy with Celiac Axis Resection (DP CAR). The modified Appleby procedure—a technique that removes roughly two-thirds of the pancreas, the spleen, and the celiac axis, which supplies blood to the liver—offers patients with pancreatic cancer another treatment option. During the procedure, the stomach is left alone. It was first described by Canadian surgeon Lyon H. Appleby in 1953 as a feasible surgical option for locally advanced gastric cancer. The procedure has been modified for pancreatic cancer in the last ten years.

After the surgery, blood flow to the liver is supplied by the pancreatic head, which has a lot of collateralized blood flow. During surgery, the distal common hepatic artery is clamped, and almost universally, blood flow will switch directions.

The modified Appleby has no specific credentialing because it's a low-volume procedure. It's a rare patient who will need this surgery, even with pancreatic cancer. Today, the number of modified Appleby surgeries performed worldwide is in the low triple digits. It's a procedure that combines all the other skill sets in performing other pancreatic surgeries. If you have the training to do a Whipple and the distal pancreatectomy, the two most standard operations, you can do a modified Appleby.

I hadn't performed a lot of modified Applebys until the last decade, and that's because we didn't have effective, systemic chemotherapy to give me the confidence that a big procedure would help a patient live longer. Most patients with pancreatic cancer don't succumb to the local disease. Seeing the tumor on the CT scan is not their biggest risk. It's developing metastasis and the cancer spreading.

Unfortunately, most pancreatic cancer surgery in the United States is still not performed at highly specialized centers. This is a tragedy in and of itself, despite at least three decades of really good science showing that results are better at high-volume centers. It's just the way our healthcare delivery system is constructed. Most patients get their pancreas surgery done at centers that perform very few each year. This is sort of a decentralized way. I'm sure there are some advantages to the way this system is set up, but it also creates a certain disadvantage. The modified Appleby is likely not even performed outside of perhaps the top ten academic or pancreatic cancer surgery centers. If your tumor is in a spot where only the modified Appleby will work and your surgeon has never heard of the technique or is unable to do it, you won't be getting surgery unless they refer you to someone who can do it. For pancreatic cancer, surgery is the key to extending a patient's life.

Best Chance of Survival: The number one factor in surviving pancreatic cancer is finding a high-volume pancreatic center. They have doctors who not only know the different procedures but can perform them, too. These centers also have top experts in oncology, hematology, and radiation. Yet most patients still get care at centers that handle only one or two of these cases a year. The modified Appleby will not be considered at a small-volume center. In fact, they may not even know it exists. So you must get to a high-volume center (center of excellence) that's seen a lot of these. Let them make the best decisions and explore all the options.

A paper published almost a decade ago by Karl Bilimoria showed a national crisis in operating on early-stage pancreatic cancer because patients were going to centers that lacked experience. They'd say, "Oh, pancreatic cancer! That's horrible. There's no hope for you." Patients who were potentially resectable were missing out on a chance of being cured. Even now, many years after Karl Bilimoria wrote that paper, the country still struggles with that same problem: most of our patients are not receiving care at centers of excellence.

PanCAN.org states on its website, "Although 20% of pancreatic cancer patients may be eligible for surgery, up to half of these patients are told they are ineligible. For eligible patients, surgery is the best option for long-term survival of pancreatic cancer." Because the Whipple procedure and the distal pancreatectomy are fraught with complication rates (besides being extremely technically demanding), surgeons who lack the experience will be reluctant to undertake them.

Each year, there are about 60,000 new cases. It's not a very common cancer compared to colon cancer, which is up in the 250,000 range. You must go to a center of excellence for a disease that's rare and aggressive.

Robotic Machines: Not only do pancreatic surgeries require a high skill level, but minimally invasive or robotic approaches demand an even higher level of training and expertise. Those services are not offered at most centers—perhaps a handful, and only at the high-volume centers.

When the robotic surgical machines came out twenty years ago, there weren't any standards for training surgeons. Nobody knew what to do. So the manufacturer offered some training courses, which led to early adopters who, even before myself, took up the platform and accumulated experience with it. Their knowledge was passed down in a "see one, do one, teach one" method. Today, thanks to one of my mentees, Dr. Melissa Hogg, we have a rigorous curriculum to train our surgeons. But fifteen years ago, when I first started doing robotic surgery, there was no standardized or rigorous training pathway. My group has published extensively on this subject. Still, we need to do a better job of training people on robotic surgery, especially considering the complex pancreatic robotic surgery, which takes a while to learn.

Credentialing Surgeons for Robotic Surgery: Since I started doing robotic surgery, I've become quite interested in how surgeons become credentialed to do it. They are not credentialed like airline pilots. In order to be credentialed and perform a robotic procedure, the surgeon only needs the local hospital to say, "Yeah, we see you have the training to do it, and we're going to say it's okay." There's nothing national, no certification, and there's no checklist. A surgeon simply goes to the hospital where they have privileges and provides whatever evidence they have to do it. The hospital then decides.

To perform open standard pancreatic surgery without a robot, the surgeon completes a five-year general surgery training program followed by two years of advanced fellowship training, usually in surgical oncology or HPB surgery. Then the surgeon is qualified to do open standard pancreatic surgery. To perform with robotics, a surgeon needs more training on top of that.

Right now, 90 percent of pancreatic surgeries are not done with robotics. It's extensively used in urology and gynecology. For complex pancreatic compatibility surgery, though, it's pretty rare. However, I'm one of the early adopters of this platform. I started doing robotics around 2008, and I've published almost 150 papers on the topic over the last decade, showing that it's safe and feasible. There are probably only five or six other people in the country who have half the experience I have.

The Future: Are the surgeon proficiencies and patient outcomes getting better? I think the hope is to convince the system and educate patients on how to select the appropriate care. Right now, there are a bunch of different people involved in this. There are third-party payers. There are insurance companies who must agree to send their patients to the top centers and not just to the cheapest place. And there must be agreements among surgeons not to succumb to the pressure to care for a pancreatic cancer patient simply because your hospital needs to fill its beds. Instead, the surgeons must be encouraged and rewarded for referring those patients to appropriate tertiary care centers of excellence. The best way is to educate patients so they take themselves to high-volume centers of excellence. I hope this book is part of the education process. I'll say it one more time: If you have pancreatic cancer, you must get to a center of excellence because that will give you the best shot at curing the disease and living longer!

In the last ten years and for the first time in my almost thirty-year career, I have more optimism than ever. I see my patients living longer and doing better than ever before. The two new chemotherapy regimens are game changers because we know they work and actually can shrink these tumors. Before that, we had one chemotherapy called gemcitabine, which was pretty ineffective.

The second thing that gives me hope is that we now *time* the chemotherapy differently. When I started in this field, surgery was the only hope to help somebody live a long time. Even now, if we have a hope of making somebody a long-term survivor, pancreatic cancer surgery must be involved. But what we know now that we didn't know about pancreatic cancer twenty to thirty years ago is that almost every patient, even if they have a normal CT scan, already has microscopic cells in their bloodstream. How do we know that? Because back in the day, when we just did surgery alone and took out everything we could see on the CT scan, 95 percent of those patients would have a tumor show up in their body at some point in the next two to three years, and certainly within five years. We used to tell patients, "Oh well, your cancer came back." But that's not what was happening because those cells were there when we first met the patient. They just happened to remain dormant until reactivating at some point later. So we took out the cancer we could see and felt confident we did a good job until later when those cells started to grow. It was tough on us since we wanted to cure the patient.

Today, we have effective chemotherapy to apply before surgery. This allows us first to treat the entire body, including the tumor you can see. With this change in sequencing, there's hope we can sterilize the dormant cancer cells *before* they get a foothold.

If you do the traditional approach, which is surgery first and then chemotherapy, that's called "adjuvant therapy." There's data that adjuvant therapy works but concern that it's not as effective as it could be because it gives micro-metastatic cells an unfair headstart. So many of us, if not almost every major pancreatic cancer center in the country, have adopted the chemo-surgery-chemo approach. It's really a sandwich approach—giving chemotherapy before the surgery to try to get rid of those micro-metastatic deposits and shrink the tumor, then surgically remove the parts you can see on the CT scan and come back and give a little bit more chemotherapy in case any cells survived. I believe the preponderance of data currently available suggests this is the best approach.

Finally, I believe the minimally invasive approach with robots allows for a much easier recovery for the patient. I'm proud that I've contributed substantially to this area of pancreatic cancer.

Chemo Combo: Just so we're clear, the chemotherapy one-two punch that sandwiches the surgery is FOLFIRINOX or gemcitabine and Abraxane first, surgery next, then FOLFIRINOX or Gemcitabine and Abraxane again. It's interesting to note that until about a year ago, everybody thought FOLFIRINOX was a little better than gemcitabine and Abraxane. This was based on one study. Then another Southwestern Oncology Group study came out a year ago and showed that if you randomized people to either gemcitabine and Abraxane or FOLFIRINOX, the response rates in survival after surgery were essentially the same. So that's been interesting.

Art vs. Science: Anytime you have a disease where the five-year survival rate is roughly 10 percent, which is what it is if you look at the American Cancer Society's annual statistics, nobody has the right answer. So if somebody had a definitive pathway to treating this that was superior, then everybody would be weathervaning to it. Though I wouldn't call this an art form, I would say there's plenty of room for trying new things. It would be great if doctors did this as part of an organized clinical trial and not just as one-offs on each patient.

Today, the standard way of administering chemo drugs is pretty straightforward and much the same across the country. A patient receives FOLFIRINOX for two weeks on, two weeks off. Gemcitabine and Abraxane are three weeks on, one week off. What is not clear is how many cycles of chemo I give you before surgery. Three? Four? Six? Do I give you total neoadjuvant (six cycles) before surgery and then none afterward? That has not been completely tested, and there are no randomized trials.

There are still some centers holding out on giving chemo before surgery. There's a lot of overwhelming non-randomized data that chemotherapy before surgery is better, but there has not been a randomized trial. There's actually a randomized trial going on right now but it's having trouble accruing patients because most surgeons and oncologists don't have the equanimity to randomize somebody and order their surgery without chemo first. There may be a small subsegment of pancreatic cancer patients who can benefit from surgery up front, but I believe most patients would benefit from chemotherapy first. So when you consider art versus science and see variations, it's usually about how many cycles to give the patient because that's far from decided.

Cycle Definition: A surgeon's view of a chemo cycle is usually one month. A FOLFIRINOX cycle has two doses of the drug—two weeks on and two weeks off. Gemcitabine and Abraxane generally have three administrations of the drug in one month, so it's three weeks on, one week off.

Immunotherapy: Immunotherapy is what excites every oncologist. The ability to unlock the body's immune system is probably the only solution that can truly lead to a cure for cancer. Unfortunately, pancreatic cancer has consistently been resistant to the first wave of immunotherapies that have come out in the last ten years. Yet cancers like melanoma, skin cancer, lung cancer, and kidney cancer have been very responsive to immunotherapy. For whatever reason, the first wave of pancreatic cancer immunotherapies did not work. Still, multiple studies are going on right now for the second generation of immune therapies. We're hopeful that we can see progress for pancreatic cancer and figure out why it's so resistant to immune therapies. Waiting for the research on pancreatic cancer immunotherapies will probably be the breakthrough that leads to the longest and most impactful survival for patients with the disease.

Early Detection: Finding pancreatic cancer early is another potential breakthrough waiting to happen. Because it's a rare disease, we can't screen everybody for it like we can with breast cancer and prostate cancer. It's not financially feasible. But if you're at risk and have a genetic disorder or family members with pancreatic cancer, then screening those folks can be helpful.

Disease Profile: Again, it's such a rare disease that there's not one profile for a standard patient. However, we know it's slightly more prominent in African Americans and men than women. It's definitely a disease of the sixties and seventies, age-wise. There's a slightly higher risk if you are a smoker or you've had chronic pancreatitis. Then there are a number of known inherited genetic disorders that are predisposed to pancreatic cancer. For example, the BRCA gene predisposes women to breast cancer and is also associated with pancreatic cancer.

How Do Doctors Cope? I'm a hopeful person. When dealing with a disease with a 10 percent survival rate in five years, I try to balance my optimism with realism. Yes, some people beat this cancer, but of course not as many as we'd like. And yet, with excellent treatment from me and my colleagues, some people can extend their lives for two, three, four, or even five years. This is time they wouldn't have had if we had done nothing.

Often, when I meet a patient, there's no standard blood test, no common profile where I can say, "Oh yeah, *you're* going to respond to the treatments and do well, and *you're* not." Everyone has a unique case and can respond differently. I approach every single patient with the idea that I will do my best to ensure this person can beat this disease. But when dealing with the individual, statistics don't have that much meaning; we're either going to make it or not. So I try to look at it from that standpoint.

Minimize Chances: Tobacco use is the only environmental risk factor we know with pancreatic cancer. So obviously, avoid tobacco use. Thankfully, rates of smoking are declining in our population. Alcohol provides a little more risk, too.

Research/Academic Medical Centers vs. Traditional Hospitals: I don't use the distinction of a research hospital because I don't find it all that helpful. A lot of hospitals train medical students and residents; they're all learning centers. I believe the most important aspect is the level of expertise at that center. For pancreatic cancer, that has to do with volume. You need a high-volume center that has seen cases like yours. I think most academic medical centers tend to be the places with the highest volume of pancreatic cancer patients and research.

Radiation: Thirty years ago, some trials said radiation seemed to help. Then another series of trials came out of Europe that suggested radiation didn't help. And right now, radiation is used in a limited number of patients who tend to have tumors involving the major vasculature. That's where most major centers are now, outside of research protocols, using radiation. Here at UT Southwestern, we treat about 10 to 15 percent of pancreatic cancer patients with radiation.

Without a Pancreas: We can remove the entire pancreas from a patient, and that patient will still live, but this makes them diabetic, which we treat with insulin. So we can live without a pancreas. However, the extent of pancreatic resection is not what limits survival in pancreatic cancer. It is when the cancer cells leave the pancreas early in the disease and spread. This happens in pancreatic cancer more than any other cancer we know about. So even though it might seem like a simple solution appears to be to remove the pancreas, we know there's a high chance that those cells are already spread somewhere else and lying dormant. We just can't detect them. That's why we aggressively treat the cancer with chemotherapy, reaching every nook and cranny of the body. Radiation and surgery are great for taking care of what we see on the CT scan, which means we must be able to see it. But pancreatic cancer is a micro-metastatic disease that's spread through the blood system, and this spread is what ultimately most patients succumb to.

PET Scans: Tumors gobble up sugar faster than the surrounding healthy tissue. We inject a sugar solution into a patient and let the PET scan measure how quickly various tissues take it up. The faster it does, the more it shows on the PET scan. However, the data so far shows that almost 40 percent of pancreatic cancers won't light up on a PET scan. Because of this, a doctor can easily miss pancreatic cancer. Thus, a PET scan just hasn't shown itself to be that effective.

Sugar and Cancer: Since tumors take up sugar faster than healthy tissue, it seems logical to cut out all sugar from your diet. There are books and books and tons of internet websites set up for this sort of thing. And if you put a tumor in a test tube and deprive it of sugar, it won't do well. But because of several hundred thousand years of evolution, your body has learned to keep its blood sugar in a very tight homeostatic range. If you stopped eating sugar altogether, your body's blood sugar would still be relatively normal because your liver would start making sugar. It's almost impossible to lower your blood sugar to a meaningful place by diet.

Now, if you're a diabetic, having high blood sugar is probably not good. Making sure you're tightly controlled so that you don't have excess sugar is a good thing. But you could go on the lowest sugar diet known to man and you're not going to appreciably lower your blood sugar below a certain level because your body won't tolerate it.

CA 19-9 Marker: CA 19-9 is the best marker for pancreatic cancer we currently have, but it's not perfect by a long shot. It's a protein that's made and secreted by the tumor. Yet even if you know you have pancreatic cancer, 15 percent of the population won't make CA 19-9. That's a limitation right there. So 15 percent of the population can never use CA 19-9 as a marker. But if you're one of the 85 percent who can make CA 19-9, and it's high, it's an excellent predictor of response to therapy.

As an analogy, there is the HIV story. Infectious disease doctors kept waiting for AIDS to appear so they could figure out a way to beat it. Then they stopped waiting and started measuring the patient's viral load. That's when they came up with the HAART therapy of using a combination of drugs to stop the virus from making copies of itself and spreading through the body. When the virus stopped duplicating, the patients didn't get AIDS and, of course, survived the disease that was pretty much 100 percent fatal. Like the viral load count for HIV, the CA 19-9 gives us an advanced warning so we can begin the next round of treatment before it's too late.

Final Thoughts: For newly diagnosed patients with pancreatic cancer, get yourself to a center of excellence and take advantage of all the current medicines and treatment therapies. I can't say it enough.

I also advise balancing what you read on the internet. There's no librarian on the internet, so you don't know the credibility of these sites. Sure, some of them have real science behind them, but they're not completely tested. Again, at risk of sounding like a broken record, it's yet another reason to get into a center of excellence and have a group of doctors you trust so you can bounce anything you hear or find online off of them.

I also want to say there is now much hope with this disease. We have made a lot of progress, and there are people who've beaten it. But you must go into it being hopeful.

Dr. Muhammad Shaalan Beg, MD
Hematology Specialist

Background: *Dr. Beg received his medical training at the Aga Khan University and Aga Khan Medical College in Karachi, Pakistan. He then performed his Internal Medicine residency and a fellowship in Hematology Oncology* *at the University of Cincinnati in Cincinnati, Ohio. With that completed in 2011, he moved to UT Southwestern as a faculty member and completed a master's in clinical sciences. He was with UT Southwestern for eleven years before moving to Prime Education, where he is an associate professor of Hematology and Medical Oncology as well as the medical director of the Clinical Research Office.*

Dr. Beg's pancreatic cancer clinical research journey began through a collaboration with a basic scientist, David Boothman. The two men obtained several grants from the Pancreatic Cancer Action Network to move some of Boothman's discoveries from his lab to the clinic. The money funded one of their first trials based on Boothman's science. With that project, Dr. Beg found himself squarely in the pancreatic cancer space. Since then, his clinical and research focus has been predominantly on identifying and developing new treatments for pancreatic cancer and caring for people with pancreatic cancer.

Dr. Beg is an oncologist, exclusively seeing people with abdominal GI cancers. However, 80 percent of his patients have pancreatic cancer.

Chemotherapy: Chemotherapies are a class of medications that attack cancer cells' unique vulnerabilities. The medicine looks to exploit those vulnerabilities and kill only cancer cells, not normal cells.

There are many different types of chemotherapy treatments that target different components of the cancer cell. Over the years, many clinical trials have tested different chemotherapy treatments for various cancers to learn which type of treatments work better for which cancer. Each approved drug goes through phase one, phase two, and phase three clinical trials.

In phase one clinical trials, scientists primarily look at the drug's safety and side effects. Efficacy is a secondary consideration. In phase two trials, the focus is on seeing how active those medicines are in a specific cancer. And in phase three trials, scientists want to know how effective the treatment is for a given cancer. If it all looks good, the drug goes to the FDA and hopefully becomes approved.

In essence, chemotherapy is a class of medications looking to attack and kill cancer cells, but there are newer treatment options that don't fall squarely into the chemotherapy box. Those are targeted treatments attacking specific mutations that can be present in cancer cells.

Another type of treatment is immunotherapy, which looks to activate the body's immune system to attack the cancer better. Targeted and immunotherapy treatments haven't made as much of a dent in pancreatic cancer as in other cancers, but there are many programs and trials right now working hard to find additional therapies to attack and defeat pancreatic cancer. Currently, though, the primary treatment for pancreatic cancer is chemotherapy.

Neoadjuvant Chemotherapy: Neoadjuvant is the administration of chemotherapy *before* surgery. In the past, everything was done *after* surgery. Research has shown that by giving neoadjuvant chemotherapy, the chances of a successful surgery are improved because the medicine can shrink the cancer and maximize the chances that the surgeon removes 100 percent of it, not (for example) 97 percent. Therefore, the purpose of the chemo is to find the cancer cells wherever they are and kill them.

For pancreatic cancer, the chemotherapy goal is six months. With a combination of neoadjuvant and adjuvant, our goal is to get people through those six months of chemotherapy. Some doctors use the term "cycle." There are different cycles depending on which combination of drugs is given. Some cycles happen every two weeks, while others are every three weeks. Some can go every four weeks. For some patients, there are a series of three infusions that combine into one cycle. Colloquially, patients often refer to their "cycle," but rather than confuse patients with six or eight cycles, it's better to use a length of time, like six months, so the patient knows when it will end.

Adjuvant Chemotherapy: Adjuvant therapy is any type of therapy that follows the primary treatment. So, adjuvant chemotherapy takes place *after* you've had first-line treatment, such as surgery to remove a cancerous tumor. The main goal of adjuvant chemotherapy is to lower the chance that the cancer will return and to improve the outcome of the first-line treatment.

Combination: The goal for pancreatic cancer patients is to provide them with a combination of neoadjuvant and adjuvant chemotherapy for six months. Neoadjuvant chemotherapy will hopefully shrink the tumor, kill a part of it, and stop it from spreading. The surgeon then cuts out the tumor, achieving clean margins. Afterward, adjuvant chemotherapy is administered, reducing the chance of the cancer returning. We've learned that cancer can come back in the area where previous cancer existed. Cancer can also appear in other parts of the body since microscopic cancer cells can circulate throughout the body. Adjuvant chemotherapy can be effective before it clings to the liver or lungs.

A pancreatic tumor before neoadjuvant chemotherapy looks different than one after the drugs. A post-chemo tumor sample will have some dead cancer cells in it. There is data showing that regardless of what the tumor looked like, patients who had neoadjuvant chemo are more likely to have clean margins than those without it. This is one reason driving the current thinking for doing chemotherapy before surgery.

Chemo Radiation: There are a couple of different ways of doing radiation. The term "chemo radiation" means receiving radiation concurrently with chemotherapy. In the past, this lasted for six weeks. Patients would come in every day and take a chemo pill. From Monday through Friday, they would receive a small dose of radiation. This dose would slowly build up to higher levels. Some centers don't give an oral chemo pill and instead give a different medicine as an infusion every week while the patient receives radiation. At UT Southwestern, our program is amongst the leaders who can provide stereotactic radiation, also called SBRT or SABR. The treatment gives all the radiation a patient would've received in six weeks over a period of five days. When we do that, we don't do chemo radiation; we just give the radiation during those five days. So we hold the chemo and they just get radiation.

Getting the Chemo Right: Clinical trials guide what chemotherapy certain patients should receive. For pancreatic cancer, it's a combination of three chemo medicines called FOLFIRINOX, which is composed of fluorouracil, irinotecan, and oxaliplatin. That regimen is the most effective in patients who are having pancreatic cancer surgery.

Other trials are looking at how to best sequence the chemotherapy regimen, but they're all using the FOLFIRINOX regimen. And all patients come before the tumor board to ensure the doctors agree with the choice of chemo, the need for radiation, and the possibility of surgery. Between the current published guidelines and literature, the tumor board, and the doctors' experience, patients can be assured they are receiving the best and proper treatment for their cancer.

Gemcitabine and Abraxane are two other medicines used for pancreatic cancer. For patients about to have surgery and receiving neoadjuvant chemo, gemcitabine and Abraxane are not used unless there's an extenuating circumstance, such as the patient can't tolerate FOLFIRINOX or FOLFIRINOX is not available.

5-FU: This is fluorouracil. It is administered slowly via take-home fanny packs because there are fewer side effects when given that way. Plus, a bigger dose can be better tolerated by spreading it out. Back in the day, patients would be admitted to the hospital and receive 5-FU via infusion over two days. When the fanny pack was developed, patients were free to go home where they were more comfortable.

Second-line Chemo: FOLFIRINOX is the first chemo weapon we use against pancreatic cancer. If the cancer returns, we can use second-line chemo like gemcitabine and Abraxane. This may be done because the cancer has likely adjusted or become resistant to FOLFIRINOX, so we need something it doesn't recognize, and gemcitabine and Abraxane can be effective for a while for many patients. If the cancer comes back yet again, it's not that there are no treatments available for them; it's that those treatments would not be considered *curative*, or treatments that get rid of the cancer. All they can do is control it, prevent it from getting worse, and help people to live better and longer.

The Pancreatic Cancer Armor: A lot of studies suggest pancreatic cancer has a shell called a stroma. The cancer causes a lot of inflammation that forces this stroma to develop. Researchers haven't figured out whether that stroma is good or bad. There was some thinking that the stroma is bad and should be destroyed. When a few clinical trials looked at developing stromal-disrupting drugs, it turned out that some patients died faster than they would've because the stroma was also controlling the cancer. The current thinking is that the stroma is more than a shell, it's a living, breathing organ that's dynamic and not static. So when we think of an eggshell, we think of it as a static barrier, but the pancreas cancer stroma has a specific balance, and we haven't really figured out how to exploit that to make our treatments better.

CA 19-9 Marker: Ninety (90) percent of patients secrete CA 19-9. Because cancer cells shed CA 19-9, an elevated score provides some evidence of how much pancreatic cancer a patient might have. But the CA 19-9 is not a perfect test. The relationship that CA 19-9 has with the tumor is not linear. If a CA 19-9 doubles, that doesn't mean the cancer has doubled. There is data suggesting a very high CA 19-9 means a very high chance of metastatic disease inside the body that's not visible on the scans. The CA 19-9 marker is used to identify patients who are better candidates for surgery, which is not considered unless a surgeon is confident they can get all the cancer out.

The second aspect of CA 19-9 is to see how well the treatment is working. CA 19-9 scores are used in conjunction with scans and how a patient is doing physically. It also helps identify patients whose cancer has been behaving itself.

The Pancreatic Cancer Difference: Every cancer is unique in its own way. As an example, breast cancer and pancreatic cancer are from different spectrums. They're not all cut from the same cloth.

But the real question is why pancreatic cancer is harder to treat. The answer is that the mutations in pancreatic cancer don't have drugs associated with them. The main mutation is called KRAS, and it does not have good treatment options against it. So it's a cancer that is fairly recalcitrant, and it resists chemo treatment, so that's what gives it its notoriety. Chemo medicines have made some progress for pancreatic cancer, but not as much as lung cancer, kidney cancer, or melanoma. A good example is Jimmy Carter's melanoma. If he had come down with melanoma two years earlier, he would've been dead. So the melanoma field has made a lot of progress, and there is hope that we will start seeing the same progress for pancreatic cancer.

But the other aspect that makes pancreatic cancer so tough is early detection. There aren't good early detection or screening strategies. By the time pancreatic cancer is diagnosed, it's either inoperable or it's spread to other parts of the body, so finding ways to detect it early is the best way to defeat pancreatic cancer right now.

The good news is that today, many different approaches are being tested to see if we can identify pancreatic cancer at an earlier stage, when it's smaller or resectable. And genetic testing is evolving to the point where we might be able to identify patients at high risk of developing pancreatic cancer due to genetic mutations or family history. These are extensive studies that have enrolled, in one example, a million people with new-onset diabetes and are trying to develop markers to see who will develop pancreatic cancer. This study provides us with some hope.

There's also a company called GRAIL, which is working on developing a reliable blood test for the early detection of different cancers, including pancreatic cancer. Currently, the innovation in surgery and radiation has plateaued. I feel the best chance of progress will be in systemic treatments, including chemo and immunotherapy, targeted therapy, and innovation and early detection.

Immunotherapy: This therapy supercharges the body's immune defense system to wake up and attack the cancer cells. It's been a huge step forward with other cancers, but right now, it's not better than chemo. But I'm a pancreatic cancer oncologist, and I can only wake up in the morning and see patients if I have optimism. Otherwise, it's a tough disease to manage. Right now, it's sort of game time because we're waiting for a bunch of trials to enroll. And we're already seeing not just the second generation of immunotherapy medicines but the third generation of immunotherapy medicines evolving. I think it's only a matter of time before pancreatic cancer is cracked by immunotherapy . . . and yes, in our lifetimes.

My Attitude: When dealing with real people with real problems and their families, I feel I can help make a difference for them during this challenging time. If I considered every unsuccessful case a personal failure, I wouldn't be able to last long in this field; yet if I'm not taking personal responsibility for failures, I'm not taking personal responsibility for the successes either. I view it more as a field that is evolving rapidly. We don't know why some people do well and some don't. My role is to ensure we give everyone a fair and best chance with their treatment. And fortunately, I've worked with many people for whom we've made an enormous difference. It's those folks who keep me going.

Angi Courtney, M.S., PA-C

Background: *Angi received her bachelor of science in zoology. She then went into the master's program at Baylor College of Medicine for two and a half years before passing a certifying board exam to become a physician assistant. She's required to recertify every ten years. Currently, she is the Lead Advanced Practice Provider for Vascular Interventional Radiology. One of her primary duties is to place ports in patients' chests.*

Terminology: The terms "implanted port," "port-a-cath," and "mediport" are all the same.

Purpose of Ports: Ports are used in patients so we can infuse medicine into their bodies without sticking their veins each time. Patients who receive chemotherapy need ports for this purpose. Also, IV fluids can be given through ports, and blood draws can also be made. It's important to only allow someone who has properly been trained to access your port.

Who Installs Ports? Currently, the majority of ports placed in patients are done by physician assistants.

Size of the Port: It's about the size of a half-dollar coin.

Where Does the Port Go? It sits on top of a rib, right beneath the collarbone. We tunnel underneath the skin and make a pocket for the port to sit in. There is nothing hanging outside of the patient's body. The catheter is then inserted into a vein, not an artery. This is important because veins carry blood back to the heart and lungs after the oxygen is dumped into the cells. The vein is not even an inch in diameter, so the catheter sits just inside the vein through a tiny pinhole. We need a larger vein because these chemotherapies can make the smaller veins unusable, so we use the vein in the neck called the internal jugular vein.

As far as which side of a patient's chest the port is installed, it's all very patient-dependent. It depends on their anatomy. For example, if it's a breast cancer patient and they've had a mastectomy on the right side, we will place the port on the left. Or if we know that they will receive radiation to that same side of their chest, we would place it on the other side. If they have known stenosis or narrowing in the vein, that condition may determine what side we put it in. I would say we mainly place it on the right side because, anatomically, the internal jugular vein drops straight into the superior vena cava. If we put it on the left side, we must come across the chest for it to drop down. So it's easier anatomically for us to place it on the right. As long as the catheter is in the proper vein, the medicine ends up in the same place. Either way, the functionality makes no difference at all.

Sometimes, if the patient is having surgery, they'll place the catheter during that surgery. When a surgeon does the placement, they do it in the subclavian vein. Interventional radiologists will always place it in the internal jugular vein. It just depends on who is placing the port as to which vein is being used.

Once it's installed, we give the patient IV antibiotics to avoid any infection.

Port Pain: During this procedure, the patient will be sedated. It's not a lot of pain, but enough to need sedation. We use moderate sedation, which is a combination of fentanyl and Versed. Fentanyl is a drug that people have been abusing. We use it in a very safety-controlled environment in the hospital. The other medication, Versed, helps you relax while causing amnesia. The combination of those two medications works very well to make patients relaxed and comfortable during the procedure. On top of all that, we also use a local anesthetic called lidocaine. When the patient wakes up, they may have a little discomfort just from having a pocket made under the skin, but it certainly doesn't last long.

What Material Makes Up the Port? Some are made of titanium and some are made of a flexible polyurethane polymer called ChronoFlex, which is a mixture of polyurethane and barium sulfate. The Bard Power-Port is an example.

Other Ports: Some patients with leukemia who need a stem cell transplant will receive a non-tunneled catheter similar to a dialysis-type catheter. This will then be used for stem cell harvest and transplant. They may receive a tunneled line with three ports for chemotherapy and transplant. The ports are basically the same for all cancers, even though different companies might manufacture them.

Not For All: Not all patients receiving chemotherapy get a port. It depends on how often they're getting chemo. Some patients don't particularly want one. However, I think those who do have it will find that it's beneficial for them just from not having to be poked all the time and not having to get a new IV access for each infusion.

Testing the Port: When we place the port, we access it with a Huber needle, the same type of needle that the chemo nurses use. We connect it to a syringe and pull back to aspirate so we get some blood. Then we push forward and put some heparinized saline in there just to make sure no blood clots form within the port itself. By seeing blood going in and out of the port, we can be confident it's working. If we are still unsure or want to double-check, we can X-ray the area.

Removing the Port: Removing a port is done on an outpatient basis in the clinic. We don't use sedation unless a patient is incredibly anxious. But if we give plenty of lidocaine and allow it to sit and work, the port comes out very easily. We still make an incision through our previous incision as some scar tissue will have formed around the port. That scar tissue keeps it in place, so we have to dissect it. Then we irrigate the pocket and re-close it with sutures. The entire procedure takes about thirty minutes.

Flushing the Port: The port is flushed every four to six weeks if it's not used. We do that to prevent blood clots from forming. If there's nothing going through it, you don't want it to clot off. If the port is being used constantly, we flush it after each chemo use.

Patient Feedback: If a patient has had a tremendous amount of weight loss and doesn't have much subcutaneous tissue or fat, they may feel it more. But I don't hear a lot of complaints that it's really painful. For most patients, it doesn't bother them at all. In fact, they can play tennis, jog, and run. They can hunt so long as we place it on the opposite shoulder of the gun butt. And they can swim after the first few weeks of placement. We put a skin glue, Dermabond, on top. Soon, it will flake off. After that flaking, you can submerge the port in water. Until then, we need to ensure all the sutures and everything underneath the skin are going to be healed up before soaking it. Dermabond allows you to shower within twenty-four hours of having the port placed. We just ask that you have your back to the shower and let the water run over your front side. When you step out of the shower, pat the port area dry as opposed to really scrubbing on it with a towel. In about ten days or so, the skin glue will have sloughed off, and it's fine to submerge in water. You can even sit in a jacuzzi. But until then, we ask patients to take regular showers.

When having the port installed, some patients are nervous. But I think the overall concept of having cancer is shocking enough to them that this port is part of their treatment and what they need to make things a little easier for themselves. Overall, most patients are eager to have the port installed so they don't have to get stuck with a needle repeatedly.

As physician assistants, we really take the time to talk to patients and make them comfortable. Even when they're sedated, I still ask them to choose the music they want to be played in the room because I'm confident they're still aware and know what's happening. So I treat them as if they're wide awake. I think the music helps to calm people and make them more comfortable, which creates a better overall experience for them.

How Long? There are no typical lengths of time that patients keep their ports in because their chemo treatment and responses vary. I've had a patient who's had their port in for twenty years. Providing it doesn't get infected, it can stay in indefinitely. Many oncologists, however, would like to have it removed after completing chemo. That's so the patient doesn't run the risk of having a potential infection or blood clots. Ideally, once you're finished with it, the port should be removed.

PICC Line: This is a peripheral line that goes into your arm. It ends up in the same place as the port, but you have two little lumens hanging outside your body. The port itself is in a pocket underneath the skin. The PICC line is temporary, while a port is permanent.

Risk vs. Benefit: Ports are not risk-free. They can become infected. They can develop a blood clot around them. But overall, the benefit certainly outweighs those risks. Still, it's a personal choice for the patient and their oncologist. Their oncologist may say, "You really need a port because the chemotherapy I'm giving you will require it." I think good communication with their oncologist and interventional radiologist, whether an APP, a physician, or their surgeon, is necessary.

If you develop an infection, you will experience some tenderness and redness. You may even have some pus coming from it. If you are what we call "bacteremic" and have discovered bacteria in your blood, they may find the port a potential source and ask for us to remove it. Patients usually know when something is not quite right. And certainly, if you're very ill in sepsis, where there are bacteria in your bloodstream, the doctors may look at the port as the potential source of infection. If this happens, we remove the port and you will go to a PICC line until we can clear the bloodstream and the infection. Once that's cleared, we can place another port on the other side if needed.

Final Comments: I'm a breast cancer survivor, so I've been on the other side of the table. Currently, I'm doing well. That experience led me to care for all my patients passionately.

Dr. Lamani Finau
Board Certified Gastroenterologist

Note: We have changed the name of Dr. Finau at his request.

Technique: Access to the pancreas is technically challenging. The pancreas is located in the core of the body, surrounded by large blood vessels and vital organs. The safest and least invasive method to reach the pancreas involves a procedure called an Endoscopic Ultrasound (EUS). The scarless, minimally invasive procedure is performed under sedation. A small endoscopic probe is passed through the mouth and esophagus into the stomach and small intestine. This is essentially following the same natural pathway as food so there are no incisions or scars created. Fortunately, the stomach and small intestine are located next to the pancreas. The sound waves sent from the ultrasound probe create an image of the pancreas and surrounding organs, allowing us to visualize this area in great detail and provide complete staging data. This allows us to see if there are involved blood vessels, lymph nodes, or whether growths are close to other organs.

If we identify concerning growths on the pancreas, we then proceed with Endoscopic Ultrasound with Fine Needle Aspiration (EUS–FNA) or put another way, we biopsy the growth. During this part, we pass a small needle into a channel (i.e., a small tunnel) within the scope. This technique prevents any injury to the patient when passing the needle. Then, using live-ultrasound technology, we pass that biopsy needle into the targeted growth, providing a real-time view of what we are sampling.

Is It Cancer? Is It Benign? A pathologist can be present in the room during this procedure so we can obtain a preliminary answer and make sure we have sufficient specimen for analysis. Final results generally take several more days for the pathologist to complete a full analysis.

The entire procedure can take an hour to image the pancreas and obtain enough samples. After the procedure, we review the results in the recovery room. I always request that patients have a family member with them if at all possible. Anesthesia can have an impact on a patient's memory and reactions right after a procedure. The comfort of a loved one close by really goes a long way.

If there are signs of cancer, we start the process of seeing an oncologist and a cancer surgeon. Each patient is discussed in detail between the surgeon and the oncologist. The decisions on the next steps will include a thorough review of the CT scan, EUS reports, and the final pathology results.

The Device: The endoscope is about one-half inch in diameter with a small ultrasound probe. This is small enough to pass through the mouth, esophagus, and stomach without difficulty.

The device has all sorts of features. There's water to clean the camera lens. There's a suction device to clear thick secretions. Additional Doppler technology can locate blood vessels and pancreatic and bile ducts (i.e., tubes of those organs). The image quality is of incredible detail. We can measure growths down to a millimeter in size and sample them safely.

My Thoughts on CT Scans vs. EUS: EUS and CT scans complement each other. Both are used in staging and diagnosis.

CT scans

- Provide a full bird's-eye view of the patient's abdomen, allowing us to see if cancer has spread far away from the pancreas
- No biopsies are performed
- No anesthesia

EUS

- Provides precise, detailed view of the pancreas, allowing us to see if cancer has spread locally around the pancreas
- Biopsies are performed
- Anesthesia required

Not all growths on the pancreas are cancer. So, if you are told you have a growth on your pancreas, BOTH of these modalities may be used to better characterize that growth.

Final Thoughts: Find locations that often deal with pancreatic cancer. It's helpful to look for centers specializing in pancreatic cancer. Several large organizations maintain lists of pancreatic cancer centers across the country. Additionally, make calls and ask your primary care doctor (PCP) for assistance, as they may be familiar with referrals for cancer and can be a good resource. PanCAN.org is a website that has valuable information to find high-volume centers close to where you live.

Dr. Todd A. Aguilera M.D., Ph.D.
Radiation Oncologist

Background: *Dr. Aguilera attended graduate school at UC San Diego School of Medicine, where his work focused on engineering and validating activatable peptide-based probes to target the tumor microenvironment. He earned his M.D. and Ph.D. through the University of California at San Diego's Medical Scientist Training program. Dr. Aguilera completed his residency in Radiation Oncology at Stanford University Medical Center. Currently, he's an Assistant Professor of Radiation Oncology at UT Southwestern Medical Center. He's* *also a physician-scientist trained as a radiation oncologist and has expertise in molecular engineering, molecular imaging, the tumor microenvironment, and tumor immunology. He treats patients with gastrointestinal cancers with radiation while developing laboratory projects in pancreatic and rectal cancer.*

Radiation Oncology: From early on, I knew I wanted to work in cancer medicine. I joined the M.D. Ph.D. program at the University of California at San Diego and conducted fascinating research into developing targeted agents for cancer by engineering different molecules and testing them. That's when I was exposed to cancer from the perspective of imaging, which led me to radiation oncology, yet another way to treat cancer complementing chemotherapy and surgery.

Radiation oncology is a highly technical, sophisticated field. It keeps my intellect challenged no matter what. We're deeply engaged in the lives of cancer patients and do our best to help cure them of their disease. So, even if I weren't going to be doing research, radiation oncology provides a constant intellectual challenge and personal touch that fulfills me.

The field of radiation oncology is technologically amazing. But even within medicine, not many doctors understand the duties and abilities of a radiation oncologist. We treat just about every type of cancer with radiation. Therefore, we must learn about cancers from the head down to the toe. That requires mastery of a lot of information.

It's so rewarding that we get to specialize in certain types of cancers in the big academic centers like UT Southwestern. I can focus all my attention on a few cancers and perform deep research. On the other side of things, many of my colleagues who work in private practice are generalists and treat many kinds of the more common cancers.

Radiation can damage or destroy every kind of cell in our bodies. However, tumor cells are more sensitive to radiation than normal cells, so this is our secret weapon. We use radiation to destroy or damage tumor cells to the point where they can't be repaired.

Being seen as the definitive curative treatment means radiation plays an essential role in the standard of care for many types of cancer. This standard has been molded by clinical trials over the years and then defined through the NCCN (National Comprehensive Cancer Network) Guidelines.

At UT Southwestern, I'm the primary radiation oncologist who specializes in pancreatic cancer, but I also treat other gastrointestinal cancers. Depending on the size of the medical center, radiation oncologists will focus on different disease types, often anatomically bound, like lung cancers, breast cancers, genitourinary cancers like prostate cancer, gastrointestinal cancers, or brain cancers. We have twenty or so faculty members in our department, and we each have different specialty areas. I focus on gastrointestinal cancers, which include the esophagus down to the anus. Because we have an excellent high-volume pancreatic cancer program, it's perfect for me because I can focus my clinical duties and research in this area to advance the field and improve outcomes with our treatments. Currently, 80 percent of my time is dedicated to cancer research and the other 20 percent is focused on my care for patients with cancer.

Our Training: During our training, we learned how to treat every disease but eventually narrowed down our specialty area. (It's hard to keep up, push the field forward, and be the best in everything!) There's a lot that's required of us to keep up with the newest technologies and best practices. Specializing at a high-volume center allows us to hone our craft to deliver the most sophisticated treatments and clinical trials on a consistent basis that an average radiation oncologist may not be prepared to offer.

Pancreatic radiation is one of the most technically advanced types of radiation treatment that we perform in our field, so it's crucial to have a team that regularly treats this cancer. The risk is high regarding the potential damage to the intestine that is essentially wrapped around the target. We must be precise and work as a team to ensure the dose of radiation goes exactly where it needs and avoids tissue that could result in major toxicity if imprecisely targeted.

The Process: When someone is diagnosed with cancer, they typically see a medical oncologist or a surgical oncologist first. At that time, a full assessment is performed. Based on the stage of the disease and potential treatment plan, if radiation is indicated, I will receive a referral. At UT Southwestern and many places across the country, this happens as soon as the patient receives their diagnosis.

In cases of pancreatic cancer, the patient is assessed in our multidisciplinary clinic and discussed in the pancreatic cancer tumor board conference after all the workup is completed. At that time, the multidisciplinary team assesses and determines for each patient the extent of the disease and cancer stage, then recommends the best treatment approach.

This board is comprised of radiation oncologists, medical oncologists, surgical oncologists, pathologists, radiologists, gastroenterologists, and interventional radiologists. At UT Southwestern, we often recommend radiation therapy as part of the treatment plan because our team is incredibly interdisciplinary and sees how each therapy can impact our patients for good. I will then see the patient, explain our recommendations, educate them about the role of radiation in their care, discuss the overall outlook and prognosis, and then proceed with radiation when it's time. This visit may also include a discussion about the physics of radiation and the medical linear accelerators (LINACs) we use to perform the treatment. The LINAC is the primary machine used, but they come in many forms. I will explain more in a bit.

For pancreatic cancer, there are several steps before we start radiation. I often ask my gastroenterology colleagues to put gold fiducial markers into the tumor. We do this so we can see the tumor's motion in real time. When someone breathes, their pancreas moves up and down with each breath. For this reason, we typically treat patients when they're holding their breath. One of the best ways to know where the tumor is at any given time is to use X-rays to see these gold markers.

After the gold markers are placed, we perform the radiation mapping session, or "simulation." We perform high-resolution CT scans and sometimes MRIs with the patient in their treatment position. These scans have coordinates specifically for our treatment machines, which help create a virtual radiation plan to enable quick, precise delivery on the day of treatment.

Once all this is in place, we usually begin live radiation treatment a week later. At the simulation we teach the patient how to perform breath holds to achieve consistency. When we feel a patient has reached a consistent breath and can hold it from thirty to forty-five seconds, we take CT images to find the exact location of the gold markers. If we supply oxygen, some patients can hold their breath for at least forty-five seconds. It's pretty fantastic. We can even help patients in their late eighties or nineties get through the procedure successfully.

When the radiation plan is ready and the patient comes in for treatment, we set up patients in the position from the simulation day and perform CT scans and X-rays on the machine. This ensures we can reproduce the position of the patient's tumor precisely where we expect it to be. This method allows us to be accurate within millimeters. Once the patient is comfortable with this process, we turn on the radiation beam and begin treatment. The gold fiducial markers are in the radiation field, but they do not impact the effectiveness of the radiation. It's solely to give us a precise and accurate delivery location in three-dimensional space and time.

The radiation machine—the linear accelerator (LINAC)—is a scientific marvel. It generates electrons and speeds them up with radio waves, which surf the accelerating wave. After about a meter, they have enough energy to generate therapeutic radiation. At this stage, the electrons are redirected downward at the patient with magnets and kept tight like a herd of cattle through a narrow gate until they collide against a heavy metal target (mostly tungsten). This collision generates high energy photons, or X-rays, 100–1000 times stronger than a typical X-ray. This occurs above the patient's body in the head of the machine. The photon spray is mostly in the forward direction toward the patient and is blocked in all directions except for where it comes out of the machine, allowing a precisely shaped beam of radiation headed straight for the tumor. The X-rays are like a spotlight, where the machine controls the shape dynamically. It works much like a nozzle on a garden hose to open wide or narrowly focus the beam down to a pinhead, depending on the treatment plan. We can sculpt the beam into different shapes that conform to the tumor inside the patient.

As the patient holds their breath and remains still, the LINAC can rotate 360 degrees while dynamically adjusting the beam shape to optimize the dose at the center of the target tumor and avoid the surrounding tissue. With this process, we can safely give higher doses to the tumor while avoiding the small intestines, kidneys, liver, and spinal cord.

For pancreatic cancer, the most important objective is to deliver as high a dose as possible to the tumor while limiting the radiation to the small bowel. Pancreatic tumors are often very close to the part of the small intestine called the duodenum. If too high a dose is delivered to this structure, it can cause an ulcer, bleed, or even create a hole in the bowel. So, the stakes are high for my team to develop the best plan possible.

It's a phenomenal technology that many are never exposed to unless they need their cancer treated with radiation.

PULSAR: We have a new approach called PULSAR, where we give a fraction of ablative radiation spaced out by one or more weeks. This has some advantages but is still in the early development phase. In all approaches, we try to optimize the ability to control the cancer while taking advantage of the biology of the tumor and surrounding tissues. Five or fewer high-dose treatments are called ablative radiotherapy.

Dosing and Treatment Plans: When you're receiving standard conventional radiation, you're typically given 20–30 fractions of low dose. When I recommend five high-dose radiation treatments, we call it Stereotactic Body Radiation Therapy (SBRT) or Stereotactic Ablative Radiation Therapy (SABR), two names for the same strategy. We use it when the goal is to have the greatest anti-tumor effect possible. Our center specializes in SBRT/SABR, which can be given for many types of cancers throughout the body, depending upon the medical indication.

A radiation plan for pancreatic cancer can last between 1–28 treatments. In the case of Lisa Stough, I recommended and planned a five-fraction treatment course with ablative radiotherapy. A fraction of treatment is defined as one trip to the machine typically done a day apart. In the case of SABR, we do two fractions a week. Each faction takes about an hour with anywhere from eight to upwards of thirty breath holds.

Obviously, patients can become tired toward the end, but we're very careful to plan out how much they can tolerate. After the first fraction is completed, the patient goes home, knowing four more are left.

There are many different reasons why you might do one of the different approaches, depending upon what type of cancer you have, where it is located, how big it is, etc., so it's very personalized to the patient.

Tumor Board: We have multiple tumor boards for gastrointestinal cancers at UT Southwestern. Each week, the pancreatic cancer interdisciplinary team meets. This means all new patients and patients with reassessments during the treatment course, usually six to ten, are presented at the weekly conference. These meetings are vital to optimize the coordination of care, which can often be very difficult.

We can be efficient and complete the meeting in an hour. It helps that at least one of the team members has seen the patient and completed the required workup prior to presentation. By the time we meet, our expert team of radiologists has reviewed images, which makes presenting the details of one's cancer efficient.

Every patient is different and unique. Some cases are complicated and require a lot of discussion, especially if they're on the borderline of possible surgery or if the patient has medical comorbidities that impact our ability to offer standard treatments. That's why we have a diversity of expertise in that room; we discuss each patient to develop the best plan.

Radiation Technology: Every few years, some upgrades and modifications make these machines even better, faster, and more precise. And roughly every five to ten years, new machines come out with substantial changes. Each one improves the delivery of radiation to the patient.

In 2021, we opened up a brand-new building with four different types of new machines. Each machine costs millions. But each machine treats many patients a day. Over the years, it ultimately pays for itself.

Some of our machines have been around for only a few years. There aren't many of them in the world. One machine combines the linear accelerator with an MRI. Another combines the linear accelerator and a PET scanner. The PET scan combo uses radioisotopes to identify the tumor based on its metabolic activity. This machine can precisely deliver radiation to the active disease. We imagine one day that we will use this for a biological delivery rather than an anatomic one. These different technologies help us be more accurate and allow for a personalized, dynamic treatment.

Proton accelerators are another type of machine we use. Luckily, proton centers are relatively common. There's one in Dallas/Ft. Worth, at least one in Houston, and over forty other centers across the country. To install these machines costs anywhere from $50–$300 million because a building must be constructed around the machine, including one large room.

The treatment machines must be well-maintained by a team of physicists as well as engineers from the companies that manufacture them. For most of the machines in our department, we have an identical one right next to them. If something happens with one machine, we can still treat our patients on the other while we get the first one back online.

Treatment at a Research Hospital: There is always a debate regarding better treatment at academic research facilities versus non-research hospitals. For me, it depends on the scenario and the disease. At UT Southwestern, we have amazing colleagues who are quite specialized in our field, but there are incredible colleagues who can provide excellent treatments close to one's home, particularly if the recommended treatment is relatively standard.

If you're in a small town and need treatments for breast cancer, there might be a doctor in that town who can treat your breast cancer with up-to-date recommended practices. Being close to home is critical for many patients, especially if you must receive twenty-five treatments. Driving into Dallas five days a week or a total of twenty-five visits can be very challenging, so having good doctors in small towns is important.

If you come to Dallas, there are many doctors, hospitals, and facilities to choose from. The main benefit of an academic research institution like UT Southwestern is that we have a lot of experience with uncommon and complex cancers. In addition, it's a priority for us to run clinical trials and be on the leading edge of how new treatments are being implemented. If a technology can provide an advantage for a particular cancer, being treated at our center makes sense because we're at the forefront of that technology and treatment.

When it comes to radiation, a lot of it is relatively standard. Any board-certified radiation oncologist can do it. Small towns may have capable doctors with the right machines to treat most cancers. However, they may only see one pancreatic cancer patient each year. If that's the case, they are often happy to refer the patient to a center like UT Southwestern, which sees these patients every week.

For uncommon or complex cancers like pancreas cancer, it comes down to volume and expertise. When it comes to treating pancreas cancer with radiation, you want to be with someone very experienced and focused on that exact cancer.

Another aspect of being treated at top research facilities is that they have a head start on new treatments. If MD Anderson in Houston runs a clinical trial and finds success with a particular drug, a patient can try to get in on that trial even though the doctors are still researching it. They will generate a protocol that they think works. It might be the final protocol released a few years later when the new drug is fully approved, or we find out later that the drug is not as effective as we wanted, so the patient may have to endure the problems and risks of not having a fully approved treatment. The big question is whether the head start is a few months or ten years. It can vary widely. Still, it's something to check into and be aware of.

The other aspect of using a big institution is that they may not be the best at everything. It's hard to be the best at everything. There might be a center that's not necessarily way ahead in a particular disease, but another institution down the street could be further ahead in that area. The subtleties can be difficult to identify and navigate.

Clinical Trials: In general, when you're thinking about clinical trials and moving the field forward, big academic medical centers are often trying to support trials whenever possible, as we are for pancreatic cancer. And with a disease like this, there is a good reason to be in a clinical trial if you can.

Chemoradiation: Chemoradiation is the combination of chemotherapy and radiation. This approach evolved over several decades. Our previous chair, Dr. Hak Choy, was one of the pioneers of this approach. Back then, it was observed that chemotherapy sensitized tumors to conventional fractionated radiation given over weeks, thus making radiation more effective.

Several clinical trials combined daily radiation for five or more weeks with chemotherapy and saw better patient outcomes. For pancreatic cancer, if you do the standard radiation (which would be around five weeks), we add chemo, which makes the treatment chemoradiation. With a short course of ablative radiation, we don't give chemotherapy because we've learned that with these high doses spread out over time, the benefit of chemotherapy is lower. This is because, biologically, radiation is more effective when given in bigger doses at one time. So one might say chemotherapy helps make up for ineffective standard radiotherapy.

Ablative Radiation: Delivering standard radiation in small doses per fraction can damage all tissue—the tumor and normal cells. Yet the normal tissue can heal much more effectively than the tumor. So that's where we get the therapeutic index of radiation. If you give multiple treatments over many days, more tumor cells die while the normal tissue recovers between each treatment.

The idea behind ablative radiation is that we have pinpoint precision to deliver higher doses to the tumor while maintaining a relatively low dose to the normal tissue. This allows us to give a dose of up to fifty times higher directly to the center of the tumor while protecting the normal tissue with a low dose. We call it *ablative* because it completely changes the biology when we deliver a large dose to that tumor in one or a few sessions; it changes what happens to the tumor and how it responds, and thus is more effective.

One hundred years ago, we knew that a higher dose in one treatment was better. However, the problem was that the high-dose/one-treatment led to worse toxicity to the normal tissue. You can burn skin and damage vital organs. We first learned about fractionation when they were sterilizing rams with radiation. If they gave one big dose of radiation to the ram's testicles, the skin became red and burnt. A mad ram is bad. But when they delivered a lower dose in more treatments, they avoided skin toxicity, and the rams were sterilized.

Our new chair at UT Southwestern, Bob Timmerman, is one of the pioneers of this ablative radiotherapy approach, which started with lung cancer. We found out that with this type of treatment, we are almost as good as surgery for getting rid of the tumor. So, you may not need surgery if you've got early-stage lung cancer. It's been a true game-changer.

Factors in Treatment: When we deal with pancreatic cancer, we determine three things:

1. Location
2. Size
3. Degree of spread or presence of metastases

When adding radiation into the treatment, we decide to give the patient either Radiation Machine A or Radiation Machine B. Then we decide the dose, pattern, how many times we send the beam, how many days we do it, and how much time in between treatments to allow the healthy tissue to repair itself.

In pancreatic cancer, if there's a big tumor and it involves the small intestine, I won't do ablative radiation. I will do a more standard, extended treatment, maybe twenty-five fractions. This is because the dose I need to kill that tumor is a dose that could potentially make a hole in that small intestine; this poses risks. It may also be that the tumor is already invading the small intestine. Therefore, the risks are higher. So, when you administer the lower dose of radiation, even though you're hurting those cells, you're not ablating or damaging that tissue the same way as when you deliver a higher dose.

We've learned over the years how much radiation different organs can tolerate. We have guidelines for that. My goal is to follow those guidelines and keep the risk as minimal as possible while still delivering the maximal anti-tumor effect.

Side Effects: The side effects of radiation oncology are highly variable, depending on what you're doing. For breast cancer, which is very close to the skin, there's a high risk of skin burns, ulcers, and pain. It's the same with head and neck cancer, which can burn the neck and create dry mouth and loss of taste.

With pancreatic cancer, when I do ablative radiation, the side effects are minimal. I tell patients that there are four things they need to be aware of:

1. Almost every patient develops fatigue, particularly each day of treatment and probably the next morning when they wake up. The experience of fatigue is different for everyone. Sometimes it's profound for a couple of hours and it brings down their normal energy level. But when they take a nap and wake up, they feel better, not necessarily 100 percent, but maybe 90 percent.

2. Nausea, vomiting, and indigestion. For that reason, we sometimes give antiemetics prior to treatment. I don't have every patient take these medications because around 10 percent get nausea. However, it can be significant for some patients.

3. Abdominal pain, cramping, and diarrhea. This occurs because radiation goes through some of the bowels, and they can be aggravated. It can cause bowel habits to change considerably. I would say less than 5 percent of the patients experience this. We can treat them with antidiarrheals if necessary. Overall, we don't see it that often with this standard approach.

4. The least common but most severe is damage to the small bowel. A high dose of radiation can cause a painful ulcer that could bleed. In the worst-case scenario, it causes a hole or perforation in the intestine, becoming life-threatening. It could even require surgery. Patients needing to be on anticoagulating medications can significantly confound this risk.

Side effects (1) through (3) can occur during the first two weeks of treatment. They gradually get better in weeks three and four. The risk of the ulcer, though, is usually weeks and months after the treatment, so I always tell patients to keep this in mind and stay in touch with me. If something like that is happening, we can help prevent a more significant complication from developing.

The Future: Because I'm a radiation doctor, I'm excited about combining new therapies with radiation. In using the new technologies, we are learning so much more about what happens in patient tissues after therapy. Therefore, we can better understand how the body responds to it.

Another significant leap forward is immunotherapy. Early in the tumor's development, there is evidence that the immune system attacks it, but for some reason the immune system shuts off or no longer responds to that tumor. Thus, the tumor grows. With immunotherapy, we jump-start the immune system to see that tumor as a threat and attack it. I'm excited that by combining therapies, we can aid the immune system to get back into the fight. Melanoma, for example, is very immunogenic, and we are making major advancements with immunotherapy, but that hasn't yet panned out with pancreatic cancer.

Pancreatic cancer presents some difficult challenges. It's a very tough cancer. Often, it evolves early to become aggressive and metastatic. We find half of patients with pancreatic cancer have metastatic disease when they're initially diagnosed. After it's metastasized, it's harder to attack and get under control.

Some cancers, like rectal and colon cancer, have mutations that make them very immunogenic. In those cases, we're finding immunotherapy is all you need. For other cancers, it's going to be a little more complicated. But I'm enthusiastic about several different drug approaches that combine with chemotherapy or radiation and get us better results and more bang for the buck.

When trying immunotherapy, you can always use chemo and radiation later. Although this is very promising, it's also very complicated. Like the COVID pandemic, it's complicated for the public to fully understand why it's so hard to tackle the problem and how we can sometimes make incredible advancements for one cancer but only move the needle a little for another. With some cancers, it may seem we're banging our heads against the wall.

Cancer Survivor: I'm a cancer survivor. This personal history motivates me every day, which is why I care for cancer patients now. And it's a key part of how I interact with patients. Everyone has their experience and motivations that drive their work. A personal history of cancer is not necessary, but for me, the connection with a patient is natural, even if the patient doesn't know my history.

I don't talk about my testicular cancer very often. Many of my patients don't know that I had cancer, but hopefully they know I'm there with them and I care. I hope that every doctor has some way to communicate and relate to their patients because when the human connection comes through, it means something bigger than ourselves.

My cancer was very curable if you catch it early enough, and thankfully, it appears that we caught it in time. All I needed was surgery. But what was challenging was that after the surgery, they assessed that there may have been somewhere between a 20–50 percent chance that the tumor would come back. I was given a choice to undergo another more extensive surgery to lower the recurrence risk, or I could enter into a surveillance phase and watch very carefully. If the cancer returned under surveillance, then we'd immediately treat it with chemotherapy. The outcomes in that scenario were still pretty good, but there was considerable risk to fertility with surgery and chemotherapy.

At the time, I was in college. It made sense to do surveillance for a young man, given the fertility risk. So, after I went through an existential transformation per se, I owned the decision and haven't looked back. Living with that risk was kind of liberating because the meaning of small things changed dramatically. So now, just over twenty-one years since my surgery, I'm still cancer-free and have two wonderful children.

Pancreatic Cancer and Radiation: Many people in the country don't think radiation plays a role in helping control pancreatic cancer when it's localized the way it was for Lisa Stough. But then, some centers give radiation to all patients, even if their tumor is readily resectable. There is justification for both sides, and each center will have its own approach.

The synergy of having strong medical oncology, surgical oncology, and radiation oncology teams leads to a dynamic where all players are looking out for the patient's best interests. Since there is no simple standard, we are all committed to learning from every patient and helping contribute to this body of knowledge.

When we are considering surgery, we don't irradiate every patient. We irradiate the patients who have a higher risk that the whole tumor may not be entirely removed through surgery. The goal is to have any tumor left behind be dead from the radiation. In this situation, it's when the tumor involves the blood vessels, mainly the arteries or the major veins, to the extent that increases the risk of the surgery and the risk a tumor may be left behind.

Lisa Stough's tumor was a scenario where many surgeons wouldn't operate because of the involvement of the arterial vessels. When tumors are touching those blood vessels, we can't always cut everything out with negative margins. Therefore, we call tumors "unresectable" when there's a high risk that that tumor will come back in that same spot. This is the reason we do radiation beforehand. By treating the areas at risk for microscopic extension and the tumor, there may be a better chance the tumor will not recur.

I have to say, these last few years have been a great collaboration among our team members. We've done this for a lot of patients and have had good results. We are gaining more experience and learning from every patient while trying to publish our experiences to show them to the world.

The way we are delivering radiation today is different than in years past, so it's hard to get robust trial data to show the value because the technology moves so fast. By the time a trial reads out, we're already doing things differently. This is a big challenge in medicine. But we must remain as rigorous as possible to ensure we are recommending treatments that work. I'm encouraged by the outcomes of our approach and the success we've had with Lisa Stough.

Dr. Shubham Pant, M.D.

Background: *Dr. Pant is a professor of Gastrointestinal Medical Oncology and Investigational Cancer Therapeutics at the University of Texas MD Anderson Cancer Center in Houston, Texas. His specialty areas include pancreatic cancer and early-stage clinical trials. He's also the Director of Clinical Research for the Sheikh Ahmed Bin Zayed Al Nahyan Center for Pancreatic Cancer Research at MD Anderson.*

He was born and raised in New Delhi, India, and attended medical school there. He came to the U.S. and attended the University of Oklahoma for his residency. Then, he attended Ohio State University for his fellowship. Finally, he returned to the University of Oklahoma and was eventually recruited to MD Anderson in 2016.

My Work: I love medicine and enjoy being a doctor every day. I've been blessed in my life to have had an opportunity to work in outstanding cancer centers and collaborate with amazing doctors and researchers. The best part of my day is interacting with my patients and caregivers, who always uplift me and teach me about fortitude and strength in the face of adversity.

What Do Doctors Who Work In Clinical Research Do Each Day? We conduct clinical trials with patients to evaluate promising new treatment approaches. My practice specializes in patients with gastrointestinal cancers, especially cancers of the pancreas and biliary tract (also called cholangiocarcinoma and gall bladder cancers). I follow patients who are on trials or on standard-of-care therapy. My team and I also enroll patients in clinical trials, follow them for side effects, and see if they respond to therapy.

The other branch of research, which is very critical, is basic science research. These doctors and researchers work in labs and conduct studies on cancer cell lines to identify targets that we can translate to humans. This is of the utmost importance, as this is where we learn what works or does not work to stop a particular cancer from growing.

Can You Talk About the Staging of Pancreatic Cancer? There are different stages of pancreatic cancer. For simplicity, let's call them early stage (which has not spread to other organs) or advanced stage (which has metastasized). In some cases, with early-stage disease, it is possible to surgically resect the disease and provide therapy afterward to prevent the disease from coming back. In patients with advanced stage, the cancer has spread out of the pancreas to other places like the liver, lung, or lymph nodes.

Lisa has early-stage pancreatic cancer. That means she had a resection, she received therapy, and now we're trying to target micrometastatic disease, which are microscopic cancer cells that she might have but aren't visible on scans.

The KRAS Mutation and What We're Doing About It: The KRAS mutation is one of the most commonly mutated genes in cancer. It is present in 90 percent of pancreatic cancer patients, 40 percent of colon cancer patients, and a smaller percentage of lung and ovarian cancer patients.

Mutant KRAS used to be called "un-druggable" as we could not develop drugs to target it. Think of the KRAS protein as a smooth, shiny metal ball. To kill cancer cells, we develop sticky bombs (drugs) and attach them to the cells. Most mutations have a groove that allows us to fit the drug to it, leading to the death of the cancer cell. Unfortunately, the KRAS protein has no "groove," making it challenging to target this mutant protein.

In Lisa's case, she participated in a KRAS vaccine trial that is trying to stimulate her immune system to attack and potentially inhibit the growth of the micrometastatic disease before these tumor cells travel to another place in the body and start growing.

Does This Trial Deal Only With Pancreatic Cancer Patients? This trial was open to patients who had disease which was surgically removed and had a KRAS G12D or G12R mutation. However, as these mutations are more common in pancreatic cancer, a number of patients who enrolled in this trial had pancreatic cancer, and there were a few patients with colorectal cancer.

In Healing and Eliminating Pancreatic Cancer and All GI Cancers, Are Vaccines the Cutting Edge, or Will Immunotherapy Be the Magic Bullet? Vaccines are a type of immunotherapy, as they work to potentially train your immune system to create antibodies against certain cancer cells. Over the past decade, there has been tremendous success with using different forms of immunotherapy for many cancer types. However, not all patients currently benefit from these treatments.

Therefore, when you hear the phrase "magic bullet" for cancer therapy, this can potentially be misleading. A drug might be a magic bullet for some, but we must be humble in targeting cancer, as it is a formidable foe, and no single therapy fits all patients.

How Do Pancreatic Cancer Patients Learn About Clinical Trials Available at MD Anderson? Patients and caregivers can explore available trials at MDAnderson.org/ClinicalTrials or call to speak with our teams for further guidance. For other pancreatic cancer-specific clinical trials, the advocacy group Pancreatic Cancer Action Network (PanCAN) is also an excellent resource.

Are There Any Other Trials Available that Target the Recurrence of Pancreatic Cancer? Yes. There are a number of trials active or in development to try and decrease the chances of recurrence.

What Direction Are the Trials Taking to Treat Pancreatic Cancer? Are They Going to Targeted Therapy, Immunotherapy, or Radiation? We are targeting pancreatic cancer with all the above options. We are conducting trials with targeted therapy, immunotherapy, vaccine therapy, and antibody-drug conjugates, which are akin to smart bombs. There also are a number of agents being developed targeting the KRAS mutation specifically, so it's truly an exciting time to move the needle and improve survival for patients with this disease.

Are All Phase One Trials Dose Escalation Studies? A majority of Phase I trials are dose escalation studies, which help to identify the optimal safe dose for patients. Over the years, as we have more targeted agents, we have also tried to get a sense of how these therapies may result in anti-tumor responses for patients.

Which Trial Participants Receive a Placebo? Phase one trials do not have a placebo arm because these trials are designed to evaluate if a drug is safe and tolerable for patients. Placebo-controlled trials in which patients are not receiving any active therapy are very rare in the U.S., but patients are encouraged to ask their physicians and trial staff this question when discussing any clinical trials.

What Percentage of Pancreatic Cancer Patients Participate in Clinical Trials? Less than 5 percent of patients with pancreatic cancer participate in clinical trials.

Why Is It Important for Patients to Consider Clinical Trials? If available, we recommend patients discuss clinical trials with their care team. Therapies that are approved to treat pancreatic cancer have resulted from testing these therapies in clinical trials. Not only could these trials potentially help patients who enroll, but they also help doctors and researchers understand more about the side effects and responses to the therapy.

Each patient who goes on a trial is helping another patient with pancreatic cancer. I often have patients who tell me they participate because it might help someone else down the road. This altruistic attitude from patients, even at a challenging time, continues to amaze and inspire me.

What Are Your Thoughts Regarding ctDNA Testing for Pancreatic Cancer Patients? Circulating tumor DNA (ctDNA) is an exciting new area of development for patients with pancreatic cancer. In some patients, we are unable to get a good tissue sample to do genomic testing and identify mutations that can be targeted. In this case, ctDNA may help clinicians identify these mutations. ctDNA tests are also being evaluated in clinical trials to see if they can be used to predict disease recurrence after resection of the tumor. This research is ongoing.

You're the Author of a Bestselling Book, *Food Matters*. Can You Talk About That? One of the most common questions I get asked is about nutrition during cancer therapy. The care of the cancer patient should be holistic, including cancer-directed therapy as well as pain control, psychological impact of cancer and therapy, nutrition, and the overall health and well-being of the patient. I wrote the book, commissioned and published by Harper Collins, to help patients and caregivers navigate nutrition during their cancer journey.

What Do You Think Causes Pancreatic Cancer? Some of the common risk factors for pancreatic cancer include smoking, genetics, obesity, and history of inflammation of the pancreas (also known as pancreatitis).

So How Do You Minimize Your Chances of Getting Pancreatic Cancer? We recommend a healthy diet—nothing in extremes—maintaining a healthy weight and avoiding smoking and tobacco use as effective approaches to reduce your cancer risk.

Is Pancreatic Cancer Trending Up or Down? Approximately 60,000 people every year are diagnosed with pancreatic cancer in the U.S. It is rare to see this disease before the age of 45, with a majority of patients diagnosed after 60 years of age.

Most Physicians Emphasize Modern Medicine and Don't Talk Much About Diet When Treating Patients. Do You Believe There Should Be More Discussion About Lifestyle and Diet? Definitely. This is even more important for pancreatic cancer patients as they lose weight and lean body mass, in addition to being deficient in enzymes normally secreted by the pancreas. So, it is important to modify the diet toward more lean protein, like chicken or fish, balanced with vegetables and fiber intake. When available, a nutritionist is an excellent team member to guide patients and caregivers. Patients should also try to get in simple exercises, like walking half an hour a day and doing resistance exercises to maintain lean body mass.

When Should a Pancreatic Cancer Patient Receive Genetic Screening? Genetic screening is recommended by guidelines for all patients with pancreatic cancer, as approximately 10 percent of pancreatic cancer cases can be hereditary.

We Want to Provide Hope in This Book for Pancreatic Patients. Can You Give Us Any Hope of Where We're Headed? Pancreatic cancer is a challenging disease, as a majority of cases are at an advanced stage when they are diagnosed. However, there is hope for the future from new tests being developed for early detection so we can catch cancer early and remove it surgically.

In addition, there are ongoing clinical trials in targeted therapy and immunotherapy, and we can personalize therapy for individual patients through next-generation sequencing tests. In the last couple of years, there has been a lot of excitement, interest, and enthusiasm around targeting the KRAS mutation, which could potentially change how we treat pancreatic cancer. Progress can only be made by a team effort. It takes a village of researchers, doctors, nurses, pharmacists, and, most importantly, patients and caregivers to improve outcomes and find more cures for pancreatic cancer.

Disclaimer: Views are my own and not for medical advice. Any medical diagnosis and treatment are based on patient-specific factors and treating physician preferences. This should not replace medical judgment.

Disclosure of Conflict of Interests: Shubham Pant has a consulting or advisory Role with Zymeworks, Ipsen, Novartis, Janssen, AskGene Pharma, BPGBio, Jazz, AstraZeneca, Boehringer Ingelheim, USWorldmeds, Nihon Medi-Physics Co, Ltd, and Alligator Bioscience. In the past two years, he has received research funding (funding to institution) from Mirati Therapeutics, Lilly, Xencor, Novartis, Bristol-Myers Squibb, Astellas, Framewave, 4D Pharma, Boehringer Ingelheim, NGM Pharmaceuticals, Janssen, Arcus, Elicio, Biontech, Ipsen, Zymeworks, Pfizer, ImmunoMET, Immuneering, and Amal Therapeutics.

Dr. Dan Zhao, MD, PhD
Department of Gastrointestinal Medical Oncology
Division of Cancer Medicine

Background: *Dr. Zhao is an assistant professor of Gastrointestinal Medical Oncology at the University of Texas MD Anderson Cancer Center in Houston, Texas. She received her M.D. from Tongji Medical College, Huazhong University of Science & Technology at Wuhan, in 2004, and her Ph.D. in*

Oncology from the Cancer Hospital at Peking Union Medical College and Chinese Academy of Medical Sciences (National Cancer Institute) in Beijing.

Her postgraduate training included a research fellowship at the National Cancer Institute and National Institutes of Health in Frederick, Maryland, from 2009 to 2012. She then did a research fellowship at Mass General Cancer Center in Massachusetts General Hospital and Harvard Medical School in Boston, Massachusetts, from 2012 to 2014. She performed a clinical residency in Internal Medicine at Brookdale University Hospital Medical Center in Brooklyn, New York, from 2014 to 2017. She then completed a clinical fellowship in Hematology/Oncology at the City of Hope National Medical Center/Harbor-UCLA in Duarte, California, from 2017 to 2020. In 2020, she joined MD Anderson.

My Practice: I am a GI medical oncologist specializing in pancreatic cancer. On my clinical days, I exclusively see pancreatic cancer patients, but I treat patients with other GI cancers as part of clinical trials. I am the co-leader of the cellular therapy program for GI Medical Oncology at MD Anderson, and I lead a variety of cell therapy, targeted therapy, and immunotherapy clinical trials. I also conduct translational research, collaborating with the talented laboratory and data scientists at MD Anderson.

Can You Tell Us About the Resources Available at MD Anderson? Is There a Specific Pancreatic Cancer Department? How Many MD Anderson Oncologists Treat Pancreatic Cancer? We have a large and talented group of experienced providers available to care for patients with pancreatic cancer. It takes a village to provide safe, high-quality care, including surgical oncologists, radiation oncologists, radiologists, interventional radiologists, gastroenterologists, medical oncologists, palliative care doctors, nutritionists, social workers, integrative medicine, and a research team, all specializing in pancreatic cancer. Our multidisciplinary team is experienced not only in treating the disease but also in addressing the psychosocial needs of the patients. Life can be very stressful and emotionally heavy for pancreatic cancer patients and their family members, and we want to provide the best care possible for them.

What Is a Clinical Trial? Can You Talk About the Differences Between Phases 1, 2, and 3 Clinical Trials? What Should Patients Expect? Cancer clinical trials are studies to evaluate new treatment approaches.

Phase I trials are designed to evaluate the safety and tolerability of a new agent. Their goal is to determine if a new treatment is safe for patients, to identify side effects, and to determine the recommended doses for future clinical trials. Safety is the number one priority in Phase I trials. We only progress from one phase to the next when the toxicity and side effects are either not seen or are not a concern.

Phase II trials are designed to evaluate the efficacy of the therapy and further evaluate the safety in a broader group of patients. Phase III trials are designed to determine if the new treatment is more effective and/or less toxic compared with the current standard of care. These trials usually include large numbers of patients and a control arm.

In some trials, we combine the tested treatment with the standard of care. In other trials, we are only testing investigational agents. Some trials may require biopsies, blood, tissue, or stool samples for analysis to understand how the cancer responds to or resists the treatment. Some studies require frequent visits or lab work.

Trials can also be observational, or they may be designed to study new diagnostic tools, interventions in nutrition, exercise, and other modalities in cancer treatment, such as radiation, surgery, and interventional radiology (IR). MD Anderson has many available clinical trials to enroll pancreatic cancer patients across multiple departments and specialty areas.

Unfortunately, we have struggled to find new treatments that can offer significant benefits for patients with pancreatic cancer. Still, the future is bright with the KRAS-targeting agents and new immunotherapy strategies.

Can You Tell Us About the Clinical Trial in Which Lisa is Participating? She Became Eligible After a Circulating Tumor DNA (ctDNA) Test Showed a KRAS Variant Was Detected. What Are Your Thoughts Regarding ctDNA Testing for Pancreatic Cancer Patients? When Should They Be Used? ctDNA testing after surgery in pancreatic cancer is something new. It can show the presence of the mutant *KRAS* DNA from the tumor, which has been shown to be associated with worse survival in pancreatic cancer. However, ctDNA testing is not approved by the FDA for pancreatic cancer yet, and we still need to collect more data on the dynamics of ctDNA in pancreatic cancer patients to determine the accuracy and reliability of this test in pancreatic cancer.

Lisa is participating in a clinical trial testing a vaccine targeting mutated KRAS. We hope this vaccine will prevent or delay the recurrence of cancer.

Can You Talk About Immunotherapy in Pancreatic Cancer Patients? Immunotherapy is approved in patients with pancreatic cancer if they have tumors with high microsatellite instability (MSI-H), deficient mismatch repair (dMMR), or high tumor mutation burden (TMB) levels. These patients can benefit from the currently approved immunotherapy agents, but only about 1 percent of patients are indicated for immunotherapy. Otherwise, the majority of pancreatic patients don't benefit from current immunotherapy options.

We need to find the right targets or approaches to overcome the immunotherapy resistance of pancreatic cancer. So far, we have not been successful, but there is a lot of research on this issue, and we are making progress.

How Can Pancreatic Cancer Patients Learn About Clinical Trials Available to Them at MD Anderson? Those interested in clinical trials for pancreatic cancer can explore available studies at MDAnderson.org/ClinicalTrials or call to speak with our teams for further guidance.

When Should a Patient Consider a Clinical Trial? As early as possible. Once you have been diagnosed, talk with your treating physician about clinical trials. We have different types of clinical trials at MD Anderson, some of which may only be appropriate for patients who have had no prior treatments.

What Are Your Thoughts for Caregivers? Caring for patients with pancreatic cancer is a difficult job. These patients face not only physical distress but also a lot of emotional and spiritual challenges. Many patients are diagnosed at late stages, and it can be difficult to cope with a poor prognosis. The treatments have complications, too, and this is not an easy journey. Pain control and symptom management are very important for patients' overall well-being.

What Causes Pancreatic Cancer? It is not clear what causes pancreatic cancer, but the risk factors are very well known. Smoking, genetics, family history, diabetes, and chronic pancreatitis all can increase pancreatic cancer risk. However, there are a lot of unknown causes. For example, some patients who eat a healthy diet and don't drink or smoke still get pancreatic cancer.

How Do You Mentally Deal With Patients Who Have Serious Diseases and Potentially Fatal Outcomes? It's not an easy job. If you see patients and their families suffering, you are affected too. I try everything possible to make sure I'm in a good state—physically, emotionally, and spiritually—to provide high-quality patient care. For me, that means reading a lot. I also talk with my friends and colleagues, and I attend workshops about caring for the psychosocial or emotional needs of cancer patients. I exercise, travel around, and have some hobbies. I also have a good support group. These all help.

In the oncology community, we help each other. One of the benefits of MD Anderson is the large and experienced network of providers. Our palliative care teams, pain management teams, and social workers help a lot. If a patient has emotional distress, an onsite social worker can speak with the patient right away. Referral for therapy with a psychologist or social worker is not uncommon, either. I have several patients whom I've referred to therapists, and they are happy with the process. It takes time for patients to be open and accepting of the help they need.

Do You See Any Future Advances in Treating Pancreatic Coming Down the Road? Chemo? Pills? New Equipment? Treatment advances for pancreatic cancer are long overdue. We have made huge progress in other cancer types, but we still have work to do in pancreatic cancer.

Targeted therapy options currently only benefit a small fraction of patients (<1 percent) who have NTRK fusions, but targeting the KRAS gene mutation is in clinical development. More than 90 percent of pancreatic cancer patients have KRAS gene mutation, and targeting these mutations is a very promising field area of research.

The other exciting area is immunotherapy. There are so many ways to modify the immune response in pancreatic cancer patients. We have more tools we can use to understand the immune response to pancreatic cancer and hopefully better treat patients using immunotherapy.

I am also conducting cellular therapy trials, which use immune cells to attack a cancer. Now we have many clinical trials using T cells, natural killer (NK) cells, and other types of immune cells. I'm confident we will have breakthroughs in pancreatic cancer treatment in the near future.

Patients Eligible for Surgery Have a Much Better Chance of Survival. You Can't Just Give Chemo and Radiation and Keep Them Alive Without Cutting It Out. Can You Talk About That? Patients with early-stage disease that can be treated with surgery usually have better outcomes. Unfortunately, more than 80 percent of people diagnosed with pancreatic cancer don't have the option for surgery. Right now, surgery is the only way to cure pancreatic cancer, but treatment with chemotherapy and radiation can still yield relatively good outcomes if the cancer hasn't yet metastasized.

Can You Talk About the CA 19-9 Biomarker and Its Reliability? CA 19-9 is a glycoprotein related to pancreatic tumors that can be detected in the bloodstream. However, some patients don't produce this protein, and thus, it won't be helpful as a tumor marker.

CA 19-9 levels also fluctuate with many conditions, such as other GI diseases, including biliary obstructions which cause CA 19-9 to be elevated. These are the downsides of CA 19-9, but it's currently considered the best marker in the clinic to monitor pancreatic cancer for now. Because it's not that reliable, we still rely on CT scans to determine the cancer stage and treatment response.

Any More Thoughts on Giving Hope to Pancreatic Cancer Patients? I feel like this disease makes me humble. We currently have limited treatment options. However, with the progress in science and technology, it's hard to visualize what will happen in ten, fifteen, or twenty years.

Yet thirty years ago, who could have imagined the changes in people's lives today? A lot of cancer treatments did not exist thirty years ago. Even ten years ago, immunotherapy was not considered a mainstream cancer treatment option. And now, look at how much cancer treatments have advanced—all the sequencing technologies, genetic editing tools, computer science, cell engineering, and immunotherapy. Nature has this amazing way.

There are a lot of unknown things in biology and genetics. We have not found the key yet. I'm sure there is an answer for pancreatic cancer; we just haven't found it yet. But the time is coming.

As I mentioned before, targeting KRAS has shown promising results in pancreatic cancer in early-phase clinical trials, and we've seen signals for synergy with immunotherapy. We have new immunotherapy strategies that could potentially overcome the immune resistance in pancreatic cancer. With the new tools in drug discovery and development, we're close to a breakthrough point.

Disclaimer: Views are my own and not for medical advice. Any medical diagnosis and treatment are based on patient-specific factors and treating physician preferences. This should not replace medical judgment. I hope this interview provided helpful information for pancreatic cancer patients and their family members. However, with the evolving cancer research and treatment landscape, the information discussed here may have errors or omissions. I will not be liable for any injuries or damages from its use.

Disclosure of Conflict of Interests: Dan Zhao has clinical trial contracts with Mirati and CARsgen and is a member of the advisory board for Affini-T.

Survivor Stories

Survivor Story: Wesley S. Semple

IT ALL STARTED ON MARCH 25, 2005, when I was diagnosed with pancreatic cancer. I had a rash on my chest, which sent me to a doctor. He suggested cortisone and Benadryl. I started applying the stuff and thought nothing more about it.

A week or so later, it was a Friday and I was at lunch. I'm a teacher. In our usual group, the school nurse sat next to me as we all ate. Suddenly, she stared at me and said, "I'm going to look at your eye." She examined me at the table and frowned. "I see a little yellow spot in your right eye. Let's go to my office right now."

We did. She studied my eye closer and stepped back. "Call your doctor right now."

I did. Right after school, I arrived at my doctor's office. They performed some blood work and said they would be in touch.

The following Monday, I went to school. I had not slept all weekend, a reverse reaction to Benadryl. I was exhausted, so I took Tuesday off. That's why I was at home when I received the phone call that changed my life.

"Pack a bag and drive straight to the hospital," they told me.

I went to the local hospital about ten minutes away from my house and checked in. They started doing their standard tests. Eventually, they said, "Here, read this." It was a paper about a test called ERCP—Endoscopic Retrograde Cholangiopancreatography. "We're going to do that tomorrow."

Wednesday morning, a doctor performed the ERCP procedure. By this time, based on my symptoms, we thought it was a gallbladder issue. I was downstairs recovering while my wife waited upstairs in my hospital room. Then a doctor appeared. He wanted to talk to her. "Your husband needs surgery. We'll provide you a referral to a surgeon."

My wife said we would like to have Dr. Elias do the surgery. I'd had a hernia repaired by him and really liked the guy. His personality and mine matched.

"He'll have to have somebody helping him," they told her. It turned out to be Dr. Draper. Because this all happened so suddenly, I had no time to check out any of the doctors.

On Thursday, Dr. Draper came into my room and explained what they were going to do. They would operate on my pancreas and take out a growth they were concerned about. They were going to do a procedure called the Whipple.

"I'm a very visual person," I said, trying to hold back the anxiety. "Can you make a drawing of what you're going to do?"

Dr. Draper drew a picture on a piece of paper, giving me the before and after. "We will see you on Friday," he said when he was done.

On Friday afternoon of March 25, they wheeled me into the operating room. Six and a half hours and two surgeons later, they had completed the Whipple. After the surgery, Dr. Elias came out to see my wife. "We're not sure what it is," he said. They wanted to wait on the biopsy because it could be anything, maybe even cancer.

A couple of days later, at 5 a.m., a strange doctor appeared in my room. I was groggy from the pain meds they had given me. This doctor stood at the foot of the bed and announced, "You have pancreatic cancer."

I let out a long breath. "I got one of the worst ones, didn't I?"

"Yes." With that, he walked out. To this day, I have no idea who that doctor was. I lay there in bed, the automatic dripline sending fluids into me, thinking about a colleague who had come down with pancreatic cancer. She died within two years. I was 62 years old. *Is this how it ends?* I wondered.

I spent twenty-eight days in the hospital, twenty-one of them with no solid food, only a feeding tube. I had a nurse's aide in and out of my room. Her brother had had the same surgery about a week before me at a different hospital. She continually updated me on his condition and compared our recoveries.

Finally, on the twenty-second day, they offered me food, but it had to be soft. I ate mac and cheese, mashed potatoes, oatmeal, and cream of wheat three times a day. On the twenty-eighth day, they discharged me.

The surgeon chose my oncologist. By the time I left the hospital, I had an appointment to see him a week later. At the first meeting, the oncologist examined my records and directed the chemo formula he wanted to put in me, called 5-FU. He sent me to a radiologist because he felt that I needed to be radiated too.

I sat and watched as a nurse stuck a giant syringe—eight inches long—into my vein and slowly injected the solution. They prescribed nausea pills and said, "If you're going to throw up, you're going to throw up at eight o'clock tonight."

They immediately sent me to another office to get tattoos to direct the radiation to the right spot. The radiation would come from under my back, up and around, to shoot at me from above. I came home from all that and ate dinner. Then I did a few things in my yard. Out of nowhere, I felt nauseated. I glanced at my watch, and it was a couple of minutes before eight, so I ran up to the house and threw up in the bathroom.

The next day, I had an appointment with the doctor and told him what had happened. "Oh good," he said.

"You wanted me to throw up?" I asked.

"Yes, because now I can prescribe these super-expensive anti-nausea pills. Your insurance won't pay for it unless you threw up."

This is a crazy system, I thought.

In the beginning, on Week One, I took the chemo on Monday, Tuesday, and Wednesday. The next dose of chemo was on the same days during Week Four. As for radiation, I had it Monday through Friday for Weeks One through Six. I got the chemo only if my blood numbers were at acceptable levels. I handled it reasonably well but was tired, especially at the end of the week. By Monday, I felt decent again, right before receiving the next round. At least I was never nauseous, except for the first day. The super-expensive pill worked wonders.

Finally, the sixth week arrived and I completed my last round of radiation. We set up the first post-surgery/chemo appointment with my oncologist. I started seeing him every three months for the first two years, where he examined me and ordered scans, blood work, and anything else I needed. The first meeting was in September, and I went back to teaching. After two years were up, my appointments shifted to every four months. This went on for the next two years. At six years, I was moved to every six months. Now I'm at seventeen years.

Right after surgery, I started having some digestive issues. When they took out the head of my pancreas, I lost the digestive enzymes it generates. It was hard to get any nutrients or calories from food, so I was put on a drug called CREON to provide the missing digestive enzymes. It took some time, but we finally figured out the proper dosage. I took two CREON pills at breakfast, lunch, dinner, and bedtime. Each morning and at dinner, I took a Prilosec pill, which shuts down the acid pumps in your stomach. Prilosec helps the digestive enzymes work. My wife said, "Whoever came up with all this is amazing."

Even today, I get up in the morning and take a Prilosec plus enzymes for breakfast, then two enzyme pills for lunch, and two more enzymes plus Prilosec for dinner because they work for twelve hours. I also take two enzymes at bedtime. Since 2005, I've been on this regimen so I can eat and maintain my weight. Anyone with pancreatic cancer will be on drugs like these.

I did have some residual issues from the surgery. I've had bowel blockages due to the scar tissue. Food doesn't want to go through the intestinal tract, so I've had a lot of scopes in both directions because of it.

This past September, I woke up at 11 one night, physically shaking. My temperature was 101. My wife had fallen asleep downstairs, so I went into my son's room and woke him up. He's a paramedic. "Call 911," I told him. "I have to go to the hospital. Something's going on."

The doctors couldn't figure out what was wrong with me, so they took bottles (not tubes) of blood to culture it. They finally discovered I had a massive GI infection—on the verge of sepsis—due to the scar tissue blocking the bile duct. It took a while for them to come up with a treatment plan. I took pills twice a day for ten days and didn't have to endure an IV or PICC line. Thankfully, we defeated the infection.

The previous year, I also had an interventional radiologist put a catheter through my liver, down through the bowel duct, and into my small intestine. This opened everything up so it could drain. Apparently, my bowel duct is a weak spot compromised from my original surgery.

◼◼◼◼◼ ◆◆◆◆ ◼◼◼◼◼

Your CA 19-9 marker is an important data point to track. Right after surgery, I learned my CA 19-9 was 4. Any number below 34 is what you want. Before the surgery, I didn't have a test because I didn't have all the classic symptoms. But since I've been doing this support work, I've seen people who are bright yellow before their surgeries with a CA 19-9 of 7,500. Randy Pausch from Carnegie Mellon University in Pittsburgh, who wrote *The Last Lecture,* had a CA 19-9 of 10,000. Mine never got higher than the one time it hit 38, which was sometime after my surgery. Since I've been in remission, it's been at seventeen.

◼◼◼◼◼ ◆◆◆◆ ◼◼◼◼◼

One surprising component of my treatment was a cancer psychologist who the hospital had set up for me. I went to see this doctor during my entire chemo/radiation treatments and a little beyond. I believe that's one of the reasons, besides how fast they did the surgery and the other treatments, that I'm still here. I suggest that anyone who has this diagnosis talk to a professional and get some outside emotional support because they're going to need it.

When you first get hit with a diagnosis of pancreatic cancer, you're just overwhelmed. You need to be able to talk to somebody else who has gone through it. My best advice for pancreatic survivors is to get into one-on-one support with a psychologist or support group. With the Pancreatic Cancer Action Network, or PanCAN.org, I've been doing one-on-one support across the United States and by email to Spain and India. I help people understand what's happened and explain what I can. The staff at PanCAN contact me and ask me to get in touch with people who need some support. They try to match you up with people around your age. I've talked to both men and women.

When I started a pancreatic cancer support group in Pittsburgh, we publicized the location. My wife was a little concerned. "Are you going to be disappointed? How many people do you think will show up for this meeting?" I told her I'd be happy with five people but guessed we would probably see ten.

At the appointed time, I showed up to a room the size of a small bedroom with eight chairs. Then twelve people showed up and we had to move to a larger room. Everyone went around and introduced themselves. To my surprise, one woman was a forty-year survivor of pancreatic cancer. We almost fell off our chairs. It gave me a lot of hope. Now, I'm eighty years old and I'm grateful to have gotten this far. And it's only because of all my doctors and how fast they tackled it.

One man I talked to had reached the one-year anniversary of his Whipple surgery. He had a four-month checkup, and it's a big emotional event with this diagnosis. He'd never heard of the word "scanxiety." Scan anxiety is undergoing the tests but being anxious while waiting for the results. I explained that such anxiety is normal.

I also advise pancreatic cancer patients to obtain their operative reports. When you have any type of surgery, the doctor creates an operative report, which explains everything they did during that surgery. When Dr. Elias did my hernia surgery years earlier, I went to see him and said, "I need my operative report." He left the exam room and returned with a report, but he was reading through it. I asked him why, and he replied, "Well, I have to make sure I didn't make any spelling errors. You're a teacher, and I know what you're going to do. You're going to go home and get out your red pen, and you're going to grade my report." I started laughing because he was breaking the ice. When I got my operative report after the Whipple surgery, it was four pages, edge to edge, single-spaced. You must get your operative report and keep it handy in case future doctors need to look at it.

A few years ago, I was in the hospital related to some GI issues. A surgeon came in, a newer one from that practice, and he said, "The scan shows your pancreatic cancer is back. We're going to have to do exploratory surgery to check it out because, unfortunately, we can't find the operative report." Hospitals only keep them for so long. I looked up at the doctor and said, "I have mine at home." He was shocked.

My wife brought it in the following day, and he studied it. Then he said, "I'm glad you had that because it just saved you from having exploratory surgery. We thought the cancer was back, but this report explained what we saw in the scans."

When you have any procedure, even scans, keep a copy. I did get rid of the old blood results but kept everything else.

———————

My diet has changed as a result of this cancer and subsequent treatment. I need to watch what I eat. I can't digest beef. If you give me a steak, I could eat it, but you don't want to be downwind of me because it generates an incredible amount of intestinal gas and distress. My wife can hear it gurgling all night long, disrupting her sleep.

I can eat pork, fish, chicken, and turkey. I'll eat salads but not a lot of heavy or rough types of food because I'll get a lot of gas. I try to eat lean foods and not a lot of fat. Occasionally, I'll treat myself, but then my digestive tract says, "Hey, you aren't doing what you're supposed to do."

———————

The big change now is genetic markers. If you have that done, the doctors can see if you have certain genes that will need a specific treatment.

People also seek out alternative medicine. Go see an acupuncturist. They can help you. One of our survivors had blood work and learned his white blood cell count was low. The doctors couldn't give him his treatment. He went to an acupuncturist, and soon, his white blood cell count was up. It allowed him to receive his treatment. So, you need to be open to other things, but definitely do your research.

———————

In 1999, I had open-heart surgery for the widow maker, a blockage on the left anterior artery. I survived a double bypass and went through cardiac rehab. Afterward, the doctors approached me and asked, "How about you come in to talk to patients after their open-heart surgery?" I told them I couldn't do it because I wasn't a doctor. "But you're a teacher," they said. "We'll train you on what to do. You just need to talk to them." I agreed, and they trained me. Of course, in the beginning, they went with me to make sure I was explaining things correctly.

One of the first patients was a man sitting in a chair who looked me up and down and asked, "So there's life after this?" I said, "Yes, there is.

But you're going to have to watch your diet and exercise." I was shocked when I was allowed to go into the intensive care unit and talk to people. That's where some of the patients need to talk the most.

I saw patients for about fourteen and a half years. Helping people is one of the most rewarding things I've ever done. It's why I do support work for PanCAN.

———————— ⊙⊙⊙⊙ ————————

When I finally got my mind straight after the chemo and radiation from pancreatic cancer, I started going to Washington to lobby Congress. From 2009 to 2019, I was there every summer lobbying.

I joined the local PanCAN group, went on awareness walks, attended health fairs, and appeared on local television a few times to talk about pancreatic cancer. There are also PanCAN walks to get involved with. I've done everything I could to get the word out.

If I can give back to somebody and make their life easier, I'm thrilled. That's why I've been doing this with PanCAN, helping people. When people say *thank you,* I tell them, "That's all you have to say to me because if I can clear your mind and get you through this, get you over some of the bumps in the road like hospitalization, I want to do it."

———————— ⊙⊙⊙⊙ ————————

Once, in the middle of the night, two and a half weeks after my open-heart surgery, I went to the bathroom. Suddenly, I had a strange experience, like I was floating and gasping. I woke my wife up and she called an ambulance. At the hospital, they found that I had a pulmonary embolism. A blood clot had gotten stuck between my heart and my lung. It almost killed me. The rest of the clot was in my leg, about twenty-seven inches long.

After that, I read about something called the "Factor V Leiden" blood-clotting disorder and told one of my family doctors about it. He poo-pooed the idea, saying, "You just sat around and didn't listen to the doctor. You didn't walk around. You didn't exercise." I told him that I did all these things. He didn't believe me, so I finally gave up.

I had the Whipple on March 25, 2005. On March 30, I had trouble breathing. I had two drains that looked like little softballs on either hip and they were filling up with blood. The surgeon said, "You probably broke a stitch. We have to go in, open you back up, and see what's causing the blood to come out so much."

They wheeled me in, knocked me out, and when I woke up, I was back in my room and able to breathe. Dr. Elias, the main surgeon, came in and said, "They found a little problem inside there—a blood clot in your abdomen the size of a cantaloupe. It was about two liters of blood."

My oncologist, who's a hematologist, said, "We're going to do DNA testing for Factor V." I told him I'd argued with my family doctor about that previously. He came back days later and said, "Guess what? You've got Factor V." Instead of making a tiny blood clot, my body keeps clotting until it's a gigantic one. I've been on blood thinners ever since. My son and my siblings all had to be tested, but I'm the only one who has it.

At the time of my cancer surgery, there were no major pancreatic cancer surgery specialists in Pittsburgh. Dr. Elias, my lead surgeon, was originally an Army MASH doctor. Occasionally, he went back to the Army and was overseas for a month or two. My wife and I agree that his military background saved me and made my surgery successful.

Update: As of July 2023, Wes is 81.5 years old and an 18.25-year cancer survivor. Take that, pancreatic cancer!

Survivor Story: Paul Suntup

I WAS A STAND-UP COMIC FOR TWENTY-FIVE YEARS. But let me tell you, pancreatic cancer is no joke. In 2017, I was 67 years old. I had never heard about the pancreas. I didn't know what the pancreas did. I didn't need to because it was never an issue. Yet, all of a sudden, I was getting very sharp pains. It turned out to be pancreatitis.

As the doctors treated my new condition, they told me that having pancreatitis increased my chances of developing pancreatic cancer. This can happen because the tissue is damaged in the attacks. The more attacks you suffer, the more damaged tissue you have, and this tissue is more likely to mutate and develop abnormally. The doctors recommended I keep an eye on that part of my body by having CT scans every three months, so I did.

Fifteen months later, a scan picked up a dot that hadn't been there three months earlier. A doctor performed an endoscopic ultrasound with a fine needle aspiration and biopsied the pancreas. The collected tissue was sent to a pathologist who diagnosed it as neuroendocrine.

I soon learned that pathology can be a fine line. Looking at the same slide, several pathologists might come to different conclusions. And apparently, that's what happened.

My doctor sent the tissue to another pathologist, who diagnosed it as acinar cell carcinoma. This is one of the rarest forms of pancreatic cancer. About 1 percent of patients have this kind of cancer.

Ironically, I would've never had that scan if I had not suffered from pancreatitis. Yet the attacks are what most likely led to the cancer.

A doctor explained the findings to me over the phone. To my surprise, it wasn't a big discussion. "I want you to see a surgeon," he said, giving me a name. "This guy is very highly rated. The hospital thinks of him as a God."

I took his words seriously and didn't question them. So I went to see this super surgeon, Dr. Gunasekaran, who works out of Mount Sinai Hospital in Manhattan but does surgeries worldwide. His specialty is liver transplants.

Because I had acinar cell carcinoma, my CA 19-9 was irrelevant. This type of cancer doesn't produce the enzymes to trigger that blood test. Instead, lipase, another enzyme produced by the pancreas, is the marker for acinar cell carcinoma. A reading of over sixty is considered out of range and elevated. My lipase was within limits.

I met with the surgeon in his office. He put up my scan and showed me the location of the tumor. We went over the size and the procedure he would use to remove the tumor from my body. "It will be a distal pancreatectomy splenectomy," he told me. "Because the tail section of the pancreas is directly attached to the spleen, I'll have to remove the spleen, even though that organ doesn't show any signs of cancer. It's a precaution because we take margins from each side of the tumor to get to healthy tissue." Then he added, "I'll probably remove around 40 percent of your pancreas."

By this point, I had done a lot of reading. If they removed my entire pancreas, I knew I'd automatically become the worst diabetic because I'd have no insulin production. So I was concerned. I asked, "Is this going to make me a diabetic since my pancreas secretes insulin?"

"I don't think that will be affected," he said. "I think you'll be fine when it comes to that. I should be able to get all the tumor, and if you want, I can do it laparoscopically. No major surgery, just a few small holes. I will have to make a little larger incision to remove your spleen because I can't take it out through a little hole." He told me I might be in the hospital for five days but he didn't discuss what would happen afterward or the outcome. He just said, "I can remove this tumor and we'll talk about the other details after I get inside and check everything during the surgery."

Up to this point, no one mentioned my odds of surviving this.

The surgery was delayed because the surgeon works out of two hospitals, one on Long Island, very close to me, and the other in Manhattan, which would be a schlep. I decided if I was going to be in a hospital for five days and if he was only at the Long Island hospital one day a week, I would have better care in Manhattan. And Mount Sinai has a better reputation. Even though it was farther away, my surgeon was there often so he could check on me more.

My surgery was on December 13, 2018. It took about five hours and everything went perfectly. He removed the four-and-a-half-centimeter tumor. I believe they said I was Stage 2 because of the size. He came into my room and said, "I did it laparoscopically, just like I promised. And I took some lymph nodes to see if the cancer has spread. We will wait to see what the pathologist says."

Right after the surgery, I was walking. I was never in my bed when they looked in on me. They'd say, "Oh, just go out in the hallway. You'll find Paul somewhere."

I walked a lot because I needed to get rid of the gas from the laparoscopic surgery. The gas pained my shoulder. It was quite uncomfortable, so I walked five hours a day, and I was out of there in three days.

Ten days after the surgery, I was back in my apartment and called the surgeon for my biopsy report. They connected me to the physician assistant, who didn't want to give it to me. "Come on, man," I begged him. "This is a birthday present for me if it's good. Can you please give it to me?"

He hesitated and said, "Oh well, I planned to give you this report next week after the first of the year, but I'll read it to you now."

As the words left his mouth, I started to cry. It was the best postoperative report that any patient could ever ask for. All my margins were clear. There was no sign of cancer anywhere in my body. They had tested twenty-two lymph nodes and all were negative. It was remarkable. Suddenly, life was good.

Once I returned home, I had a visiting nurse come to my apartment once or twice a week to check the bandages and ensure everything was healing correctly. She also checked a drain the doctor had installed in my chest. I emptied it out every day or two. Each time she visited, she said everything looked good. Ten days after the surgery, the drain was removed.

Right after the surgery, a tumor board met to discuss my case. A tumor board consists of doctors at a particular hospital who meet weekly to discuss various cases. On mine, they took a vote as to whether or not I should have follow-up treatment like radiation or chemo. A majority of the doctors felt that no treatment was necessary.

I thought about all this. *Why have chemotherapy if we can't find anything specific that needs to be killed?* To be sure, I talked to my surgeon. "So if you're telling me my lymph nodes are clear, and the margins are clear, why kill everything, including my good cells, with chemotherapy for no reason? There's no visible tumors or cancer, right?"

My surgeon nodded. "I'm one of the doctors who voted you shouldn't have it."

I pondered this. "The folks who voted that I should have chemo, are they the same doctors who always vote to have chemo, no matter what?"

"Absolutely," he replied.

"So let's discount those," I said, "because that's always their train of thought." I put their concerns aside and decided not to have any follow-up treatment except CT scans every three months. I wanted to keep an eye on my body. That was my post-op decision, and it was final!

Thirty days after surgery, my surgeon set me up with an oncologist so we could check a box and say I'd talked to one. This oncologist felt that there was no documentation showing that having chemo would be beneficial to me. Once again, this confirmed what my surgeon and I had already decided.

Three months later, March rolled around, and I had my first CT scan after surgery. Sure enough, the scan was completely clear, with no cancer anywhere. Life was still good!

Sometime after this scan, I decided to deal with a health issue I'd been suffering with for ten years. I had thin skin like rice paper and bruised very easily. Yet I wasn't on any blood thinners. This puzzled me.

I talked to my surgeon and he recommended a second oncologist, someone closer to my apartment. I sat in his office, and he walked around to his chair, plopped down, leaned back, and said, "Okay, so let's schedule your chemotherapy treatments."

"Whoa, whoa, whoa," I said. "I'm not here for chemo. I'm here because I bruise easily and I'd like to see if you can do some testing to find out why I bruise." I had been reading about the healthcare system and saw some reports about the money being made in hooking everyone up to bags of chemo. It was a massive business, one I didn't want to participate in.

"Okay," the oncologist said. "We can do that. I can run some tests and see what pops up." He leaned forward and narrowed his eyes. "Look, you decided not to have chemo, but I just want you to know that if you have one microscopic cell that nobody sees and it travels somewhere else, you could be in trouble down the road. One cell can metastasize somewhere and chemo can kill it before it gets started."

"I know," I said, holding up my hands. "I'm aware of that, but I choose not to have chemo because there's nothing visible." I could tell this was a guy who had probably voted for chemo on the tumor board.

"I hear you," he said, "but microscopic means you can't see it. So I just want to make you aware of this." He paused, but I said nothing. "Have you ever had genetic testing?"

"No," I replied.

"Well, I recommend you have that now because knowing your genetic makeup might be important down the road."

It took about a month to get the results and learn I had the BRCA2 mutation. Because I'm an Ashkenazi Jew, I had a 25 percent chance of developing this mutation. Today, every doctor highly recommends patients have genetic testing so they and their family members can be aware of any disease they might be prone to. My brother was tested and learned he is also BRCA2 positive. Now he gets scans once a year, more often than most people normally would, to keep an eye on anything that might develop.

Knowing I had the BRCA2 mutant gene but was cancer-free, I decided to treat myself to a vacation. The first week in May, I traveled to Costa Rica and checked into an all-inclusive resort. I proceeded to eat and drink as much as I could because my weight was down to 120 pounds when it had been 155. Each morning, I ate bacon, eggs, omelets—whatever I wanted. Sitting in the sun, I downed a lot of Pina Coladas. I drank two glasses of wine with dinner, sometimes four. I didn't think anything of it.

In June, I had my next scan about five weeks after my Costa Rican holiday. When the results hit my computer, it was Father's Day weekend. I'm not a dad, so my two nephews are the closest thing I have. We spent a fun Sunday in the city, which exhausted me by Sunday night, so I didn't look at the report. On Monday morning, I finally pulled up the CT scan and began reading. Buried in the nouns and verbs was the word "metastasized." My heart sank. I started crying. It was a cruel blow.

Two days later, I sat in my surgeon's office. I brought my cousin with me and asked if I could record the visit because I often forgot what was said. I wanted someone else to listen, too.

He said my pancreas was clear, but twenty to twenty-five tumors had metastasized on my liver. The liver is an essential organ for life. It does a lot of things. But the fact that the tumors were on my liver and not my pancreas turned out to be a godsend.

"What now?" I asked.

"I can't operate," he said plainly.

"Can you do a liver transplant?" I asked. That made sense to me. Get rid of my diseased liver and give me a new one.

"No," he said, explaining that I could wind up with more cancer if things went wrong. I also figured they didn't want to risk a precious liver on a losing cause. He directed me back to the oncologist who'd warned me about not having chemo. "Don't worry," the surgeon said. "They've had a lot of good results with various drugs and chemotherapies out now."

Fighting back the tears, I hung my head and stared at the floor. "I'm dreading asking you this, but how long do I have?"

I heard him rub his hands together as he sucked in a breath. "I'm not putting a timeframe on it. I'm just telling you they've got a lot of good things going on with various treatments. So hurry up and see your oncologist."

I went to see the oncologist the next day. To his credit, he never said, "I told you so." He put me on FOLFIRINOX, one of the strongest chemotherapies out there.

"I could give you a lower dosage," he said, "but these tumors are real tough. We've got to throw our most powerful weapons at it right now."

As you can imagine, I was now agreeable to anything that came out of his mouth. Still, I decided to have one of those conversations you might see on TV. This time, I stiffened my back and stared directly at him. "I need to have a serious discussion. Can I live with what I have for ten years?" I decided to start high and negotiate downward until I got the truth.

"Doubtful," he said before I could mentally prepare myself for the answer.

I gripped the chair hard, my knuckles turning white through the thin skin. "Can I live *five* years with what I have?"

"That's doubtful," he replied instantly.

I heard William Shatner on a Priceline commercial urging me lower. "Can I live *three* years?"

"Look," he said, raising a hand and turning his head, "let's stop there. Let's not go with these numbers. I have patients who do very well with FOLFIRINOX. They keep training. They even run marathons. But I'm not overselling this because FOLFIRINOX will make you feel like crap. You really will. This stuff is strong."

"Will I lose my hair?" I asked, leaving the death sentence questions behind.

"Your hair will thin," he said. "Probably twenty-one days into the treatments."

I ran a hand through my soon-to-be-gone hair. Then I thanked him for his time and left.

The next day, they put me in the hospital to install a power port in my chest. This port would deliver the chemo. When they were done, I went home and read some test results on my computer. Everything seemed in order until I read a recent blood test. I felt my anger rise and headed straight to my oncologist's office, where I made a scene.

"What's up with this?" I said, holding the blood test result.

The secretary looked at it. "Oh, I don't understand. Normally when the lab sends this back and there's a result like this, they'll call us. They'll also highlight it so we can't miss it."

"None of you have said a word about this, and I find that very troubling," I said loudly. Several nurses came and joined in. As this noise level increased, another doctor in the practice came over and tried to diffuse the situation.

"Hey, what's bothering you?" he asked me.

I thrust the blood test in his face. "Nobody told me that my lipase was 6,200! That's not right. It's supposed to be below 60."

He studied the test. "Okay, I agree," he said, to my surprise. "Have you had a biopsy done?"

I put my hands on my hips. "You're asking the same question I have. Why am I not having a biopsy? Why aren't we confirming that whatever's growing on my liver is the same type of cancer as my pancreas? Won't that determine the kind of treatment I have? What if it's not acinar cell? What if it's something else? What if it's adenocarcinoma?" I learned that acinar was not as aggressive as adenocarcinoma, which is the most common kind of pancreatic cancer. I wanted to make sure that this was still acinar.

Over the next few days, I had to fight and push to get a biopsy scheduled *before* I started chemo. I didn't want to delay chemo but wanted to be sure FOLFIRINOX was the right weapon. Eventually, they scheduled me for a biopsy seven days before my first chemo treatment, but I had to do much of the work myself. I collected my medical records and CT scans and hand-delivered them to the doctor performing the biopsy. Then I had the procedure and waited.

Seven days after the biopsy, I was literally hooked up to the chemo bag, about to receive the drugs, when a preliminary biopsy report came in. Sure enough, it was the same cancer as my pancreas, so my scheduled chemo treatment went ahead as planned. This was important to know, and it was just in time.

After my first FOLFIRINOX treatment, they fastened a device to my belt and sent me home with it. This device delivered the chemo to me on a time-released basis. Being single, I had slept alone for so many years, but now I had company: the 5-FU pack. I'm sure there are some jokes about the name, but I can't do them. It's just too easy.

During the second day of carrying that pack around, it ran out of drugs and commenced beeping loudly. I called the office and asked, "How do I shut this off?" The nurse said, "You have to come in." It was crazy. I walked into the lobby of my building, beeping loudly. Everyone was disturbed, wondering why I didn't just shut it off. Some folks were getting pissed.

I drove to the doctor's office, the pack beeping in the elevator all the way up. When the nurse looked at it, she said, "Oh, you just press the stop button three times in a row." I was dumbfounded at how they had failed to tell me this. It seemed like such a simple instruction to give.

Once they removed the pack from my belt, I was done with chemo. I decided never to get it again. It wasn't the side effects, which weren't bad (though they weren't pleasant), but I knew they would become worse with each treatment. Instead, I went back to the research I'd done about the money made in the chemo business. My oncologist billed Medicare $21,000 for the chemo treatment. I spoke to a couple of people taking alternative treatments and learned they were doing well. There was a center in Suffern, New York. I decided to go there and see what they could do.

The center gave me high doses of alpha-lipoic acid, or ALA, through my port, in conjunction with a low-dose pill, naltrexone, or LDN, which is often used in high dosages to help addicts come down and beat the habit. I started with .5 milligrams and worked up to something tolerable: 4.5 milligrams.

LDN is supposedly a wonder drug for so many things, including arthritis. The story goes that some patients in New Mexico were dying from pancreatic cancer and sent home to die. Instead, they came to this doctor, and in some cases, he cured them. Supposedly, the doctor presented in front of the National Cancer Institute in Washington, D.C. There are online videos of him presenting in front of some of the biggest names in cancer research, during which he shows CT scans of patients who had complete tumor coverage of their livers and pancreases. After treating them, their scans showed no visible tumors. I said to myself, "Oh my God, what cancer patient would not be excited about this?"

I drove up there two days a week for infusions. At night, I took the pills. The only side effect of the pill was very vivid dreams. I asked the nurse, "Vivid dreams don't have to be bad. They can be good, too. Right? Should I go to bed with a bowl of popcorn?"

I did have some vivid dreams, and some were not so good. Eventually, they settled down and were tolerable. There were no side effects from the ALA infusions except time and money. Each infusion took ninety minutes and cost $185. Of course, these visits aren't covered by Medicare or insurance. I also paid for visits with the doctor at the center before I started. He laid out what he thought was best for me, and his time cost $400. Also, every two weeks, I had a high-dose Vitamin C infusion for $185. Despite the time and money, I felt it was worth a shot.

In mid-July 2019, right before I began the alternative treatments, I went to see a third oncologist, Dr. Allyson Ocean. She works at Weill Cornell Medical Center in Manhattan and is world-renowned. She has an open mind. I took my scans and records to her and explained I'd had one round of chemo and wanted to try an alternative center. Most oncologists only think straight ahead: chemotherapy. That's what they know. "What do you think about me going to an alternative treatment center, and do I have the time, where I won't die if this doesn't work?"

She looked at the scans and said, "I think you have the time because I don't believe you're dying in the next three months. Give it eight weeks, maybe ten, to see if it benefits you. If not, you need to start back up with chemo. And by the way, tell them you might want to do a high-dose Vitamin C infusion." I was excited, especially with the extra advice she gave me about adding the vitamin into the formula.

I went to the alternative treatment center in upstate New York for three weeks until I found a place closer to home on Long Island. The alternative doctor there happened to be an oncologist hematologist. He knows about chemotherapies but also does alternative medicine treatments. The guy is a genius. He knows everything about everything, which was comforting. I went there through the end of 2019.

Three months into my alternative treatments, I had a CT scan. Sure enough, my tumors were shrinking. Unlike that *Seinfeld* episode, shrinkage is a terrific word. It's what cancer patients long to hear. However, there was an issue. We'll never know if they shrunk because of the alternative treatment or the one round of chemotherapy. Or perhaps a combination of the two. Still, I was happy.

In late 2019, I had a CT scan that showed the tumors were growing again. At that point, I needed to do something. I was still trying to avoid chemotherapy like the plague. I'm not a big fan of it because I know a lot of patients die from chemotherapy rather than the cancer. It just destroys your body. It's a poison, and it doesn't differentiate between killing good and bad cells. It kills them all. I didn't want to be reduced to nothing from chemotherapy. But at that point, as they say, timing is everything. There's a pill that's a PARP inhibitor. You'd have to look up everything it does, but these pills have been on the market and had clinical trials like the POLO project. I remembered the oncologist who'd started the first round of chemo had said, "We also have in our back pocket a PARP inhibitor that we can try in conjunction with or on its own at some point. We've had great success with people who have BRCA mutations."

When I celebrated my birthday on December 28, I had the best seventieth birthday present I could ever ask for: LYNPARZA, a PARP inhibitor previously approved by the FDA for ovarian and breast cancer, was now approved for pancreatic cancer. And this approval had come the day before!

In the first week of January, I had an appointment with my oncologist, Dr. Ocean, to discuss various possibilities of what I would be doing next. She said, "I would like you to start this PARP inhibitor LYNPARZA," which was music to my ears because it was exactly what I was hoping she would say. Within ten days, I had that pill delivered to my home.

On January 10, 2020, I started taking two pills twice daily. The side effects can be numerous, but initially, I only felt nausea, throwing up once. After taking those pills for eleven months, every scan showed my tumors shrinking. Some disappeared. It was incredible!

Unlike with chemo, I felt pretty good. I played golf and did everything I usually did. What more could I ask for?

In December 2020, I had a tumor on my liver that started to grow. We thought perhaps the LYNPARZA was either not working at all or not working as well as it had been. We had to decide what to do next.

I started researching how to destroy tumors on my liver. I read about a procedure called "radioembolization," specifically Y90. The Y stands for Yttrium on the periodic chart. It's an amazing procedure about ten to twelve years old. A catheter is inserted into the blood vessel that's feeding the tumor. Then the machine sends millions of radioactive isotopes through the catheter and hammers the tumor. Instead of blood coming into the tumor, it's radiation. Unlike typical radiation, which comes from above and outside the skin, this stuff is like a Trojan Horse. It kills the tumor from the inside.

After reading all I could about radioembolization, I called up my alternative oncologist on Long Island, Dr. Richard Sollazzo, the walking encyclopedia. I'd been keeping him in the loop and sending him my CT scan results so he would know what was going on. Before I could tell him what I had found, he said, "Paul, I want you to write this down." I pulled out some paper, and he said, "Write down Y90." I freaked out and told him I had been reading about it.

"That's the thing you should do," he told me. "I've sent patients down South through the years, but more hospitals up here are starting to do it. There's basically no side effects, and it works almost every time."

I thanked him profusely and decided to get a second opinion from Dr. Ocean, my oncologist. Due to COVID, many of my visits were via video. She looked at the scans and said, "Based on what I'm seeing on this CT scan, I think you should have a procedure called radioembolization or Y90."

"Do you see the smile across my face from ear to ear?" I said. "That's because I have two geniuses who have not talked to each other and just recommend the same exact procedure that I've been researching and praying I would be able to have."

Dr. Ocean said she would send my records over to Dr. Steve Lee, the physician doing the procedure. Dr. Lee called and we spoke for an hour on a video chat. He went over the procedure and how it's done and did not rush me. He provided everything you'd want from a doctor. "This is normally a procedure you do over two days," he explained, "but because of COVID, we don't want any extra visits, so we're going to do this in one day." That was fine with me.

I had the procedure in December 2020. It was a long day. I was in the hospital for twelve hours. During the first part, they mapped out my body to find the blood vessel feeding the tumor. I relaxed on a table while they scanned everything. They asked me questions and played music in the background. We kidded around. At one point, they inserted the catheter and injected albumin, a protein made by the liver. Then they put me under a machine similar to a CT or PET scan. This allowed them to see that albumin was delivered to the tumor and didn't go anywhere else. I was under the machine for forty minutes until it confirmed they had the right spot.

Then I went upstairs and hung around the recovery room because someone else was being treated in the same room. When they finished with that patient, they called me back down and hooked me up to everything again. They called downstairs and a guy delivered the Y90 after they'd put on their lead suits and gloves. It was like in the movies.

"We've got to be real careful," Dr. Lee said. "If anything drops here, we've got to close this room down for thirty days and can't use it."

"I understand," I said. "I won't tell you any jokes or make you laugh."

They injected the Y90 into the catheter ever so carefully and gave my tumor a pleasant surprise. When that was over, I went downstairs to the gamma camera so they could make sure the radioactive stuff went to the tumor and nowhere else in my body.

It was six o'clock in the evening. I'd been there since six in the morning. Dr. Lee had his backpack on and was ready to leave. He bent down to this tiny opening in a room that shielded them from the radiation and showed me his phone. "Look at that," he said. "Your tumor is bright yellow and glowing, pulsating too. We got that sucker right there, and all the radiation went right into the heart of that tumor and nowhere else."

"That tumor is going to be pissed," I said.

"I hope it's going to be dead!"

I got off the table, took the subway to the Long Island Railroad, and drove my car home. This radioembolization is amazing technology. And they only billed Medicare $110,000! The bad news from all this is that my body is now radioactive, and I have to live in Chernobyl. (Just kidding... I think.)

In January 2021, thirty days after Dr. Lee's attempt to turn me into a Marvel superhero, I had a PET scan. It showed the tumor was shrinking. In March, another scan showed more shrinkage. In June, a scan confirmed more shrinkage but also showed five more tumors on my liver. Dr. Lee said I was still a candidate for more Y90 treatments because he could find the blood vessels feeding these tumors and blast them with radiation. Also, the liver can regenerate itself, but too much radiation would permanently damage it, so a person can only have three or four Y90 treatments.

"I won't know until we map it out and look, but I'm probably going to have to do this over two treatments," Dr. Lee informed me.

"If that's what you have to do, that's what you have to do," I told him. On June 2, I had a second Y90 treatment. Dr. Lee felt he'd gotten about 60 to 70 percent of the area he needed to treat. Two weeks later, I went back and received radiation on the remaining new tumors. Again, there were no side effects, and I took myself home each time.

In July 2021, I got a PET scan that showed no live tumors in my body. Everything we'd zapped was dying. In October, a CT scan showed some of the tumors had disappeared, and two others were half the size or less. Even my blood work produced an acceptable lipase range of 39. Anything less than 60 is normal. This was good news because my lipase increased as each tumor grew. Then it jumped to 73 and I was somewhat concerned about that. But I was also taking a digestive enzyme, CREON, which correlated with the increase in lipase. So I hoped the increase was from the extra lipase in that pill and not from the tumors growing. I also read a clinical trial study published six weeks earlier, in which people who'd taken CREON experienced higher lipase numbers. But that only happened for them during the first thirty days they were on the pill. I was only into my sixteenth day so it made sense that my body would acclimate to it. But if the numbers kept increasing, I'd need a CT scan to see if something was growing.

Life was good into 2022, with Dr. Ocean, my oncologist, providing an uplifting comment during a video call. I asked her, "If you looked at my latest scan but didn't know it was me, what would you think?"

"I would not think this person had ever experienced cancer," she said. That brought a smile to my face.

Then, in June 2022, my scan showed two tumors on my peritoneum. The peritoneum is a lining—a sheath—covering the stomach and internal organs. Dr. Ocean looked at the scan and said, "It's a little unusual because normally we see a popcorn effect, with tiny tumors spreading out along the peritoneum. Yet your tumors are in one spot, which puts them close to the liver and where your tumors were obliterated."

"What do we do?" I asked her.

"I think it could be systemic, and if it's systemic, I don't think radiation should be the number one thing we do because, yes, it'll probably work well on these two tumors, and it's the latest technology, but if it's systemic, we'll only kill the tumors in the peritoneum. What if there are other cancer cells floating around your body and it's going to manifest somewhere else? The targeted radiation won't kill all that. But chemotherapy will."

I wanted to avoid chemo like the plague. Then I remembered something I'd read. "What about metronomic chemotherapy?" Metronomic chemotherapy is relatively new. It's a lower dose of chemotherapy given more often. Some studies have found that it works as well as stronger chemo but without considerable side effects. "Am I a candidate?" I asked my doctor. "Would you be willing to administer metronomic chemotherapy to me?"

"Yes, of course," she replied. "I don't think that'll be a problem."

I started metronomic chemo at the end of July 2022, receiving an infusion of oxaliplatin, the only part of FOLFIRINOX she recommended. Oxaliplatin is a platinum-based drug that has been effective in patients with the BRCA mutation. I also took a pill, capecitabine (or Xeloda), twice a day. This entire regimen was two weeks on and one week off for two months. During that time, my lipase never came down much. Then, it started an upward trend, so I wasn't confident this stuff worked. I cautiously waited for the scan results. Sure enough, my two tumors were larger. Not only that, I had developed a third one. That chemo regimen had been a complete failure.

As my doctor explained the results, I said, "It's time for the radiation!" This meant the SBRT (stereotactic body radiotherapy). They mapped out my body and hit the tumors for five straight days. My tumors moved from day to day, so they had to map them out each time. The great thing about this was no side effects. It all ended in November 2022.

Before, during, and after the radiation therapy, I was put on an immunotherapy drug called Keytruda. Earlier, I had my blood tested by a company called Guardant 360 and learned I had a tumor mutational burden (TMB). This result qualified me for the Keytruda drug infusion once every three weeks. The doctors feel that Keytruda enhances the radiation treatments to work better. But it's not without possible side effects. It can affect your thyroid, and sure enough, I developed hypothyroidism and had to take Levothyroxine. It took three months to figure out just what dosage I needed.

Another side effect of Keytruda was lightheadedness. Then in December 2022, the shit hit the fan. I started getting pain in my arm where I'd experienced it before, usually when I played golf. Now, it was every day—at my elbow and wrist—yet I wasn't playing golf. It reached the point where I couldn't hold a pen, touch my thumb to my pinky, or even rotate my wrist to see my palm. I went to an orthopedist who took X-rays. He said, "Yeah, you've got a nodule in your elbow floating around. You've also got arthritis."

I had an MRI the next day, which was my birthday, December 28. My orthopedist said, "Don't you have a better way to spend your birthday?"

"If you can help me figure out what's going on with my body, then it's a great birthday present."

The MRI showed the nodule in the elbow as well as a partially torn rotator cuff, which doesn't bother me. It was possible I'd torn the rotator cuff while undergoing radiation because, while in the MRI tube, I had to keep my arm extended behind my head for over an hour without moving. Then, this pain in my right arm traveled to my left arm. I was stunned. With both my arms, elbows, and wrists in pain, I discovered my legs hurt. They felt like tree trunks weighing a thousand pounds each. And my bony knees swelled to the point I couldn't see them. I had trouble walking downstairs.

With all this going on, I took a trip to Hawaii in late February. My friends had been begging me to come. I got a tan, saw some beautiful sights, and spent some quality time with my friends. Once I was back home, I was put on prednisone, a steroid. I took those pills for over two months. They worked but I still felt pain. At least I hit two homers with the Yankees. (Doctors don't want you on steroids because you can get ulcers, brittle bones, and shatter MLB's homerun records.) Thankfully, the pills allowed me to use my elbows and wrists, and my quality of life improved. With some pain in my body, we decided to leave me on two pills that would allow me to use my joints.

At my next scan, one tumor was completely gone and the other two had shrunk. Plus, nothing new had appeared anywhere. The radiation had worked. It was the great news I needed.

In late March, I put some sunscreen on and felt a bump protruding from my chest. "What is that?" my friend asked.

I studied it carefully. "It looks like a golf ball. I fear it's only a matter of time before I see the word Titleist across my chest." But it wasn't a joke. Every week it grew larger. I had an ultrasound, which showed it to be solid, not liquid. This meant it was most likely a tumor.

I got a scan and it showed the tumors on the peritoneum were stable or perhaps had shrunk slightly. The scan did pick up the new growth in the rectus muscle of my chest, however. Even after the ultrasound, the doctors weren't sure what it was. It could be scar tissue or the post-treatment from the radiation. They said it might be a lot of different things and not necessarily a tumor. We discussed it, and the radiation oncologist said, "I could kill it if it's a tumor. But why do anything if it might be gone on your next scan? It's only one centimeter. If it's scar tissue or whatever, or if it moves or it doesn't get larger, we can just leave it."

I agreed.

Another issue I'd been dealing with was lightheadedness. Back in the middle of January, we stopped the Keytruda infusions, hoping it was the cause of all my problems. Yet five months later, my lightheadedness was worse, so maybe it wasn't the Keytruda. The doctors didn't know.

In May 2023, I had another scan and found the new spot on my chest had grown. Now we knew it was a tumor. "I'd like to get a biopsy," I said, "so that we know what we're dealing with to make sure it's the same kind of cancer and not a different kind."

I had the biopsy, and sure enough, it came back malignant for acinar cell, the same cancer I had. This was actually good news; it was not a new strain I'd have to deal with.

Dr. Ocean suggested SBRT since it had worked back in November. The radiation oncologist saw it and said, "Yep, this is right on the surface. I can kill this sucker. It'll work just like it worked on your peritoneum tumors. And this is even easier to get to. It's right there, begging to be zapped." Then I started thinking about all of this and said to myself, "Maybe surgery can just cut this thing out. I mean, it's right there."

I mentioned this to the radiation oncologist, and he said, "Whatever you want. If you want the SBRT, I'll do it. If you want to have surgery, talk to a surgeon."

I didn't want to wait months to see it hopefully shrink when I could visibly see it disappear after surgery. I floated the idea to Dr. Ocean. At first, she said, "No, I think you're better off having the SBRT because we know it's worked before and there are risks with the surgery." Still, I pursued it and spoke to a friend with a medical background. He said, "The surgery sounds like it'd be a quick fix, and I can tell you the guy to go to because he saved my life when he did my surgery years ago, where another surgeon would've closed me up and sent me home to die. He did what he had to do."

"That's the guy I want!" I declared.

I set up a video appointment with the surgeon a few days later, and he said, "I probably could remove it, but I want you to get a PET scan."

I went back to my friend about this PET scan, and he said, "Surgeons have their own protocol before they operate. They want to know if there are any other active tumors nearby."

The PET scan showed my chest tumor as active and was a little murky about the other two tumors still on my peritoneum. He was a little hesitant to do the surgery. "If your oncologist, Dr. Ocean, is okay with it, then I'll be okay."

I hit Dr. Ocean with wave after wave of arguments until she finally agreed to it. I had the surgery on June 30, 2023. In recovery, I was certain I'd been hit by an eighteen-wheeler. The surgical site still seemed large, perhaps with fluid. I hoped it was not an alien coming out of my chest.

The surgeon had cut out the entire tumor and that was good news. Now I just have to wait until the chest heals and goes down. Sometimes I feel like I'm playing Whack-a-Mole as new things pop up. I'm 73 and will reach my five-year anniversary of getting pancreatic cancer in November. So my best advice is to live your life and survive by kicking that can down the road, like the James Bond movie *Die Another Day*.

Through all this, I've developed some bullet points for folks in my situation:

- You are your own best advocate. No one cares more about your health than you do.

- Do your own homework. Do your own due diligence. Read everything you can. Do all the research you can.

- Don't take the first opinion as gospel. Ask somebody else. Go to another doctor.

- Ask a lot of questions. Don't worry if someone gets upset that you keep asking questions. Ask them because the doctors might not think of them, or they might not be giving you answers to things that you need to ask. Just write them down ahead of time. Have them there.

- Everyone's body is different. There's no one-size-fits-all treatment plan. You could have one hundred people and give them the same treatment, and you can get ninety-nine different results. The same thing that works for one person might not work for another, and therefore, you have to try to find something specific for what you have.

- Don't blindly accept what's being pushed at you by the doctors. Ask why it's being pushed.

- Look for therapies targeted to your body and situation. More doctors are deviating from standard care to targeted therapies. I found out they now have platinum-based chemotherapies that are more successful in patients with the BRCA mutation.

- Which brings me to the next item: do genetic testing. You don't know what you don't know.

- There might be perks when you have cancer. Play the cancer card and it can get you a couple of things or a little better treatment than somebody else. Maybe you'll be pushed up the line for whatever you need. Hey, it can't hurt to try.

- Consider volunteering. I work with the Pancreatic Cancer Action Network or PanCAN.org. This is an organization people should be aware of after diagnosis. The people they have sent to me have allowed me to give them advice or tell them what I've been through, which makes me feel good. If I can help one person positively with anything I do or say, that makes my day. It puts a smile on my face. It's very rewarding. PanCAN does great work!

- Finally, keep a positive attitude. Don't get down. Try to maintain a positive viewpoint on things and try to keep a smile on your face. I always tell myself there's somebody out there who definitely has it worse than I do.

I wish you the best of health and a long, happy life.

Survivor Story: Stephen Tanit

M Y NAME IS STEPHEN TANIT, and I'm a pancreatic cancer survivor. My story starts in Iran, my home country. I was the oldest of four children. When I was 8, my father died of tuberculosis. As a young boy, I was husband and son to my mother and a father to my brother and two sisters. For the next three years, I hid my face in a pillow at night and cried for my father.

I was eleven when I finally got over my father's death. Then, my mother, 26, passed away due to heart failure. I had to earn money to support my siblings.

In my late teens, I decided a career in the military was the best option. I attended the Air Force Academy in Iran, completing pilot training at a U.S. Air Force Base. Since the United States had sold us the planes, they taught us how to fly their equipment. Eventually, I was offered a job by the U.S. Air Force. Because I speak five languages, they wanted me to be a translator, an intelligence officer, and a liaison in the Iranian Air Force and the Middle Eastern area. I agreed and received my commission.

I earned a master's degree in aeronautical engineering while flying F-4s, F-5s, and C-130s. Most of my missions were as a fighter pilot, serving different countries and, eventually, Iran.

Then one day, a revolution occurred and our government fell. A religious faction took over. This led to a hostage crisis and a distrust of the United States. Due to my connections with the U.S., the police investigated me and found reports I'd sent to McDonnell Douglas. These reports detailed the performance of planes while alerting us to potential maintenance items before they broke. The uneducated government officials didn't understand that a manufacturer of such an expensive piece of equipment would want to learn how to improve the product and understand any crash or failure so they could ensure it wouldn't happen again. With these papers, I was accused of spying, arrested, imprisoned, and an execution date was set. Since F-4s have two-man crews, my copilot was treated just like me. Four other flight crews were arrested and charged. Three of these crews were quickly executed. Of the remaining four pilots, two men had American wives, so they were executed and their wives freed. That left my copilot and me.

I was in solitary confinement for two years. During that time, they tortured me. When torture didn't work, they imprisoned my wife and son, who was so young, he learned to speak in prison.

One time I saw them and almost broke down. But I didn't. The guards released them after twenty-three days.

Life in an Iranian prison is medieval. I'm six feet tall, and the cell was six feet by four feet. When sleeping, my head hit the door and my toes tapped the other wall. My hands would touch the two side walls. It was rough.

Since the cell didn't have a camera, the door had a small hole with a flapper outside. This allowed them to open the flapper and check on me. At the bottom of the door was a slot to slide food in and out.

The cell had a little light on the top corner, but the light had been dirtied intentionally or through a lack of cleaning. It cast a dim light throughout the cell and made it hard to see anything. With no window or access to the outside, I never saw the sun.

I was in two different prisons. The main difference was the toilets. The second prison cell had one, but the first cell did not. They provided a large bowl as a toilet. The prison staff would blindfold us each morning and take us down the hall to a common restroom. I carried my bowl down there and had to wash it out blindfolded. Then I filled the bowl with drinking water and carried it back to the cell. That was all the drinking water I received for the day.

During the morning, the staff came and served us our food—a big spoonful of rice—into the bowl. The trick was to drink the water and eat the food fast, then use the bowl for my toilet. The Iranian guards and staff were barbaric.

Men and women were in the same prison, but each had a separate cell. One night, I was trying to sleep when I heard a woman crying. It was midnight. She said, "Why are you doing this? Don't you know I'm seven months pregnant? Aren't you ashamed of yourselves?" They raped her as she screamed and cried.

Often, they took me out during executions. I was chained to another person and led blindfolded up to the roof. They would shoot the other guy, and his body would fall to the ground, threatening to pull me down the steps or off the roof. This happened over and over again. On one of these trips, I returned to the cell with brains splattered over my shirt.

I remember sitting in my cell when the guard opened the door. "Are you going crazy?" he asked.

"Why do you say that?" I replied.

"I've been watching you for over an hour. You're just sitting there, looking at your hand and playing with your fingers."

"Come in, let me show you something." I held up my hand. "See the beauty in these fingers? They move, yet humans have not been able to make a machine that does it so well. If you think the One who created this hand will leave me alone here and let you do what you want to me, you're wrong. I've been talking to Him."

The guard shook his head and slammed the door shut.

Since that moment, whenever I feel something negative, or the pressure piles up on me, I look at the One who made this extraordinary hand and try to find His wonders within me. That washes out all the negative, giving me hope that I've got someone to take care of me even though I'm supposed to care for everyone else in my family. It gives me that feeling. And if you can get that same feeling, you can survive anything, even pancreatic cancer.

Then, a miracle of sorts happened: Iran went to war with Iraq. Most of the fighter jets had been sitting around gathering dust, and they realized that by killing the pilots, they didn't have enough experienced pilots to fly these war machines. And right before the revolution, Iran had purchased some laser-guided bombs, but they couldn't make heads or tails out of these bombs. Suddenly, I had value.

One day, they came to see me. Of course, I had absolutely no idea what had been happening in the outside world. I especially didn't know Iran was at war with Iraq. I had been in solitary for two hard years. The officers said they wanted me to train their new pilots on using the laser-guided bombs. I asked about my sentence, and they said, "It's going to remain pending until the end of the war. We'll see what happens then."

I accepted the opportunity and came out, training numerous pilots while flying 131 combat missions over Iraq. Since I was now a high-ranking officer, I led a lot of missions. However, during all this, they put me back in prison twice. The first happened when the former president of Iran escaped. I had been on alert status and was scrambled to shoot down the Air Force tanker but it was too far ahead and I lost it. Back in prison, the guards continued torturing me with hot water pipes in my rear and other unspeakable crimes. Once they stopped the torture, they asked if I would lead missions again. The choice was simple.

When I was incarcerated a second time, I thought, *Enough is enough. I need to escape from this nightmare.*

With help from some U.S. sources, I escaped via the Persian Gulf and ended up in Dubai, U.A.E. Three days later, I landed in Germany. But my wife and two boys were still in Iran. They had to hide because the government would arrest and execute them. With some help, six months later, they escaped through Istanbul, Turkey, and rejoined me in Germany. It had been a close call.

With my flying experience, I was able to get a job as a pilot for a major airline. We moved to Texas and spent most of our money changing my private pilot's licenses to commercial. When I showed up for work with my thick accent and permanent dark tan, the chief pilot explained, "As long as I'm here [racial epithet], you won't be flying here!" I was crushed. We had used up our money for me to get this job and now had none.

I had a helicopter pilot friend who ran a used car department in Texas. He called and said, "Stephen, why don't you come here and sell cars until you find out what you want to do." I knew nothing about cars other than how to drive one. "I'll teach you," he said. "It's easy."

He was right. And he treated me well, so I became a car salesman for two years before rising to management. I was a manager for eight years and then started my own business selling luxury automobiles.

I had twenty people working for me and sold nice, clean cars. I looked in the mirror and had a great business, good people to work with, a healthy family, and all in America. My life couldn't get better.

Then everything changed.

After seeing my father die of tuberculosis, I learned that the disease could sometimes stay in children and show up after many years. Throughout my life, whether in the Air Force in Iran or selling cars in America, whenever I had any kind of chest pain or discomfort, I rushed to a doctor and said, "Check me."

It was the summer of 2009. I had a minor pain under my ribs radiating into my back on my right side. I raced to my doctor again and said, "I've got a pain right here."

"Okay, lay down," he said, making a joke about it. He checked me out and took X-rays, informing me that my lungs were fine. Then he studied my pained face and touched my stomach. My body arched with each touch. "Let me do some blood work on you," he said.

The next day, I was at my dealership when he called. "Have you had lunch yet?" When I told him no, he said, "Don't. You can't eat anything. I've got you checked in as an emergency. Go to the hospital right now. I'm going to meet you there."

I drove to the emergency room to find him waiting for me. "You've got a severe case of pancreatitis," he said.

I had heard the actor Patrick Swayze had just died of something having to do with his pancreas; it was all over the news. While I was in the hospital, I read on the internet about the symptoms of pancreatic cancer and I had all of them: weight loss, lack of appetite, change in eye color, jaundice, and a change in stool color. When I mentioned this to my doctor, he said, "It can also be pancreatitis."

He set me up with two exams, including a lady who performed an ultrasound on my abdomen. As she rolled the sensor over my body, her eyes twitched.

"What is it?" I asked.

"Oh, nothing. The doctor will talk to you."

The hospital's doctor didn't talk to me because he didn't catch it. Instead, he said, "It's okay. You had a minor flare-up of pancreatitis." So they released me.

The next day, I went back to my family doctor and explained what the hospital's doctor had said. "No, it's more than that," he said. "I saw the ultrasound report. There is something concerning." He sent me to the best pancreas doctor in town.

The expert looked at my MRI and said there was a slight shadow on my pancreas. He wanted to do an endoscopy. He put me under and did it. After the procedure, he told my wife, "I can't see anything, but I know something is there. I feel it. I want to do a procedure, and I need your approval. I need to go in from outside of his pancreas." She gave permission while I was still under, and they did it.

When I woke up, my wife was there next to me. I glanced over to see my doctor say, "You have pancreatic cancer." Just like that, without any sugarcoating. I had figured this out earlier, so it wasn't a major surprise.

"How much time do I have?"

"Maybe six months. But I think we can resect it. That will give you a little more time."

"Who does the surgery?" I asked.

He gave me a business card and said, "He's a good doctor. I'm sending you to him." Then he walked away.

Seconds later, my phone rang. It was the surgeon's nurse calling to set up an appointment for the next morning. *Wow!* I thought. This was moving so fast it felt like I was in a whirlpool with no control.

There was no time for a second opinion or even learning my CA 19-9 level. Instead, I went home and saw my grandson sitting there. He was two and living with us because my son and his wife had separated. I grabbed him and went to the nearby park where I walked our dog. Night was falling as we sat on a bench alone together.

I don't belong to any religion, but I believe in God. That night, I talked to Him again. "You put this inside me. These doctors tell me they can't take it out, but You can. I have this kid here that I must raise. Either take it out of me and let me raise him, or You raise the boy. I surrender myself to You." Suddenly, I felt Him sitting in the park directly in front of us in the grass, listening to me. He was there, and I was comforted.

I met the surgeon, who was blunt. "I have to open you up, but I'll give you no guarantee that you'll come out of surgery alive because the tumor is very close to your aorta. We just don't know how bad the situation is or if it's attached to your aorta. It may have spread to your liver and lymph nodes."

I swallowed hard, thinking back to all the torture I'd endured in Iran. "Okay," I managed. "When are you going to do it?"

"Right now, if you'll let me."

I checked into the hospital, where I underwent a five-and-a-half-hour surgery called a Whipple procedure. The surgeon took five centimeters off the head of my pancreas and removed my gallbladder and a portion of my duodenum and small intestine. He saved the pyloric valve at the bottom of the stomach. Then he replumbed me. My spleen was unaffected.

When I woke up, I realized I'd survived the surgery. The doctor smiled and said, "Full margins! It was near a couple of lymph nodes but we don't think it spread to them. If that's the case, you may live about four or five years. If it's spread, well, we don't know."

The second day after my surgery, I came down with jaundice. They had to open me up again and clean out the blockage in the bile ducts.

Eventually, the pathology confirmed the margins were clear and the cancer had not spread to the lymph nodes. The cancer had been encapsulated so we caught it just in time. It was a true blessing.

I was in the hospital for fifteen days. When I was released, I had two tubes in my stomach sucking stuff out. I also had a small machine hanging on my shoulder. They told me to go home and lie down and rest. Instead, I walked my first mile two days after they released me from the hospital… against the doctor's orders. My son followed me to make sure I didn't fall. I pushed myself to get better and it worked.

I saw an oncologist and learned I'd been staged at 3A. He put me on gemcitabine or Gemzar four weeks after the surgery. The cycle lasted six weeks. The side effects were throwing up a lot, confusion, and disorientation brought on by throwing up. I never had radiation.

I still had my car business, which my older son, who worked with me, ran while I was gone. Once I was healthy, I returned to the business.

I took digestive enzymes for a year, then stopped. The side effects were diarrhea, upset stomach, throwing up, and stomach pain. We changed the enzymes a few times, and after a year, the doctor said, "Why don't you stop taking the enzymes? Let's see what happens." And it worked.

The main issue I have now is digesting food. My pyloric valve, which connects the stomach to the small intestine, doesn't always work. As a result, food will stay in the stomach and rot. I'll feel pain, bloating, and gas. To resolve that, I throw up, sometimes twenty-four hours later. It used to happen once or twice a year. Now it's about once a month. Fatty foods are usually the culprit because of a lack of enzymes. Acidic fruits like berries and cooked tomatoes have the same effect. I haven't found any substance that makes it better.

My diet is extremely low in fat. I eat a lot of vegetables, fruits, greens, and bland food. I was 175 pounds when diagnosed. After surgery, I weighed 130. Now I'm back to 175 but it took seven months to get there.

I also have post-Whipple attacks, which are basically pancreatitis attacks because the pancreas can't produce the level of enzymes required to digest what I ate or drank. Medication can also trigger attacks. Last week, I had an attack. My lipase should be 60 or less but it was 1,140. The IgG4, the gauge of the immune system inside the pancreas, goes up. They put me on a large dose of steroids for sixty days to solve this problem.

I have also developed ulcers in my stomach because of food staying there and burning the lining with acid.

My blood and CA 19-9 are checked once a year. If I have inflammation, they check it more often. I also have MRIs and CT scans.

Thirteen years later, I'm still here. I've had some ups and downs, occasionally having to be hospitalized, but I'm alive. And I raised my grandson until he was 10, when my son took over. God got me through it!

I've had a healthy life. I'm not a smoker. I've never touched drugs in my life. I ran five miles every day—still do. So, pancreatic cancer came right out of the blue. The doctors said it could be genetic, as it usually bypasses one generation and goes to the third generation.

When I came out of surgery, I met a nurse who said, "You know what? You should talk to these people. They can give you more information." She handed me a brochure and I talked to some folks in California with the Pancreatic Cancer Action Network, or PanCAN.org. I went to their local meetings. Since God gave me my life back, I didn't want to waste a minute. I got involved with PanCAN, volunteering to coach pancreatic cancer patients all over the nation. The patients call and we talk about my experiences, expectations, and what to do and what not to do. I don't provide medical advice but give them questions to ask their doctors. I also discuss what food works, what to do if you get diarrhea, and similar issues.

At UT Southwestern in Dallas, they have meetings every Thursday for newly diagnosed patients. A group of us travel there and meet them. I'm the only PanCAN volunteer, as the others are a social worker, dietician, and chaplain from the hospital. I gave them my phone number. So far, I've talked to 391 diagnosed patients. That's how I met Lisa and Robin Stough.

As part of my volunteer work, I also travel to fundraisers all over the country and give talks. I try to inspire people not to give up. Through all this, I've realized a lot of it comes down to a state of mind. I've seen people hang their heads and give up. They die. But for those willing to fight, it's been wonderful seeing them make it.

I can't recommend PanCAN enough! Their people and resources are the first stop you need to make. Contact them. You won't be sorry.

My wife of forty-five years has been my caregiver through all of this. It was excruciating for her to watch me crawl to a corner of the room, get into a fetal position, and cry. Sometimes I banged my head with my fist. The pain was tremendous. Since I don't like pain medication, I had to endure it. Yet she stood there like a rock, even though I've seen her crying in the closet. She'll go between her clothes and sob hard. Then she comes out, wipes her face, and looks like a rock again. And she's stood by me for these long thirteen years.

It's affected her health. Even though the kids are out of the house and we're financially secure, she recently told me that she's been thinking about being alone when I die. She's 68 and working through the depression my disease has caused her.

Caregivers need to take time for themselves. They must have a life because this disease does not stop in a day or a week.

When it comes to doctors, I feel like a machine in which they're changing a part or adjusting my carburetor or radiator. Perhaps it's too much to ask, but I'd like some compassion.

Most of the nurses showed caring and compassion. After all, I might be losing my life. I don't need pity, but there's a fine line between pity and compassion. You need to understand compassion while letting me be me. Don't feel bad for me. Let me be alive. I'm still alive. Don't look at me like, "Okay, you're dying. You're going to be dead. That's all I can do for you."

I've talked to patients all over, and that's what many of them tell me: "Don't write me off. I know I'm dying, but don't kill me before I die." Sometimes families do. Sometimes some doctors do, too, because it's the nature of their business. They can't be emotionally attached to a patient.

Most people will write you off. They don't call. They don't check on you. They ask your wife or son, "Is he still alive?" That's why I isolated myself. I didn't let any negativity come into my life. I still don't. If anybody's negative around me, I push them out. If you find a compassionate person, hang on to them.

So my advice to doctors is that every patient wants to be one of a kind. Every patient wants to be the center of attention. It's my life, after all. I only have one.

Why did I survive? God wanted to give me a chance. I made a deal with Him. Now I'm trying to hold up my end of the bargain, but it's His will. Actually, He has given me a couple of second chances in life and I didn't recognize them. But I know it now.

Despite everything I've been through, I wouldn't change anything about my treatment. I hope it doesn't come back, but I'll fight again if it does. If I fail, that's okay. I'm 72. We all die at some point. At least my grandson is with his dad—my son and his new wife. They are doing great and he's my best friend.

Update: I was suffering severe stomach pain a few times each month. This led to calling 911 and spending two to three nights in the hospital. The diagnosis was always the same: chronic pancreatitis. I also had very high lipase, amylase, and IGG4 numbers. They put me on two to three days of liquid diet with lots of antibiotics and steroids. Then I was released.

My scans have always shown a piece of what doctors believed to be a harmless piece of stitch inside the biliary duct. Eventually, scans indicated an enlargement of the biliary duct to 8 mm. The normal size is 3 to 4 mm, so this was life-threatening.

The doctors said someone needed to go in with a scope to see what was causing the blockage, but it was a risky operation. Three doctors declined to do it due to the danger of perforation and death. Finally, the GI doctor who had originally found the tumor accepted the challenge as my last chance. However, he now taught at UT Southwestern and did not actively see patients anymore. After signing my life away, I went in for the thirty-minute surgery, but it didn't go as planned.

Because of my former Whipple surgery, the doctor spent over three hours trying to find the entrance to the duct. Once he did, he had to break the large stone that had formed beyond the loose stitch and clear the biliary tube. Then he closed up and waited for me to revive.

That was eight months ago; I've experienced no more pain since. I've had no additional hospitalizations and feel healthy and great again. As of July 2023—fourteen years after diagnosis—I'm still here!

Survivor Story: Fred Belkin

FIRST, LET ME SAY THAT I'VE BEEN HAPPILY MARRIED to Rosalyn Belkin for forty years. We have one daughter who's 35 years old, single, and lives in the Washington D.C. suburbs, ninety minutes south of where we live. I was an environmental and occupational health chemist and laboratory manager for the federal government and have a master's degree in chemistry from the University of Delaware and an MBA from the University of Baltimore. I'm a scientist, retired about twelve years ago. I'm currently 78 years old.

The story begins in June of 2016. I was 71 and had some issues pop up, like loss of appetite, fatigue, and weight loss. Since I'm pre-diabetic, I saw an endocrinologist. She sent me to a gastroenterologist.

I saw the gastroenterologist, and he said, "It's been five years since you had your colonoscopy. We need to do another one." I agreed, and that came out fine, though later on, he would tell me he'd initially thought I might have colon cancer. But that wasn't the case.

Continuing his investigation, the gastroenterologist ran some tests for digestive enzymes. One result was low so he ordered an MRI, looking for a pancreatic issue. The MRI showed a slight shadow on the tail of my pancreas, but it wasn't definitive. So he ordered a CT scan. I read the report and it stated the shadow was suspicious for adenocarcinoma pancreatic cancer.

He referred me to another GI doctor who performs endoscopic ultrasound via fine needle aspiration (EUS–FNA). This allowed the doctor to take a biopsy of the mass they saw on the tail of my pancreas. The pathology confirmed it was pancreatic cancer, so the doctor told me and my wife right in the outpatient recovery room.

By this time, it was October 2016. I was hoping for a different outcome but this diagnosis wasn't a big shock. I'd been prepared for pancreatic cancer after reading the CT scan report. However, during this entire journey, I discovered that whenever I experienced bad luck, I had good luck right behind it. I'll explain.

Back in the recovery room, as I heard the doctor say I had pancreatic cancer, I knew it was bad luck. But then he said I was eligible to have surgery. I had researched pancreatic cancer and knew that surgery provides the best chance of survival. Yet only 15 to 20 percent of people diagnosed with pancreatic cancer are eligible for surgery, so I considered this good luck.

The GI doctor who'd performed the EUS referred me to a surgeon at his Baltimore suburban hospital. I met with him and learned the procedure he'd perform was a distal pancreatectomy with splenectomy. He would remove the bottom half or bottom third of my pancreas. This was not the Whipple surgery that removed the top part of the pancreas. I had the lower part to remove, which was a simpler surgical procedure. More good luck.

After sharing my diagnosis with our friends, one of them recommended I check out Johns Hopkins, an academic hospital with a better facility. I met with a surgeon who's performed over 3,000 procedures. He was close to 80 years old and is considered one of the experts in the field.

This would be a standard surgery with no robots or machines. After a high-resolution CT scan, the surgeon explained that the tumor was not up against a blood vessel and confirmed I was eligible for surgery, which I had in November 2016, right after Thanksgiving.

The surgery was a long procedure, four hours plus. My first thought was, *Well, hey, I woke up from the operation. That's good news.* I had read that a small percentage of patients don't make it through the surgery, so my first thought was about surviving. The procedure has been refined to a high level of success, so that was more good news.

Before the surgery, I had asked the surgeon how long I'd be in the hospital. He said it was usually seven or eight days. It didn't quite go that way because I had a partial blockage of the bowel. They would not release me until things were back to normal, which finally happened on the eighteenth day. What a relief! It was more good news since after my long stay I was on solid food and had no devices to wear home.

A couple of days after my surgery, an oncologist from Johns Hopkins came into my room with a resident. The oncologist discussed a follow-up treatment, specifically chemotherapy. She wanted to use gemcitabine (Gemzar) and capecitabine (Xeloda). She left the room, but the resident stayed.

"Fred, do you want to know how long you have to live?" he asked.

"Okay," I replied. "You might as well tell me."

He came a little closer. "You have two-and-a-half years."

After initially looking up pancreatic cancer, I thought I'd be a goner within a few months. But upon hearing this, I said, "Oh, two-and-a-half years. That's not too bad."

Once I got out of the hospital, I read an article that suggested it was a mistake to tell me two-and-a-half years because that was merely the average. But then I read that with the old chemotherapy of Gemzar alone, the five-year life expectancy was about 15 percent. With this new chemo combo, the five-year life expectancy had risen to 30 percent. So I had a good chance of having a five-year survival. Well, a 30 percent chance, anyway.

When I was in the hospital, I also saw a radiation oncologist. When you have pancreatic cancer, one option is radiation treatment in the abdominal area to kill cancer cells that can't be detected. We discussed it, and he was very good. Being a scientist, I asked him, "What's the evidence this works?" He said a study done in Europe was inconclusive, so based on that, I decided against radiotherapy.

One issue I had in the hospital while recovering was a bedsore (pressure ulcer) on my butt. The hospital quickly switched me to an air mattress to reduce the pressure and stop additional sores. Besides having the wrong mattress, I had lost a great deal of weight, getting down to 122 pounds. Being thin somehow contributed to the bedsores. It was bad luck to have the bedsore, but it was good luck when the hospital released me with home healthcare support. As a result, a nurse, a physical therapist, and a dietician came to my house to ensure I was healing correctly. My wife and I were grateful for the support.

One night, about a month after leaving the hospital, I began vomiting. I had weakness in my legs and couldn't stand. We called 911 for an ambulance and they took me to the local hospital, two miles from my home, before transferring me back to Johns Hopkins. A nasogastric (NG) tube was inserted to help stabilize me. After a few days in the hospital, I met with a surgeon who believed I had a fully blocked bowel due to scar tissue from the surgery. An hour before the surgery, though, I resolved the issue. A nurse who saw the result said, "I guess because you're so worried about the procedure, we scared the shit out of you."

After six days in the hospital, I was discharged. It was interesting that I had received the same room I'd had during my pancreatic surgery stay at the hospital. It was a nice room. Like the first time, Rosalyn spent the nights in a lounger bed next to me.

Let me stop right here and say thank you to my wife because having her in the room helping me get up and walk around was more good luck. She was also an advocate, ensuring I received the correct medication and asking questions about my care. And if I needed a nurse, she hopped out there and got one. So I had good luck having an advocate and caregiver throughout my entire journey.

There are a few more items I want to cover. Before the surgery, I didn't have any chemotherapy or radiation. My CA 19-9 blood test for pancreatic cancer was low, in the single digits both before and after surgery. A physician told me that about 20 percent of patients with pancreatic cancer do not have an elevated CA 19-9.

Eventually, it was time for chemotherapy. My surgical wounds had healed enough to get chemotherapy. Prior to starting chemo, I had a chemotherapy port surgically installed into my chest. While chemotherapy may be bad luck, my Hopkins oncologist said I could have chemotherapy at Upper Chesapeake, only two miles from my house, instead of driving thirty miles to Johns Hopkins. Again, more good luck! It turned out this standard of care had recently been approved a few months earlier when a scientific paper had been published. More good luck in getting the latest chemotherapy.

Rosalyn and I met with the oncologist at Upper Chesapeake and discussed modifying the standard of care. It was a high dose of chemicals, and we were concerned about the side effects. We decided to cut down the dosage and change the cycle slightly. I had six months of chemotherapy. Infusion for Gemzar was once a week—two weeks on, one week off. Xeloda was given in pill form and taken at home. Sometimes, patients can't complete the program because their white or red blood cell counts are too low. But I was fortunate that I could make it through the entire program. By the summer of 2017, I had finished the chemo. There were no complications and I had minimal side effects. I began focusing on gaining weight.

The doctors said I had no dietary restrictions except to take CREON, a digestive enzyme, with meals. I was gluten-free, which was a life choice unrelated to the disease. I also had to take insulin—first, it was long-acting (Lantus), and then I added short-acting (NovoLog).

After the surgery and chemo, I had CT scans every six months. In May 2020, they found some nodules in my lungs, including one new one. A thoracic surgeon went in and resected one nodule. My medical oncologist studied this and said, "I think we should start chemo next week, but why don't you get a second opinion."

My oncologist suggested the University of Pennsylvania might have some experience. We found a second medical oncologist who looked at my records and said, "You have a number of these nodules in your lungs. I don't think you need any chemo now because they're very small and appear to be slow-growing."

We decided against chemo and continued following up with her. Then, in October 2021, she compared a recent CT scan to the one a few months earlier. She felt two of the nodules were growing faster than they had been before. Since she knew we were traveling to Florida in December for the winter, she said, "You know what? It's not urgent. Why don't you wait 'til you go down to Florida and start the chemo when you get there?"

I started the chemotherapy in Florida in the winter of 2021, which was a combination of two drugs, gemcitabine (Gemzar) and Abraxane at the standard dose, first-line treatment. There was an infusion one day a week every other week. The good news was after five treatments, the CT scan showed a 10 to 15 percent reduction in the size of the lung nodules. Unfortunately, the chemotherapy made me so weak that I could barely walk. We stopped it temporarily, and my oncology nurse recommended I see a palliative care physician. I did and he provided an at-home physical therapist to increase my strength.

On our return to Maryland, we consulted with our Penn Medicine oncologist. She recommended that I be treated with one chemotherapy drug, gemcitabine (Gemzar). The good news was the chemotherapy was effective in stabilizing my lung nodules for six months.

In the winter of 2022, there was some growth in the nodules, so we needed to change to another chemotherapy. Since we were in Florida, my Penn Medicine oncologist recommended consulting with an oncologist at the University of Florida, 200 miles from my location. It was good luck that the University of Florida oncologist was willing to perform a telemedicine visit. The treatment plan he recommended was to use gemcitabine and Abraxane at a 60 percent reduction from the standard dose. As of now, I continue to be on this regimen with minimal side effects.

So, that's where that story is as of July 2023. And the good news was reaching the six-year survival mark on October 21, 2022. That was a lovely celebration.

Now it's time for me to give all the advice I can.

Early Detection
The faster you can discover the pancreatic cancer, the better your chance of survival. You want to discover the disease while there is a surgical option. You can get regular check-ups and see a doctor for anything out of the ordinary: abdominal bloating, pain in the mid-back or upper abdomen, weight loss, jaundice, diabetes, and especially a new or changed digestive problem.

High-Volume Center
Go to an institution that has performed a lot of pancreatic cancer surgeries and dealt with the disease, then look for their doctors who have extensive experience in this specialty. Most high-volume medical centers are located in major metropolitan cities. Hopefully, one is close to where you live. You may be able to have a telemedicine visit.

Spread the News
Tell everyone you have pancreatic cancer. When I was first diagnosed, I read an article about a woman who had breast cancer. She'd told all her friends and she said they had started treating her differently, which made her advise against telling everyone. I mentioned this to a counselor, and she said, "No, you *should* tell everyone." It was great advice because it was through friends that we received excellent recommendations for doctors and nurses and were directed to a high-volume medical center. Our friends also provided my wife and me with a lot of support. Just let everyone know you have it. Let people help you and they will.

Caregiver
You need to find a good caregiver. I had my wife, Rosalyn. She's been an excellent advocate for me and asks questions that I wouldn't have thought of.

Stay Positive
Be hopeful and have a positive attitude. Don't just look at the statistics. And don't Google things like, "What are my chances with pancreatic cancer?" You need to have hope and be informed; both of these are important, even though they might feel like opposite responses.

Advocate for Yourself
Advocate for yourself. Read up on your cancer or have someone else do it who you know has a science background and is interested in helping you navigate your disease journey. Never be afraid to ask the medical professionals, "Why are you doing [this]?" or "Why aren't you doing [that]?" Don't stop asking questions.

Join a Local Pancreatic Support Group
I joined one local pancreatic support group, as well as one in Florida and one peer-to-peer sponsored by the AmCan Foundation. I enjoy exchanging information with other survivors and caregivers.

Use PanCAN

What a blessing it was for me to learn about PanCAN. They have tremendous information on their website. And don't be afraid to call them if you have questions. They can do a search for clinical trials, find support groups, and match you with a survivor or caregiver mentor in the SCN (Survivor Caregiver Network). Each spring, there is a PurpleStride event to raise awareness and funds for research and patient support.

Second Opinion

Don't be afraid to get a second opinion from another large institution. PanCAN has a list of institutions and providers that can help you. A second opinion saved me from having chemo too early.

Get Your Genes Checked

You should have genetic testing. The first type of genetic testing is for germline genes, which are inherited from parents to offspring. The second type is the mutation in the tumor's genes or biomarkers. Physicians may be able to access the tumor by resection, biopsy, or by liquid biopsy from your blood. My tumor mutation is KRAS G12V. There is no targeted therapy for this mutation.

In our pancreatic support group, we have several members with a mutation of the BRCA gene. Most people think it's only related to breast cancer, but the BRCA mutation could cause pancreatic cancer. Treatment for BRCA may use targeted therapy instead of chemotherapy.

My germline testing (inherited mutation) found the APC gene mutation. This gene doubles the risk for colon cancer, which is typically 4 percent of the population. As a result, I opted for a five-year colonoscopy, which did not detect cancer.

Keep Yourself Healthy

It's essential to keep yourself healthy. I would recommend seeing a dietician as I've done, especially one who deals with cancer patients. She's been excellent in helping me keep up my weight and energy level. Also, don't neglect the rest of your health. I have diabetes now and see a specialist (endocrinologist). I recommend getting a COVID-19 vaccine and having your booster shots. Don't neglect any other health issues. Manage all your physical and mental health issues.

Clinical Trials

Clinical trials are very important. You may be able to participate in a cutting-edge clinical trial and be one of the first to receive a life-changing drug or treatment. If a doctor presents a clinical trial to you, investigate it. Do some research. PanCAN can be a resource for clinical trials, so give them a call.

Research

When I started my journey at Johns Hopkins, I had signed up to be in their research program. I participated in a study that took several years. They collected extra blood whenever I came in for a CT scan. They were studying circulating tumors and liquid biopsies. Scientific papers were published. As a scientist, I feel good that I've contributed to science.

Pain

It's not acceptable to be in a lot of pain. Advocate for yourself rather than suffer. There are plenty of medicines and procedures to help you, including physical therapy and acupuncture. Also, many states now have legalized medical cannabis. Of course, keep in mind that when you're undergoing chemo, you must be careful with other medicines you take, as they may interfere with your treatment.

Mental Health

It's important to have mental healthcare for yourself and your caregiver. Often, the caregiver is more stressed than the patient. The journey is very stressful because you're living your life with this uncertainty hanging over you. Take full advantage of the mental healthcare professionals out there. My counselor said, "Your pancreatic cancer is like getting PTSD. You're in shock from that and you need to realize it and take care of your mental health." I took his advice and have kept myself mentally healthy by joining a pancreatic cancer support group and being an advocate.

Estate and Financial Planning

When I was diagnosed with pancreatic cancer, we rewrote our wills and started better organizing our finances and consolidating our accounts. It was important to get our financial affairs in better order. My beneficiaries will be less stressed when they have to deal with things because we've now cleaned them up.

Volunteer

I'm a volunteer in the Survivor and Caregiver Network (SCN) at Pan-CAN. I talk to other people who have just started their journey. I give them free advice. So, step in and roll up your sleeves. Give back to someone. You'll be better for the experience.

Health Insurance

Review your health insurance. I had good PPO health insurance, but this plan did not have any out-of-network coverage. When I was diagnosed with pancreatic cancer, I switched plans during the open enrollment period to a similar plan, but one that covered out-of-network care.

Palliative and Hospice Care

Palliative care physician specialists are not always on the radar of patients. These professionals address a cancer patient's physical symptoms, including pain, as well as emotional and social stresses. We met with a palliative care physician who brought a social worker to the meeting as well, and we all discussed my pain and mobility related to the chemotherapy treatment. Don't overlook these folks.

Professional Health Resources

Besides the medical oncologists who have treated my cancer, oncology nurses provided excellent support. I had a team of health professionals to manage this serious disease: primary care physicians to manage my general health, including preventive disease management, social workers for mental and social health, dietitians for better nutrition, physical therapists for pain-specific health issues, an endocrinologist for diabetes, and a GI physician for digestive enzymes management. You can get the same team.

Standard of Care

You may want to read the publications below for guidelines.

- PanCAN "Roadmap" for treating patients with pancreatic cancer. Published in *The Oncologist* in April 2023.
- NCCN (National Comprehensive Cancer Network) Guidelines for Pancreatic Cancer Adenocarcinoma 2023.

Survivor Story: Doug Sheaffer

Background

I WAS IN THE ELECTRICAL INDUSTRY FOR FORTY YEARS, going from an inside sales associate to outside sales. At the end of my career, I was a sales manager. I mainly sold industrial automation to manufacturing plants and products like switch gear, programmable controllers, variable frequency drives, and energy management systems. I retired in 2020, the year that COVID-19 hit.

I'm married with two kids and live in York, Pennsylvania. I'm also an unwilling member of the pancreatic cancer club.

Getting Sick

In August 2018, I was 64 years old and started having some problems. I was losing weight—over twenty pounds—and had loose stools. I went to my primary care doctor, who said, "It's just old age." I'd been constipated my entire life, so completely switching to having loose stools just didn't feel right.

A few years earlier, my wife had been diagnosed with colon cancer. It was discovered during a routine colonoscopy. As a result, she was referred to a colorectal surgery practice. The doctor there performed colorectal surgery, and she had no further problems or treatments.

Now she goes for regular follow-ups and blood work. Lucky her, right?

My wife and I discussed my problem and thought perhaps I should see her colon surgeon for a colonoscopy. "Maybe they'll find something," I said.

I had the colonoscopy and nothing was found. When I told the doctor that I couldn't believe it, he suggested a CT scan to help us find out what was going on. So I had the CT scan. Both the colonoscopy and CT scan were in December 2018.

In January 2019, I met with the surgeon who had my CT scan on his desk. "What is it?" I asked him.

"I see some growths on your pancreas. It looks like pancreatic cancer." He showed me a diagram of the growths and how one was up against my portal vein. He recommended I see an oncology surgeon and talk through the findings. He also suggested seeing a gastroenterologist. Both of the recommendations were to professionals in York and Maryland hospitals.

I met with the gastroenterologist, and he showed me the doctor's notes. He had found some jaundice issues and urine blockage. It seems the tumor in my pancreas was blocking my urine flow.

The gastroenterologist suggested I have two procedures at once: a ureteral stent to take care of the urine blockage and a biliary drainage catheter to free up the bile ducts that were causing my jaundice. By now, I was turning colors, so I agreed.

They admitted me to the hospital and performed the procedures. When I woke up, I was surprised to find a tube coming out of my side. No one had told me this would happen or that it was permanent.

I soon learned that the tube drained my bile into a small bag on my side. The bag must be emptied periodically. This was a shock.

I was still in the hospital recovering when my blood pressure dropped dangerously and I began blacking out. They quickly realized that they had accidentally nicked an artery when they inserted the ureteral stent, causing one of my lungs to fill up with blood. They grabbed the gurney and rushed me down for lung surgery with a trauma specialist. I waited in the preop room, watching my wife hurriedly sign all these documents and release forms. The doctor explained that a lot could go wrong with this surgery.

As she signed form after form, the weight of this became too much for her. She was frantic. I asked the nurse, "Can you just like take her away and get her some support? This is getting to be too much!!"

They escorted her to the waiting room and found a pastor. He talked to her and prayed with her. Meanwhile, they rolled me into the operating room and stopped. "Wait," someone said. "We need to push him a little bit further."

Someone started pushing my gurney and it hit some trays. This sent glass vials and surgical instruments crashing to the floor. Everything that could break shattered. *I'm a dead man,* I thought. *This is never going to work.*

I wondered if they used the same five-second rule we have at home when food hits the floor. If the food is picked up in five seconds, it's all good. *Will they still use those instruments?*

After the surgery, I was lying in a hospital bed in York, Pennsylvania, in a weakened condition, when an oncology surgeon walked in. I hadn't yet approached any doctors about my pancreatic cancer, but word traveled fast in this hospital. "Hey, we'll be taking care of this thing for you right here in York, right?" he asked.

I had no idea. I was still recovering from lung surgery, lucky to be alive.

After I was released from the hospital and felt up to it, I saw that oncology surgeon in his office. He explained that I had Stage 2 to 3 pancreatic cancer and was a strong candidate for Whipple surgery. But he had some concerns about the tumor being so close to a portal vein. Although he'd experienced a lot of success doing Whipples, he consulted with another oncology surgeon in Wisconsin, whom I believe had been his mentor. The York surgeon wasn't sure if he could do the surgery due to the closeness of the tumor to the vein. He said I might have to go to Wisconsin to have the surgery, but he wouldn't commit to a decision yet.

The York surgeon recommended chemotherapy to hopefully shrink the tumor away from the vein so he could perform the surgery. To start this off, he installed a chemo port in my upper chest during outpatient surgery. This allowed the chemotherapy drugs to be efficiently delivered into a vein without constant needle sticks.

With my port in, I was referred to an oncologist at the local York Cancer Care Center. He didn't have much experience with pancreatic cancer but was aware of the recommended protocol. The plan was for twelve cycles of FOLFIRINOX. A cycle is defined as the drug being administered into the vein and some additional drugs to protect the stomach lining and other organs. I also received a shot to prevent an allergic reaction. The FOLFIRINOX was done every two weeks, with one week for recovery. I did only ten cycles, though, as the side effects were hard on me.

Another CT scan showed the tumor had not shrunk sufficiently for surgery, so the oncologist switched me over to a lighter chemo, gemcitabine. Again, without a surgical option, this was considered more of a palliative care option—living longer with the cancer while keeping it at bay—than a permanent cure.

I decided I really wanted to shrink the tumor so I could have a Whipple surgery. I didn't want to give up. I pressed the oncologist for a solution. He tried to get an answer from the surgeon, but they weren't communicating. Frankly, I believe that the surgeon didn't want to take the risk. He only wanted to commit to a guaranteed, successful outcome rather than just giving it a try.

My health insurance had a feature allowing me to get a person to help facilitate communication between doctors, called a nurse advocate. I started the process of bringing her to the team.

By networking and talking to family and friends, the word got out about my pancreatic cancer. I learned of a friend of a friend who had the same disease. He had surgery done at Johns Hopkins. I got the name of this very renowned surgeon, Dr. Wolfgang, and set up an appointment.

My first stop was getting all my records. I collected everything and sent it to Dr. Wolfgang. Then I went down to Johns Hopkins with my nurse advocate and had a CT scan, after which I met Dr. Wolfgang. I had no expectations that he would be able to do the surgery because I trusted the folks in York. Yet when Dr. Wolfgang entered the exam room, he said, "I could have done your Whipple surgery right when you were diagnosed. There was plenty of room to operate."

I soon learned that the more advanced hospitals have access to the latest high-definition CT scanning machines. The scan in York was not the latest technology, so the image did not show much of a gap between the tumor and the vein. This new CT image showed there was plenty of room for surgery.

"Are you in?" Dr. Wolfgang said. "Do you want it?"

"I'm in!" I said. "I'm all in."

"My people will contact you with surgical dates."

I had CA 19-9 marker tests after each round of chemotherapy. First, it was 280. Then it went down to 50 as I faced surgery. All I could do now was trust Dr. Wolfgang and his team to get the job done.

My Whipple surgery was performed at Johns Hopkins in August 2019. When it was over, Dr. Wolfgang told me it had been successful and to begin my recovery.

Five weeks later, I was healthy enough to have four more cycles of FOLFIRINOX, which I needed to neutralize the cancer cells in the bloodstream and lymph nodes surrounding the surgical site.

I continued working with Johns Hopkins and Dr. Wolfgang, along with an oncologist, Dr. Laheru. They worked together well. Each quarter, I had a CT scan on their high-definition equipment. Everything was great until December 2020, over a year after the Whipple surgery. The three-month CT scan showed a spot on the liver. In February 2021, with two spots present, my oncologist at Hopkins suggested we do four more rounds of FOLFIRINOX in hopes of shrinking or removing the spots. I had the chemo but it wasn't successful.

I explored a surgical option with two surgeons, including Dr. Wolfgang. He had transferred to New York, taking a higher position at New York University Hospital. So I used the surgeon at Johns Hopkins he recommended but that guy said no. Their protocol for doing a successful liver surgery was a maximum of three spots. Unfortunately, a recent MRI showed some additional spots developing. He determined that a resection would only be a temporary solution and could be too dangerous for a successful recovery.

I thought, *Here we go again.* I'm not one to take the first "no," so I contacted Dr. Wolfgang at his New York hospital. Originally, he seemed pretty excited about doing it. He's a gung-ho kind of guy. But after his team looked at it, they said no.

To date, I haven't had surgery on my liver. I presently have up to six spots, which are too many for surgery. And more spots continue to appear on my liver.

I'm now starting a clinical trial with Johns Hopkins. It consists of two drugs to pick up or boost the immune system and bacteria to help attack the cancer. At present, I feel terrific. My wish is that this treatment will either keep the cancer at bay or reduce the tumors. All I can hope for is time for the medical team to advance a cure.

So, after almost three years from my initial diagnosis, I'm grateful to the medical caregivers for their help in keeping my story alive.

Caregiver

My wife has had to be somewhat of a caretaker for me. When I was going through one of my clinical trials, a minister came in and asked how I was doing. Then she looked at my wife and said, "So, how are you handling all this?"

I hadn't even asked my wife that question and felt so bad for that failure. I'm an upbeat kind of guy, and nothing gets me down. I'd been plowing through this thing, never stopping to ask how my wife was doing emotionally and physically. It was an eye-opening experience.

Advice

If you hear something you don't like, don't accept it. Keep searching for a second opinion and maybe a third. PanCAN has an excellent support helpline. If you don't know where else to call, PanCAN can provide more information to get you better choices.

Before COVID, when I was receiving my chemo, there were other people physically close to me in the treatment room. It wasn't a private area. So I started talking to them. Many were often down, lamenting their situation. I'd just say, "Take a look around. There's always somebody worse off than you." I think that helped some people.

I take CREON for the digestive system and it works well for me. I've heard from many people who have had problems with CREON, but I've been very fortunate that it's worked for me.

There aren't many foods I have to avoid. Lately, it's been orange juice because of the acid. But I'm very fortunate to have a good stomach. Still, I recommend staying away from fried or spicy foods.

Alternative Medicine

I worked with a naturopathic dietician during chemo treatments. She gave me advice on protein shakes and eating vegetables (generally a healthy diet) to keep my weight up. She also recommended a few supplements for sleeping and energy, specifically for the liver. It's all helped.

Volunteer

I'm on the Survivor Council with the Philadelphia PanCAN group. I find both caregivers and cancer patients really appreciate talking to people with the same condition. There are cancer support groups out there, but pancreatic cancer has its own set of issues, so it's really nice to have folks to talk to who have the same kind of problems.

PanCAN does interviews of survivors and did one with me. My hope is that if it helps one person, it's all worth it. Obviously, I recommend you volunteer and give back to others.

Update: The clinical trial was interesting but not a positive experience on my body. We stopped it after three months and I was given three to six months in January 2022. I then started chemo again with some good results up until April 2022. My body was just getting beat up with the chemo, so my wife and I made a decision for quality of life and we stopped chemo four weeks ago.

I feel terrific, and I'm certainly aware of the consequences. I have been a survivor for 3½ years and feel very fortunate for the time. I spent a lot of time with family and did a lot of traveling, including a river cruise in Germany after the COVID restrictions eased. I have been blessed with much more than twelve months of survival.

Note: Doug passed away on June 29, 2022.

Survivor Story: Doug Dobbs

IT WAS 2021. ELEVEN YEARS EARLIER, I HAD RETIRED FROM PRO STAFF, a staffing and recruiting business that helps folks find jobs. I sold my share of Pro Staff to my partners and after thirty years, looked forward to enjoying the rest of my life with my wife, Laura. She had also retired as a project manager from the sales and IT integration industry. In the past eleven years, we'd traveled and hung out with ten wonderful grandkids. Other than the pandemic, we were having a good time.

Back to 2021. I was 71 years old and found my blood sugar spiking. The pancreas was always on my mind, especially with my younger brother's situation. He'd been a business partner at Pro Staff, so we were close. And he had Type 1 diabetes. We grew up in Minnesota, and he was active with the University of Minnesota in supporting research and transplants, islet transplants, and different treatments to address Type 1 diabetes. Seeing my blood sugar spike caused me concern. I started taking Metformin to lower it. Of course, it didn't help that I'd been eating terrible stuff during the pandemic and adding some unnecessary weight. I kept monitoring my blood sugar, but it didn't resolve.

I also began having severe pain in my gut every time I ate. I located it in the upper left quadrant of my stomach, just below the ribcage. The pain progressively worsened, and I even felt it at night. At that time, I didn't have any back pain.

I wondered what could be causing it. I had previously suffered from diverticulitis and a colon resection in 2004. The colon had become infected and caused pain in different regions of the gut. I thought this might be related to that.

I also have an identical twin brother who'd gone through gallbladder surgery. I called and asked him what the pain felt like and he told me where and how it had felt. Listening to him, I realized that my pain was different. In addition, I had floating, yellow, disgusting stools—foul smelling. Something was definitely wrong. Still, I endured it for two months.

I soon figured out the heavier, greasier, harder-to-digest foods made it more painful. At one point, my nephew came to town and we went out for barbeque, but I had to leave to go sit in the car afterward because of the severe pain. The pain wasn't as severe when I didn't eat or stuck with easier-to-digest, lighter foods. As a result, I lost a little weight.

I finally went to my primary care physician and he decided to do a CT scan. That was on June 9, 2021. The next day, my doctor called and said the scan showed a small mass and irregularities in the pancreas. He said it might be pancreatitis but was most likely pancreatic cancer. He immediately referred me to an oncologist. It didn't really sink in, as Laura and I were still in denial. We heard the doctor say it *might* be pancreatic cancer, so it still needed to be confirmed.

We met with the oncologist on June 15, 2021, seven days after the scan. She told me I had a small tumor on the body of my pancreas abutting the main artery (SMV) and celiac axis running through the stomach into the liver. She explained it was possibly operable but not necessarily easily done. She referred me to a surgeon who specialized in surgeries in this area of the body.

On the way home, the news hit us hard. We were stunned. Devastated. Our son-in-law's father had recently been diagnosed with pancreatic cancer. Four months later, he was gone. And we'd heard other pancreatic cancer stories. It was always a matter of months.

At home, the fear crept in. We pondered what kind of treatment plan I'd have to endure. We contacted our daughter. She's in medical sales and has relationships with gastro doctors. We started talking to several of them.

Until now, none of the doctors we'd seen had said anything about my prognosis. It was all, "Stay positive. Stay optimistic. Never give up hope." They also gave us general statistics but told us that each person is their own statistic. Of course, we turned to Dr. Google to see about life expectancy and possibly get more education on the subject.

Two days later, I sat in front of a surgeon. He had ordered another CT scan and was studying the results. My CA 19-9 results were all normal because I'm one of the 10 percent who don't trigger that test. He explained the scan indicated locally advanced Stage 1 to 2 nonmetastatic pancreatic cancer. This was also the first time I learned about CREON.

As we left the hospital, we decided to get a second and maybe a third opinion. The very next day, June 18, 2021, we went to UT Southwestern. I had been treated there before, so they had records on me. The staff drew blood and did the labs immediately. We met with Dr. Herbert Zeh. He called it borderline resectable or Stage 2 to 3. Before we left, I received a CREON prescription as well as samples for ZENPEP and CREON 24,000. Because the CREON is so expensive, I took the samples until we could figure out the insurance, my qualifications, and the cost.

On June 21, 2021, we met with yet another surgeon. He felt it was operable, yet had a different approach from Dr. Zeh and did not use robotics. Instead, he does open surgery with a vertical incision.

Two days later, the first hospital performed an EUS with an FNA. I learned I had the more aggressive form of pancreatic cancer: adenosquamous carcinoma of the pancreas (ASCP).

On June 24, 2021, we returned to UT Southwestern and met with oncologist Dr. Beg. He explained that they were prescribing FOLF-IRINOX as chemotherapy for twelve rounds—six before and six after surgery—with radiation after the first six rounds. If the tumor was still operable, the surgical oncologist (Zeh) would perform an Appleby surgery using robotics.

On June 30, 2021, we met with radiologist Dr. Todd Aguilera at UT Southwestern. This was when we decided to go with UT Southwestern. We felt this place offered the most inclusive treatments and had highly skilled doctors, especially those able to perform the Appleby. And by now, we knew having surgery was the key element to the possibility of a longer life.

Everything moved fast; I had a mediport installed in my chest on July 1, 2021. Throughout this entire process, I've never had any problems with my port.

My first chemo session was on July 6, 2021. I quickly suffered vertigo and had to be helped to the bathroom to avoid falling. Vertigo and lab results with low white blood cells pushed back my second round to July 26, 2021. After the second round of FOLFIRINOX, I was doing terribly. I began to worry about the long-term implications of this chemo drug. Ten years earlier, I'd been hit with the West Nile virus and had developed Meniere's disease. That gave me vertigo, hearing loss, and tinnitus. It didn't take long for me to realize that oxaliplatin had to go. For the rest of my rounds, I took FOLFIRI and each round was done on time, always with the 5-FU pack and Neulasta injector every other infusion. The chemo rounds were much easier without the oxaliplatin.

One day before my last chemo round, I had a CT scan. Then, I underwent an EUS marker procedure for radiation. I was also accepted into the Galera clinical blind trial. I received an infusion followed by radiation. The trial was to reduce radiation toxicology, allowing a stronger dose that could be more effective in beating cancer. Basically, it wanted to show that by taking the Galera drug, a higher dose of radiation could be used without damaging the organs. It also required eight rounds of chemo before radiation, so I had two more on October 15 and 29. Then I had simulated radiation on October 30, 2021, and five actual radiation sessions from November 10th through the 17th.

My surgery was on January 14, 2022, during the height of COVID-19 reinfections. Few surgeons perform the Appleby surgery, with Dr. Zeh at the top of that field. He removed two-thirds of my pancreas, leaving the head intact. He also took out the spleen because the blood supply had been cut due to the tumor, and it had atrophied. Fortunately, I had extra arteries running into the liver, which worked out well. Maybe 10 percent of people have this.

After the surgery, I felt like I would have a quick recovery, and I did. They discharged me after four days. Four days is a very short stay, but they thought it would be safer to release me and be at home with COVID-19 exploding and filling the hospital to capacity.

One week after going home, I walked a mile at a pretty good clip and thought, *Wow, this thing's going to go pretty good.* This did not last long—the recovery process, in general, was hard because of the GI issues related to pancreas function.

On March 27, 2022, they put me back on chemo for four more rounds of FOLFIRI. I completed three rounds and my last chemo session was on April 25, 2022.

On May 12, 2022, I went in for a CT scan. As we were leaving, the doctors called me to say I had to go to the ER because I had pulmonary embolisms. They put me on blood thinners to resolve the clots and I remained in the hospital for four days. But the good news from this was that my CT scan showed I had no evidence of disease (NED).

Two months later, in July, I started losing weight again. I had cramping, constipation, and diarrhea issues. I also had some acute pain. I did have some dramatic weight loss and kept losing pounds—about forty in total now—returning to my high school weight while losing lots of muscle mass in my thighs, arms, and shoulders. It took some time to identify how much CREON should be taken per meal. Once I did that, most of my GI issues resolved and I could start putting on weight. To battle the enzyme deficiency, I was put on CREON 36,000 and another CT scan was ordered. On July 26, 2022, thirteen months after my original diagnosis, I learned the cancer had spread to the liver with one lesion about 1 cm. At the original surgery site, the CT scan showed possible scar tissue. Another biopsy was scheduled for August 23, 2022.

Before the biopsy could be performed, I came down with COVID. This delayed the biopsy until I tested negative for COVID. After a delay of three weeks, it was finally done on September 14, 2022. Nine days later, I learned that the liver lesion was indeed cancer with no other spread on the liver or elsewhere. The next step was to go back into chemotherapy treatment (standard of care). This time they would try something different—perhaps changing the chemo cocktail.

I joined chemotherapy in a clinical trial. I was not randomized to receive the trial drug Pamrevlumab through Precision Promise PanCan. I decided to stay in the trial to get some free CREON and better attention along with the standard of care. So, on October 13, 2022, I received the treatment paclitaxel (Abraxane) and gemcitabine (Gemzar)—G&A. The sessions were every seven days. I completed six of them on November 23, 2022. My drug dosage was reduced because of side effects issues. We left the trial because it was too much, too often, and I wasn't doing well. There was no flexibility within the trial, either.

On October 25 and 26, we went to Houston and met with doctors at MD Anderson. Once I was established as a patient there, we received a second opinion and they agreed with everything UT Southwestern was doing. We also studied all the clinical trials at MD Anderson, and I was available/eligible for none. The doctors did give me a statistical prognosis of six to twelve months left on Earth.

On January 9, 2023, I received chemotherapy outside of the trial, but it was still a G&A drug. My fourth session ended on February 23, 2023. I also had a CT scan that day. On February 28, 2023, the scan showed growth in the liver lesion as well as additional 2 mm lesions. The scan also showed growth at the pancreas resection site, so we knew it was definitely cancer and not scar tissue. No other spread was shown.

On March 13, 2023, I started a new chemotherapy regimen and will do two rounds and then have a CT scan before the third cycle with three drugs: oxaliplatin, fluorouracil, and leucovorin.

We also met with the folks at Mary Crowley Cancer Research to see about clinical trials. We've also contacted NIH out of Bethesda, Maryland, about a trial for metastatic adenosquamous carcinoma. They are retrieving my medical records for review to determine eligibility.

I met Robin Stough through a friend who plays golf with him. My friend knew about his wife Lisa and mentioned my pancreatic cancer. Robin explained what he'd been through. Next thing I knew, Robin contacted me and we discussed different treatment options. We've been talking and texting ever since. He's been a great information resource, and I appreciate him taking the time to do it.

The one thing I learned early on was the importance of a care partner and advocate, someone to walk alongside me to keep track of this stuff and ask the right questions. Many times, my mind was cloudy and ineffective. It freed me up not having to worry about appointments or anything important, as well as having Laura do all the driving since the treatments had compromised my balance. Plus, a patient is not allowed to drive from the healthcare facility after a chemo session. As a former project manager, she's good at this stuff. And she's had to do all the chores around the house, including some that I used to do. I try not to add any burdens to her emotionally or physically. And we try to have fun and laugh and enjoy life together.

Now I've gained back about fifteen pounds. After the diagnosis, we completely changed the way we eat. We consulted with our pharmacist and eliminated all sugar and simple carbs like potatoes, bread, and pasta. Then we eliminated the grains and beans. Everything is now organic. We eat vegetables and less greasy food. And no processed foods. Even Laura has lost weight.

The FOLFIRI took a lot of my hair, but not all of it. When I went on G&A, the rest of the hair remained.

Going through something like this made us lean on our spiritual beliefs. We prayed all the time. That's been the most incredible experience through all this, seeing the amount of support, the encouragement, people praying for us, the deep, deep feelings coming out, and love from all sorts of people. Folks I haven't talked to in some time are calling me. It's just amazing. I honestly don't know how people go through this without prayer and belief in God. But know this: we did not find religion through the diagnosis. We were already Christians.

Our relationship with our children and grandchildren has become stronger as well. Plus, we have a core group of friends for support.

I don't want to say that I haven't been empathetic, but I probably have more empathy for others now. I see people who are much worse off and feel bad for them. I feel fortunate to be here, strong enough to go out and walk and exercise. I'm not saying my golf game is good, but I still go out with friends and family and enjoy the outdoors when not recovering from chemo. Each morning, I see the sun rising and appreciate things like that more.

For me, it's been narrowing down what I focus my time on, mainly family and friends and appreciating those times together. I don't necessarily want to go on any big trips or do any of those things. We were fortunate enough to be able to travel quite a bit. And I traveled a lot in business, so I don't have that urge to get out and see anything. I just want to focus on those meaningful relationships and do my best to continue to exercise, stay mentally optimistic and positive, and hope for the best outcome possible.

I would say my biggest factor has been the support, prayers, and encouragement. I also love seeing the little grandkids' basketball games or soccer games. That's a great time, a real emotional lift. That's been hugely impactful on my mental outlook. We don't know when we will leave here, so I live each day and take advantage of whatever time I have.

Laura has told me she determines my down days and modifies what we can do. You have to be flexible and know that your plan could change. We pivot a lot. And we make tentative plans while doing our best.

Laura and I have been married for twenty-three years and together for twenty-five.

My advice to people diagnosed with cancer is to educate themselves. Go with what the doctors say, but you must be responsible for yourself or someone you care for who has cancer. And you must have an advocate! It's too traumatic. It's too much information for an individual to do this alone. It would be best to have somebody you trust and can depend upon. And do your homework and get educated while seeking out information. Rely on the doctors, but rely on yourself, too.

Find the best team that suits you and your needs. We selected UT Southwestern based on everything they could offer, the surgeon, and the entire picture. It's important to assemble the team; it's life or death.

There are resources available through PanCAN.org. There are different organizations with different treatments. Don't be afraid to ask questions. Laura and I ask a lot of questions about the treatment protocol and why this is better than that. It gives us some comfort that we're headed in the right direction. But we also want to know what the options are. There's so much more available today than just a few years ago.

I would urge you to focus on the positive. People are surviving this disease and living long lives. It's not necessarily a death sentence.

And remember, you're still alive. Given the circumstances, try to live your life as well as you can. Exercise and try to stay mentally optimistic.

We've also had divine intervention many times throughout this journey. As one of the oncologists said, "Don't ever give up hope. Stay strong, and don't give up hope." That's helped me quite a bit, just thinking about that.

Be proactive with the decisions you make. It was three weeks from when I was diagnosed to when I started chemo. We were very fortunate and could dedicate all our time to that since we had retired—meeting with different surgeons, getting the port put in, getting the fine-needle aspiration, and moving very quickly in order to begin my treatment as soon as possible.

Right now, it's May 10, 2023, and I'm powering through. It's day to day, and I'm doing okay; just happy to be here. I went through four more infusions recently and a scan. The results were delivered on May 4, 2023, and showed a 13 percent progression of the cancer. Because that's less than 20 percent, I'm considered stable. Anything over 20 percent is labeled "progressed." However, I'm now scheduled for four more rounds of chemo with irinotecan added back in. And I'm coming up on my twenty-four-month survival, so stay tuned. I know I will!

Update: I'm continuing chemotherapy and will have scans in August 2023. Chemo has been tough this time. I was hospitalized for five days with severe sepsis—Group A strep bacterium—which came out of nowhere. The doctors speculate I caught it through throat sores caused by the chemo. After being released, I had two weeks of antibiotic infusions. My chemo was canceled, and the next round was lower doses since I was still recovering. My treatment was set back for a month. I've fully recovered, but sepsis is no joke. Apparently, I've used up my nine lives. And I'm still considering the NIH trial for Minnelide, a novel drug for pancreatic and liver cancer, if chemo becomes too much or I'm not responding. For the update, that's it. That's enough!

Epilogue

O N JANUARY 25, 2021, Lisa's treatments ended. Now she had a long road of recovery ahead. First, she had to deal with the weight issue; she needed to gain a bunch of it. She was about 115 before her diagnosis, around 112 when first diagnosed, and believed her ideal weight was 110. So, at the start of her recovery, she weighed in at 90.6 pounds. There were times during the treatments she was under 90 pounds, so it could be worse.

Lisa worked hard, and one year later (February 2022), she was at 102.6 pounds—a little more than a 13 percent gain in total body weight. By May 2023, she was a little over 105—only a tiny 2 percent gain in year two. She still feels she has a few more pounds to go as her body heals and evolves.

Six weeks after Lisa's last chemo session (all time periods here relate to her last chemo session), her nausea and diarrhea completely disappeared. By week 28, her bowel movements were normal.

Her diminished appetite started improving around the 21-week mark. The ZENPEP digestive enzymes were another issue. She took the enzymes for 43 weeks, experimenting with different dosages, never sure she had the right formula. She could handle protein drinks at six weeks and felt good about eating most foods by 17 weeks. At the 23-week mark, poor nutrient absorption was still a concern and focus. Lisa also started taking a wheatgrass shot each morning. They had read somewhere this could help prevent a recurrence.

Throughout her recovery, Lisa worked closely with dietician Shelli Hardy. When Lisa had digestive issues, Shelli reminded her she was detoxing from the chemo. She also explained enzyme deficiency was real and Lisa was probably experiencing it. That's why, at thirteen weeks, they upped her dosage from two to three capsules, depending on the meal. But really, it's up to the patient to experiment with the proper dosage to see what works best.

One inspiring comment Shelli made when they talked about discontinuing enzymes was, "I think that's doable because I'm continually amazed at how the remaining pancreas often regains full function."

Dr. Beg finally let Lisa stop the enzymes at 43 weeks. She watched for diarrhea or greasy, floating, or light-colored stools, but nothing happened, and she hasn't looked back since. Apparently, "a tincture of time" was the right prescription.

Lisa's fasting glucose and A1C—borderline high—were two more issues she had to deal with. She and Robin visited an endocrinologist, Dr. Amy Vora, at the 19-week mark, and Dr. Vora ordered tests for C-peptide and serum glucose. The doctor guessed that her C-peptide would be adequate since the surgery was almost a year ago (August 3) and her hemoglobin A1C had been okay.

C-peptide is a byproduct created when insulin is produced. Measuring the amount of C-peptide in the blood indicates how much insulin is produced. Lisa had the body and tail of her pancreas removed during surgery. Dr. Vora indicated the body and tail are the most responsible for insulin production, and therefore she may be at risk for low insulin production going forward.

The test was nonfasting, as Dr. Vora wanted to see how Lisa's pancreas functioned while her glucose was elevated. After getting the results, she told Lisa her C-peptide test result was 5.6, which meant the pancreas produced adequate amounts of insulin—a somewhat high but acceptable result. Lisa's nonfasting glucose was also normal. Since everything checked out well, the plan was to monitor her hemoglobin A1C every six months.

Lisa also discussed her bone issues with Dr. Vora. At 14 weeks, a bone density scan diagnosed Lisa with osteopenia/osteoporosis. The L1 compression fracture, likely caused by her fall in the bathroom, now made more sense. The risk factors included treatment during chemotherapy, specifically glucocorticoid treatment (the steroid Dexamethasone), low body mass index with low body weight and improper nutrient absorption, and being postmenopausal. Regardless of how or when it came about, Lisa needed to treat this condition.

Dr. Vora recommended the following: (a) Start calcium carbonate 800 mg daily, (b) continue vitamin D 2,000 units daily (check levels),

(c) start alendronate, more commonly known as Fosamax (weekly), as long as Lisa's vitamin D was adequate (they discussed the very low risk of osteonecrosis of the jaw), and (d) avoid Forteo, which was contraindicated due to her radiation history.

Lisa was not totally comfortable with these recommendations, so she solicited opinions from a doctor friend, who suggested taking Fosamax daily. Then Lisa went back to Dr. Aronoff. He'd been her PCP for thirty-five years and was the one who'd sent her for a CT scan back in February 2020 when this journey began. In May 2021, when Lisa first reunited with him, Dr. Aronoff was excited to see her and gave some emotional hugs. He wanted to hear everything about her journey. He examined her and reviewed her lab work. For osteopenia/osteoporosis, he liked Actonel and calcium citrate. After discussing her options with Dr. Aronoff, Lisa decided to take a 150 mg tablet of Actonal (also known as Risedronate) once a month. She ended the meeting with more hugs and then left, thrilled to have Dr. Aronoff back in the loop.

Yet another issue vital to Lisa's recovery was the physical aspect. She'd lost so much muscle that she needed to get back to working out. First, she had to increase her energy levels. That happened at the four-week mark. She was even able to stay up until 9 p.m.

By eight weeks, she was walking one mile a day and drove herself to appointments with a dentist and for a mammography. It was her first time doing any real driving in one full year. By twelve weeks, she drove everywhere by herself.

One of the driving trips was to Lisa's gynecologist. She was due for a checkup, and everything was good. The gynecologist mentioned his mother had died of pancreatic cancer. Then his nurse mentioned her father-in-law had also died of pancreatic cancer. Although both diagnoses differed from Lisa's, hearing these stories created a real mental challenge that Lisa would always need to work through.

She started working out at 21 weeks. Dr. Amanda Kayser, a physical therapist/trainer at the Four Seasons/Sports Club in Irving, put Lisa through the paces. Dr. Kayser specialized in physical therapy for clients experiencing and recovering from major medical issues, including cancer treatments. She was also qualified to help Lisa with her mental game and anxiety, which were equally important. After two weeks of hard work,

Robin said she was 85 percent of her old self and, by 27 weeks, 95 percent. Her endurance and strength continued improving.

Lisa went back to enjoying lunches with her good friends Sallie, Kim, Ray, Cindy, Rochelle, Laurie, and Karla. It was a mental boost to her recovery.

Lisa's hair was another issue. She cut it to 1/8 of an inch a few weeks after her last chemo session. It was mostly gray and continued falling out or breaking off, definitely needing a reset. Eventually, the hair became less brittle and grew back, albeit slowly. At five months, her hair started coming in nicely. It was still gray, but it wasn't brittle or falling out. By the ten-month mark, Lisa's hair was almost back to her normal color. And by the end of her first year, it was completely normal.

One strange issue that popped up was some pain behind Lisa's right rib cage and mid-back. At fourteen weeks, it came and went, then grew more severe and frequent. Dr. Zeh was concerned it might be gallstones until the ultrasound showed nothing. Then the pain went away. Perhaps it was from her compression fracture, strained or atrophied muscles, latent surgical pain, scar tissue, or stress. Dr. Beg emphasized the pain was not from cancer, as that kind of pain did not "come and go." It remained a mystery.

Lisa was asked to keep her port after the chemo treatments, and it required maintenance. It served as a reminder that recurrence was possible. First, she had to continue taking Xarelto, a blood thinner, to keep blood clots from forming. Next, she had to have it flushed with saline every four to six weeks since it wasn't being used. The nurse also drew blood to ensure the port flowed both ways. These flushes and blood draws continued for 44 weeks. That's when she had the left subclavian mediport and catheter removed by an interventional radiologist at UT Southwestern. He used local anesthesia with four initial numbing shots surrounding the port area. Lisa started feeling pain as they worked on it and received two additional numbing shots. It turned out the port had two stitches anchoring it to a nearby muscle. Those were cut and removed along with the port and catheter. She received five internal stitches and external glue to close the wound. Before they proceeded with the removal procedure, a last-minute CT scan was ordered out of an abundance of caution and showed no issues.

After the removal, Lisa had some serious bruising around the port area. Two days later, a hard lump formed near the port site. An ultrasound showed it to be a hematoma, probably caused by discontinuing the blood thinner a bit too early. It soon resolved, and everything was smooth again. It was a small price to pay after wearing it for twenty months. What a physical and mental relief for Lisa to see that port thrown away!

At fourteen weeks, Lisa had her first follow-up exam. Here's how it went down:

- Lisa reported for CT scans of the chest and abdomen/pelvis and lab work.
- She visited with the doctor.
- She waited for two possible answers: either she was good for another three months, or her cancer had returned.

Both Robin and Lisa had to deal with "scanxiety"—the stress that came with these follow-ups. The wait was torturous, and the term was real.

On April 1, 2021, Lisa and Robin celebrated their 40th wedding anniversary. Just a quiet evening at home.

On April 5, 2021, the 21st Century Cures Act added requirements that healthcare providers give patients access to all their health information without delay. This meant MyChart users could see all their labs, tests, and imaging results as soon as they become available—often even before their healthcare provider had reviewed them. Although having these immediate results was great, it could make a patient anxious before their doctor had a chance to interpret or explain them. Lisa and Robin became extraordinarily stressed more than a few times. That being said, they did prefer to receive the results immediately.

Before the new law, they had to go back the next day or wait around anxiously all weekend. Then they'd come back, stressed out again, waiting for someone to appear. They would study the doctor's expression for any signs of what he knew that they didn't. Then they heard the words "NED—you're all good." Relief and heavy sighs followed as the clock started ticking toward the next three-month follow-up. But now, Lisa could see the results superfast.

After her first follow-up exam, she heard the word NED (no evidence of disease). Relief again!

Her CA 19-9 came in at 11.0—well within normal, and the lowest reading since 11.9 immediately after surgery. The pathology report indicated a subtle increase in the size of several lymph nodes. That was concerning since the report indicated a "differential consideration" could be metastatic disease.

In a meeting with Dr. Zeh, he indicated the interval increase was not a concern. This was not the usual way pancreatic cancer metastasized, and according to him, metastasis was not "usually" found until three to six months after an abnormal CA 19-9 reading.

The next follow-up was at 28 weeks. It showed NED with a CA 19-9 of 13.8 and a fasting glucose of 93—both good numbers. Lisa's abdomen/pelvis CT scan did show a slow increase in the size of the portacaval lymph node. The lymphatics section of the radiology report read: "1.2 cm portacaval lymph node, previously 9 mm on 4/20/2021, 7 mm on 1/25/2021; indeterminate, would consider PET/CT imaging." Other than the lymph node issue, her CT abdomen scan was clean.

This enlarged lymph node concerned Robin and Lisa, so they contacted Dr. Zeh. His quick response over the weekend via email was, "The findings are nonspecific, meaning they do not provide definitive evidence of disease recurrence. Moreover, a CT scan slice is typically 3 to 5 mm, thus, there is no statistical difference between an LN 9 mm or 12 mm on two different CTs. In the setting of a normal CA 19-9, I am further reassured that there is no evidence of disease recurrence. I would recommend continued serial interval surveillance as we have been doing."

Lisa also discussed this issue with Dr. Beg's team. It centered around the interval size increase of the portacaval lymph node. Leticia Khosama, Dr. Beg's nurse practitioner, responded with their thoughts,

> Dr. Beg reviewed it and discussed it with Dr. Zeh as well. They're both in agreement to monitor with a repeat CT in three months. They do not think the increase in size of the reported lymph node is anything significant or something that requires further workup at this time. With normal tumor markers and excellent treatment response on pathology, we do not expect this slight change in size to be anything significant.

When Lisa met with Dr. Zeh, he pretty much repeated his email; he didn't believe the reported slow increase in the size of the portacaval lymph node was an issue. After reviewing the radiology reports, he wasn't totally convinced the lymph node had increased in size as it was being reported. He explained a CT scan slice and what represents a statistical difference. He also indicated that lymph nodes could increase and decrease in size over time. And he reminded Lisa and Robin that he was a big believer in the CA 19-9 tumor marker. Often, an abnormal CA 19-9 reading precedes tumor visibility on a CT scan by three to six months. To deal with these lymph nodes, Robin and Lisa discussed undergoing a PET scan, and his answer was a quick no. He indicated the possibility of a false positive with this test, and as they already knew, Dr. Zeh only recommended PET scans for pancreatic cancer in select instances. Dr. Zeh said that no immediate action would likely be taken even if cancer was suspected in this situation.

During the meeting, Dr. Zeh examined Lisa's incisions, which had healed nicely. Robin and Lisa asked if there was anything they could do to prevent a recurrence. Specifically, they asked about the "vaccine" Johns Hopkins was working on. During his time at Johns Hopkins, Dr. Zeh had been involved with the clinical trial for a similar vaccine. He indicated it "did not work." He was not aware of any other trials, and his final advice to Lisa: "Go live your life."

Subsequent follow-up exams have all continued to show NED is in the house. Then, at 41 weeks, Lisa's portal lymph node decreased from 12 mm to 8 mm. Dr. Beg believed it was evidence of a normal ebb and flow. That was good enough for Lisa.

In late 2019, before Lisa's pancreatic cancer diagnosis, she'd had a small spot on her forehead. During chemotherapy, it turned angry and red before disappearing for a time. Then it returned a few months later. At 29 weeks, she went to her dermatologist, who confirmed it was a basal cell carcinoma. It was time for Mohs surgery.

Surgical dermatologist Dr. Priya Zeikus was tapped to do the surgery. Her fellowship in Mohs micrographic surgery was earned at Harvard Medical School, where she also completed an internship. Her father was a prominent plastic surgeon in Dallas, and she spent some time working with him. Up to this point, she had performed over 12,000 Mohs surgeries.

The total process lasted 3.5 hours. Everything went well, and no evidence of cancer remained. Lisa had seven external and five internal stitches. Stitching was done vertically to keep from pulling up her eyebrow. Dr. Priya Zeikus did not feel plastic surgery was necessary or that any scar would ultimately be visible. Lisa felt some moderate pain but did well overall. Just a walk in the park compared to what she'd been through.

———————————◆◆◆◆■———————————

At 33 weeks, it was time for Lisa to repay the kindness she'd received throughout this long ordeal. She wrote a heartfelt thank you to all the friends and relatives who had followed her on CaringBridge and made comments encouraging her. Here it is:

> Being diagnosed with pancreatic cancer was like a punch to the gut. Your world shrinks to an inch in front of your face. I had no idea how I was going to get past this diagnosis. Then you came along. Each morning, seeing your messages of compassion, guidance, advice, wisdom, and support were legs that kept me standing when I was sure I was going to fall. I endured the brutal chemo sessions and surgery because of you! I want each one of you to know how much I appreciate all of you. Your prayers, words of encouragement, kind thoughts, and well-wishes meant more to me than you will ever know.
>
> I hope you never need CaringBridge for yourself, but if you do, I hope you'll have the kind of loving family and friends as me. I also want you to know how much Robin cared for me during all this. And he still does. All the research he did, phone calls to doctors and hospitals, while handling the household chores and taking personal care of me, was both incredible and awesome. It was very stressful for him, but he always came through for me and still does. He fought so hard for my survival that I don't know where I would be today without him.

He is my rock. I pray each of you is blessed with a spouse like Robin.

Recently, I received a good medical report. I am a NED (no evidence of disease). It may never come back. Or it may decide to make an encore. If it does, I know, without a doubt, you will be there for me. I just wanted you to know how good that feels. Thank you, and God bless you!

Having folks in your corner rooting you on and providing encouragement was more important than Lisa had realized. Whatever you have to do, include your family and friends in whatever you're going through.

At 38 weeks, Robin and Lisa met with her gastroenterologist, Dr. Finau. She had scheduled a routine colonoscopy with him. Because of everything she had been through, Dr. Finau wanted to talk with Lisa first. He had performed the EUS with FNA (endoscopy) on her back on February 20, 2020. That was the horrible day when they'd learned with absolute certainty about Lisa's diagnosis. They had not kept in touch with Dr. Finau, so he was amazed and elated to see her doing so well. He wanted to hear Lisa's story from the past twenty months. After bringing him up to date, he was extremely positive about her prognosis, and they left that meeting feeling really good. It was another great moment in this long recovery. And later, the colonoscopy went well.

Many folks out there can't afford the cost of healthcare like Lisa had. Robin and Lisa worked hard and had taken some economic risks and they paid off. They could afford good care. Lisa's carrier was Blue Cross and Blue Shield of Texas. Generally, it did a good job without any major surprises or concerns. Her treatments from diagnosis through February 2021 cost about $420,000. That was the first twelve months. With her deductible plus three genetic tests Robin ordered (and understood would not be covered), Lisa's share was about $20,000.

There are many questions about how all this works, but right now, Lisa can say she is blessed to have good insurance.

Lisa and Robin continued looking for ways that might prevent a possible recurrence of her cancer. During their previous visits with Dr. Zeh, Robin questioned him about vaccine trials taking place at a couple of pancreatic cancer centers, but again, Lisa still wasn't eligible for any of them. Then, in April 2022, Dr. Zeh found a trial called "A study of ELI-002 in subjects with KRAS Mutated Pancreatic Ductal Adenocarcinoma (PDAC) and Other Solid Tumors (AMPLIFY-201)." The details were at ClinicalTrials. gov with an identifier of NCT04853017. This Phase 1 (non-placebo) clinical trial was being administered at several high-volume cancer centers. One of them was MD Anderson in Houston. MD Anderson is part of the University of Texas System, as is UT Southwestern. They work closely and share information about a lot of things.

The primary goal of a Phase 1 trial is to assess the drug's safety and determine a maximum tolerated dose. It is called a dose-escalation trial. The secondary goal is to measure the efficacy of the treatment, in this case, the circulating tumor DNA (ctDNA) reduction and clearance rate.

Dr. Zeh explained this was a trial Lisa might want to consider. She would have to travel to MD Anderson in Houston and undergo testing to see if she qualified and most importantly, complete a ctDNA test through blood work. Similar to a liquid biopsy, ctDNA testing examines a patient's blood for tumor cells. Essentially, the test is looking for circulating tumor DNA. The ctDNA test is relatively new and can be more sensitive and specific than CA 19-9 or other blood tests. The measurement criteria differ from a CA 19-9 test, and the FDA does not presently approve it for pancreatic cancer. So Robin and Lisa weren't 100 percent sure how this might go.

If no circulating tumor cells were found (hopefully, there wouldn't be), Lisa would not be eligible for the trial. If circulating tumor cells were found, she'd be given a *customized* vaccine that fit her tumor's DNA. The vaccine would prevent the cancer from "landing." Everyone fully expected she would test negative.

On May 20, 2022, Lisa and Robin traveled south to Houston and visited MD Anderson to meet the clinical trial team and oncologist Dr. Dan Zhao, a pancreatic cancer specialist. The Stoughs' desire to be proactive led them to this appointment. They agreed to the meeting with MD Anderson; it was not pushed on them.

Dr. Zhao reiterated what Robin had read on the trial literature and government site. All patients exploring the trial must ultimately complete a ctDNA test. Instead of examining DNA fragments in the blood, an entire tumor cell was captured. Although it was challenging to prove, many doctors believe that circulating tumor cells can be the seeds of metastasis.

Lisa would be eligible only if she tested positive for circulating tumor cells. UT Southwestern had already shared Lisa's tumor characteristics and would send a physical tumor specimen to MD Anderson. The post-surgery testing of Lisa's tumor showed it was KRAS variant G12R. Initially, this trial was intended for patients with the G12R or G12D KRAS variant, and from that perspective, Lisa was a candidate. The trial drug or vaccine was customized for those specific variants. Theoretically, the drug would prevent a recurrence by revving up and teaching the immune system to attack and kill the circulating cancer cells, thereby preventing them from "landing." This was immunotherapy, similar in some ways to the mRNA vaccines now used for COVID.

Because they are part of the same system, MD Anderson had access to all of Lisa's scans and lab work from UT Southwestern, including her pathology report and much more. That helped speed up the process. Also, it helped that Robin had already secured a patient number when Lisa was diagnosed in February 2020. But back then, they hadn't made it to MD Anderson. Between the wait to secure an appointment and the COVID pandemic, they had decided to stay closer to home at UT Southwestern.

Dr. Zhao looked over Lisa's records. Her previous genetic testing confirmed she had a KRAS mutation. A very high percentage of pancreatic cancer patients (85 to 90 percent) had the KRAS mutation, so that was expected. In the past, KRAS has often been described as undruggable, but times were changing.

Lisa was told that simply testing for this trial could open a can of worms and cause undue concern and anxiety. Even so, she decided to proceed for these reasons:

1. She wanted to be proactive and leave no stone unturned in stopping the cancer from returning, if that was even possible.

2. She believed it was essential to pay it forward by participating in research for the cancer patients who come after her.

3. It would establish a relationship with MD Anderson, a world leader in research and clinical trials.

4. Lisa would be well studied for the next two years.

5. Lisa felt the side effects and risks from this type of treatment would be tolerable.

6. And it just might work.

For all these reasons, Robin and Lisa felt confident about their decision to participate.

UT Southwestern provided stained and unstained slides to the MD Anderson clinical trial team and Elicio Therapeutics (the trial sponsor). Unfortunately, there wasn't enough sample tissue to define Lisa's DNA characteristics, probably due to the almost complete destruction of her tumor during chemotherapy. There was another option, though. They did have Lisa's FoundationOne CDx genetic test that had been done from a physical sample of her tumor post-surgery. That was the test that showed her mutation as KRAS G12R. So, they used that test.

MD Anderson is cutting-edge for research, immunotherapy treatments, and clinical trials. Their partner in this trial, Elicio Therapeutics, is a clinical-stage biotechnology company based in Boston, and this platform was initially developed at MIT. They focus on developing novel immunotherapies for the treatment of cancer. The first patient for this study was dosed at MD Anderson in October of 2021, so Lisa was at the right place.

After meeting with Dr. Dan Zhao, her PA, and her nurse, Lisa had more blood work done. Then she and Robin returned home.

They flew down to Houston several times for blood work and testing. Lisa had to provide her blood samples at the MD Anderson Clinical and Translational Research Center. All blood draws had to physically be performed there. That was trial protocol.

After all this, Lisa was cleared to move on to the next phase to see if she qualified for this trial. Here is what she went through:

- ctDNA testing at the MD Anderson Clinical and Translational Research Center

- Comprehensive blood testing, including CA 19-9
- COVID test
- Electrocardiogram
- Consultation with Dr. Amanda Olson regarding the leukapheresis procedure. (This procedure would be part of the clinical trial.)
- Consultation with the oncologist, Dr. Dan Zhao
- CT of her chest, abdomen, and pelvis

After testing, they learned that Lisa's CA 19-9 reading at MD Anderson was 28.3. It was still under the normal of 38, but this was more than *ten points higher* than her last test at UT Southwestern one month earlier. Always skittish, the jump caused the Stoughs great anxiety, as they became concerned it could be the first indicator of a recurrence.

For their peace of mind, when they returned to Dallas, they had UT Southwestern redo the CA 19-9, which came back at 13.3. It was a huge relief. The difference could have resulted from the calibration and model of the testing machines, among other factors. They were reminded again that you must compare testing data against the same testing lab, as different results are often observed. All of Lisa's subsequent CA 19-9 tests at MD Anderson came back in this higher range, although all were under 38. Keep that in mind with tests at different labs. Dr. Zeh said his other shared patients with MD Anderson frequently showed CA 19-9 results ten points higher than reported at UT Southwestern.

Finally, Robin and Lisa received word from the ctDNA testing lab, Sysmex Inostics, that a "mutation was detected." The test showed "a Mutant Allele Fraction (MAF) of 0.098%." Although that was a low number, it meant Lisa's ctDNA test was positive, and circulating cancer cells with the KRAS mutation were detected in her blood. Based on Lisa's otherwise normal testing and good CA 19-9 reading, this was somewhat shocking to the doctors and the Stoughs. Then, they wondered about false positives. *Is the test result accurate?* Another huge jolt to the system had just hit Lisa and Robin.

Before this test, they knew Lisa had the KRAS G12R variant. G12R is the third most common KRAS mutation for pancreatic cancer and is thought to be a driving force behind 15 to 18 percent of all pancreatic cancer tumors. It's one of the target mutations for this trial, leading to Lisa's eligibility. But Sysmex Inostics said she had a G12C mutation. Only 1 percent of pancreatic patients had this variant. That was confusing and another big surprise.

The trial sponsor, Elicio Therapeutics, is located in Boston, Massachusetts, and is affiliated with MIT. They have approximately twenty-five employees. They believed the Sysmex test was accurate and the tumor may have mutated from G12R to G12C, or the tumor may now possess both characteristics. No one was sure what it meant.

Dr. Zhao was also surprised the ctDNA test was positive and more surprised about the change in mutation. She wasn't sure if the test was a false positive. Lisa wanted more clarification, so they set up two additional ctDNA tests. There were obvious questions. Was Lisa still eligible for the trial? Was this test, which the FDA had not yet approved for pancreatic cancer, truly accurate? Maybe it was too sensitive.

Robin researched Sysmex Inostics. Apparently, various technologies can be used to execute a ctDNA test. This lab used one of those technologies and has a strong reputation for detecting very low-frequency ctDNA mutations. The Sysmex Inostics platform was developed at Johns Hopkins and scored high in comparing analytical sensitivities against several leading ctDNA tests based on different technologies. They self-described their platform as the current gold standard for this field.

On July 5, Lisa and Robin flew back to MD Anderson in Houston to complete the first of two additional ctDNA tests. This first test was executed in-house at MD Anderson's Molecular Diagnostics Lab. A second test would later be completed at UT Southwestern using the testing company Guardant. Dr. Zhao wanted results from two separate companies and labs. These tests were completed for their own personal comparison. Since they were not part of the trial, Lisa could have them done at outside labs.

While Robin and Lisa had Dr. Zhao in front of them, they asked her about the elevated CA 19-9 results at MD Anderson. She confirmed that if your CA 19-9 readings rise consistently and stay out of the normal range, it could be a matter of months before the disease became radiographically evident.

They then asked, "Does disease become evident in a few months if the ctDNA is positive?"

"No one knows," she said, "particularly since Lisa's CA 19-9 is normal. There are also examples of a positive ctDNA test turning negative."

The elevated CA 19-9 readings at MD Anderson and circulating tumor cells floating in her blood certainly added to the Stoughs' anxiety level. They were aware that the ctDNA test could open up a can of worms, and it certainly did. This type of testing and treatment was new and emerging quickly. MD Anderson has a lot of resources; the facility is massive, and they have top-notch professionals. Robin and Lisa had to trust this would all work out.

Around July 15, they received the results from these two additional tests: negative for cancer cells in Lisa's blood. No circulating tumor cells were found. *What?!*

They talked with Dr. Zeh and their new UT Southwestern oncologist, Dr. Al Mutar. Both doctors reiterated what the Stoughs had previously discussed, that there were many unknowns with the current ctDNA technology. Robin and Lisa also had a long conversation with their MD Anderson clinical trial contact, Dr. Li Xu. She confirmed the trial sponsor, Elicio Therapeutics, discounted the negative tests, so Lisa remained eligible for the trial.

Although Dr. Zeh and Dr. Al Mutar had reservations, they both conceded the Sysmex test might be meaningful and were not against Lisa entering the trial. Lisa and Robin were already leaning that way and agreed with their assessment. Even though it was a Phase 1 trial, it presented a unique and most likely one-time opportunity to potentially eradicate the circulating tumor cells. There were no other known trials or treatments for circulating pancreatic cancer cells. And the trial was scheduled as a two-year Phase 1 dose-escalation trial that included eighteen patients from around the country, six in each cohort (a group of participants who shared a common treatment). Lisa would be in the third and final cohort, which tested the strongest dose. The trial was also being conducted at UCLA, Memorial Sloan Kettering, and several other prominent cancer hospitals. The trial drug (ELI-002) was designed to teach the immune system to fight the disease by training it to target the cancer cells. In part, the drug signals parts of the immune system, called T-cells, to go to the lymph nodes where they believe it will be most effective. Essentially, it was a targeted immunotherapy that has the immune system fight the cancer before it lands, and it doesn't use chemo. This was a window of opportunity to treat circulating tumor cells before they became visible in radiographic scans—a very unique trial. The bottom line was that they didn't want to pass on the trial and live with any regrets down the road. So Lisa proceeded while Robin made the travel arrangements and carried the bags.

They flew to Houston on August 15, 2022, to begin the clinical trial. Lisa completed the blood work and most of the results came back within two hours. MD Anderson has around thirty-five phlebotomists in their main lab. It was extremely busy but very organized and efficient. It was unbelievable how quickly results came out.

They returned the next day so Lisa could complete a procedure called leukapheresis. This procedure required a 15 cm catheter to be inserted into her jugular vein stretching toward her heart. It was an invasive procedure. Blood cells would then be collected as she remained still and flat on her back for three hours. They hooked her up to a machine that circulated her blood, separated her white blood cells, collected those cells in a bag, and then returned the blood to Lisa's body. In this case, the white blood cells would only be kept for study and comparison later. Lisa would have another leukapheresis procedure a couple of months down the line.

This was not CAR T-cell therapy; it was more of a vaccine trial, so the goal of leukapheresis was specific to this situation.

On the third morning, Robin and Lisa met with Dr. Zhao and her team. Once Dr. Zhao approved Lisa's blood work, she checked in at the Clinical and Translational Research Center. This triggered the staff to begin unfreezing the drug ELI-002. (It arrived frozen from Elicio Therapeutics in Boston and took hours to thaw.) Once it was unfrozen, the MD Anderson pharmacy prepped it for Lisa's injections. There was a lot of waiting.

The injections had to be subcutaneous, with the needle inserted into the fat area between the skin and muscle. She received four injections per visit: one in each arm and leg. Once she received the injections, she had to be monitored for at least one hour before MD Anderson released her. The exception was the first injection. She was required to stay for four hours after the injection and remain within one hour of MD Anderson for the next twenty-four hours.

Although the trial sponsor covered the medical costs, it was still expensive and time-consuming, especially for out-of-town patients. Thankfully, Robin and Lisa had the time and means to do it.

On the fourth day, they flew back to Dallas and began the wait to do it all over again.

Not counting the leukapheresis procedure, Robin and Lisa whittled it down to a two-day event. They'd fly down early Tuesday for lab work, and on Wednesday, Lisa would meet with Dr. Zhao for evaluation. Then she would get her injections before they flew back to Dallas. During the immunization stage, she received a total of four injections every week for four weeks, then four injections every other week over four weeks—an eight-week process. Her injections were given in each arm and leg. This was followed by a three-month observation stage consisting of lab work and scans before starting the booster stage. The booster stage was four injections weekly for four consecutive weeks. After Lisa's last dose of ELI-002, she entered a twenty-month follow-up stage.

Other than minor pain, Lisa showed no side effects. Dr. Zeh had worked on similar trials during his time at Johns Hopkins and had said early on that side effects shouldn't be a problem.

Throughout this trial, Dr. Li Xu, the administrator, and her team at MD Anderson, were ever-present. There were weekly health question-naires Lisa was required to complete.

Even though Robin and Lisa weren't given much information regarding efficacy, they did confirm everything was safe and in order. Apparently, it was normal to hold information and any interpretation of results close to the vest until the trial was further along or completed. It was frustrating for the patient, but just part of the business aspect. They did hear that this trial would likely advance to Phase 2, as safety didn't appear to be in question. Apparently, some efficacy was also being achieved. So, they counted that as promising news.

The Stoughs initiated a meeting and spoke with Dr. Shubham Pant, the MD Anderson Study Chair for this trial (and other clinical trials at MD Anderson). Dr. Pant made a presentation regarding this specific trial in June 2022 at the American Society of Clinical Oncology's (ASCO) annual meeting in Chicago. In a quote from that presentation, Dr. Pant stated, "KRAS [the main cancer mutation for pancreatic cancer] has long been called undruggable, but there are a lot of different small molecules and vaccine therapies that are trying to change the tide. I'm really excited about this trial [and there is] a lot of enthusiasm from other investigators. [It] is ongoing at our institution and multiple other institutions."

After reviewing Lisa's records and good test results, Dr. Pant commented, "I don't have much to say. Everything looks great." He did comment that he was happy Lisa was in the trial.

In October 2022, the Stoughs received results from two additional ctDNA tests Lisa had completed with Sysmex. One of those was taken before the trial began. Both were negative. In February 2023, they received two more results from ctDNA tests done in late 2022. Both of those were negative. Lisa had now taken seven ctDNA tests with three different providers.

The very first test with Sysmex was the only one where a variant (floating tumor cells) was detected. The remaining tests were negative. While that was great news, no one was ever sure the first test was believable or confident with that result. It was also possible the treatments had helped.

Lisa endured her final leukapheresis procedure. She now had scars from her leukapheresis procedure, port site, surgery, and permanent tattoos used as markers for her radiation treatments. She didn't complain and instead carries the scars of 21st-century pancreatic cancer treatment.

In December 2022, Lisa met with her new oncologist at UT Southwestern, Dr. Al Mutar. He explained he now "sometimes" administers chemotherapy to patients who have CA 19-9 readings above normal but show no evidence of disease. Thus, the treatment protocols are constantly being tweaked to fit new evidence.

Here are some interesting facts:

- In February 2023, Lisa set a personal record at MD Anderson with sixteen tubes of blood drawn from her body in one visit. At around 105 pounds, that was a lot.

- As of February 2024, a conservative estimate for the number of doctors' appointments, visits for port insertion, port extraction, chemo infusion, detach 5 FU pump, attaching the Neulasta injector, emergency nausea visits, radiation, gold seeds implanted, blood clot issues, lab draws, CT scans, clinical trial injections, multiple Zoom calls, hospitalization for surgery, and leukapheresis, not to mention their initial "interview" at UT Southwestern, totaled well over 200 for those four years.

- Through February 2024, the Stoughs have traveled twenty-five times to Houston for Lisa's clinical trial.

- Lisa will continue her clinical trial with lab work, CT scans, and other testing for the remainder of 2024 and into 2025.

- From June 23, 2020 until February 2024, Lisa had received over 8,822 visits to her CaringBridge site. She and Robin have reviewed every heart, reaction, and comment.

UPDATE July 2023:

Lisa learned that the ctDNA tests taken in November and December 2022 were both normal, and her CA 19-9 was in the normal range at 25.7. All good.

Unfortunately, her March 2023 visits and testing raised concerns, as her CA 19-9 test at MD Anderson on March 7 had come in at 41.8. That was her highest reading since she began chemotherapy three years ago and her only reading above normal since that time. An additional reading at UTSW on March 9 came in at 25.1. That was normal, although it was her highest reading from that hospital in three years. Due to these unexpected increases at MD Anderson and UT Southwestern, Lisa was recommended to complete another CA 19-9 in one month.

On the plus side, her scans were clean. That was excellent news. Yet the concern was that continued results outside the normal range might precede radiographic evidence of disease by three to six months. She and Robin knew how these tests could be and have dealt with a number of scares along the way. They hoped this would be an aberration and Lisa's CA 19-9 numbers would return to normal. Until then, they faced an anxious month.

On April 6, Lisa completed lab work at UT Southwestern in Dallas. Her CA 19-9 came in at 30.7, up from 25.1 on March 9. It was not the news she wanted, and everyone was even more concerned. Although it was still a normal number, the trend was problematic. Then there were the testing differences between UT Southwestern and MD Anderson. She knew the number would most certainly be above normal at MD Anderson. Due to this concern, an unscheduled trip to MD Anderson was set for April 11, with a follow-up at UT Southwestern on April 12. Lisa would complete another CT scan at MD Anderson and CA 19-9 and other lab work at MD Anderson and UT Southwestern. Scanxiety hit her and Robin hard.

That anxiety rose exponentially on April 11, when Lisa's CT scan showed a total of three new indeterminate subcentimeter hypodensities on her liver. April 11 was not a good 65th birthday for her.

Dr. Zeh told Lisa there was a 50/50 chance the cancer was back. He said it would be 20 percent if Lisa's CA 19-9 had not risen. MD Anderson's Dr. Zhao said there was a 60 percent chance this was a recurrence. Robin pushed them to give percentages, which was not healthy.

Dr. Zeh said if the pancreatic cancer returned, it would be in one of three ways. The first would be local recurrence near the original tumor site. It's possible that could be treated with radiation or surgery. The second would be a combination of local and metastatic. Lastly, a recurrence could be wholly metastatic. The odds of each scenario happening were equal.

Two of the spots were measured at 0.4 cm and one at 0.5 cm. They were told the spots could be artifacts where the contrast did not fill in. The spots could also be incidentalomas. When a person is scanned frequently, things show up. Most everyone has something going on. If Lisa didn't have a cancer history, these spots would probably just be monitored. Unfortunately, when spots are identified at the same time your CA 19-9 rises, it becomes very concerning.

The great news was that Lisa's CA 19-9 from MD Anderson was now down to 31.6—in the normal range. And the most recent ctDNA test from March 7 was negative for floating tumor cells. Again, fantastic news. Elicio Therapeutics (who ordered the ctDNA tests through Sysmex) said: "The ctDNA is thought to be the best marker, while CA 19-9 can be helpful but is less specific and sometimes is elevated by non-cancer processes like gallstones." Lisa's doctors didn't necessarily agree that ctDNA was the best marker, yet it brought some reassurance.

On April 12, 2023, UT Southwestern did another CA 19-9, which came in at 21.9. Again, this was down slightly and still normal.

An ultrasound and MRI were ordered to check out the liver spots. If the results identified them as concerning, it might lead to a biopsy or simply waiting to see if they grew larger.

On April 16, 2023, UT Southwestern completed the ultrasound on Lisa's liver. The report landed in Lisa's electronic file and read:

- Liver parenchyma is unremarkable.

- A 9 mm simple cyst within septation visualized in the right lobe of the liver. No solid hepatic lesions identified.

- No evidence of portal hypertension.

- Tiny gallbladder polyp. This requires no further follow-up.

In layman's terms, they could not identify any lesions/spots on Lisa's liver. This didn't come as a complete surprise, as Dr. Zeh mentioned the spots seen on the CT scan were so small that an ultrasound might not identify them. Apparently, an ultrasound is not quite as detailed as a CT scan. Still, this was not bad news.

The 9 mm cyst has been with Lisa for a long time and is common. The gallbladder polyp was news to them. Through three-plus years of scans, it was never mentioned.

A medical paper Robin read said an elevated CA 19-9 in benign disease can be explained by several mechanisms, such as "…inflammation and proliferation of non-tumorous tissue."

To be completely sure of what they were looking at, the pair flew to Houston on April 17, 2023, and Lisa had an MRI at MD Anderson. The full report popped up within hours on her MyChart and read:

"Hello Ms. Stough. The MRI only showed benign findings in the liver! I have set up a telephone call Wednesday to answer any other questions you may have."

Again, a huge relief! Lisa and Robin gave MD Anderson an A+ for understanding their stress and quickly providing the results. They do get it.

The report recognized "Subcentimeter arterially enhancing lesions in the liver, which appear benign and likely represent hemangiomas." Thus, the findings were benign and all good.

On May 3, the Stoughs completed their 22nd trip to MD Anderson in Houston. This was prescheduled as a follow-up for Lisa's clinical trial. In addition to comprehensive lab work, the testing included another CA 19-9 and ctDNA test. Once more, it was a stressful day waiting for results. Thankfully, Lisa's lab work came back normal, and her CA 19-9 showed to be 28.3. That's in the normal range and down from 41.8 on March 7 and 30.7 on April 11. Coincidentally, the 28.3 CA 19-9 reading was identical to Lisa's first CA 19-9 test at MD Anderson almost one year earlier, on May 20, 2022. No one knows why her CA 19-9 reading had briefly climbed beyond the normal range. They do know this normal reading, coupled with her negative CT, MRI, and ultrasound tests, indicate no evidence of disease. She is a NED!

As of February 2024, all of Lisa's CT scans and blood tests have confirmed she's still a NED. Lisa's doing great physically and feels 100 percent. But she and Robin can't help but think about how close she'd come to bad news since her doctors had said there was a 50 percent chance of a recurrence. Somehow, they'd beaten the Russian roulette game with a six-chambered revolver and three bullets. She doesn't want to play that game again, thank you very much.

Appendix

CA 19-9 chart

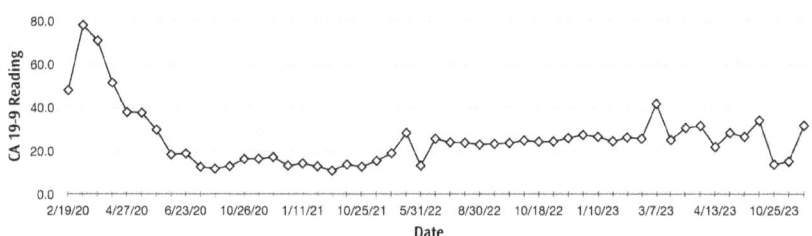

Date	CA 19-9	Location	Date	CA 19-9	Location
02/19/20	48.0	Hospital	08/15/22	24.0	MD Anderson
02/26/20	78.1	Oncology	08/23/22	23.8	MD Anderson
03/05/20	71.0	UTSW	08/30/22	23.0	MD Anderson
04/06/20	51.5	UTSW	09/06/22	23.3	MD Anderson
04/27/20	37.9	UTSW	09/20/22	23.7	MD Anderson
05/06/20	37.6	UTSW	10/04/22	24.9	MD Anderson
05/11/20	29.8	UTSW	10/18/22	24.3	MD Anderson
05/28/20	18.4	UTSW	11/20/22	24.4	MD Anderson
06/23/20	18.9	UTSW	12/13/22	26.0	MD Anderson
07/28/20	12.7	UTSW	01/03/23	27.4	MD Anderson
09/14/20	11.9	UTSW	01/10/23	26.6	MD Anderson
10/12/20	13.0	UTSW	01/17/23	24.5	MD Anderson
10/26/20	16.3	UTSW	01/24/23	26.3	MD Anderson
11/12/20	16.4	UTSW	02/08/23	25.7	MD Anderson
11/30/20	17.2	UTSW	03/07/23	41.8	MD Anderson
12/28/20	13.3	UTSW	03/09/23	25.1	UTSW
01/11/21	14.3	UTSW	04/06/23	30.7	UTSW
01/25/21	12.9	UTSW	04/11/23	31.6	MD Anderson
04/20/21	11.0	UTSW	04/13/23	21.9	UTSW
07/23/21	13.8	UTSW	05/03/23	28.3	MD Anderson
10/25/21	12.8	UTSW	07/25/23	26.6	MD Anderson
01/24/22	15.5	UTSW	10/17/23	34.1	MD Anderson
04/27/22	19.0	UTSW	10/25/23	13.8	UTSW
05/20/22	28.3	MD Anderson	12/05/23	15.2	UTSW
05/31/22	13.3	UTSW	01/09/24	31.7	MD Anderson
06/22/22	25.7	MD Anderson			

Photos

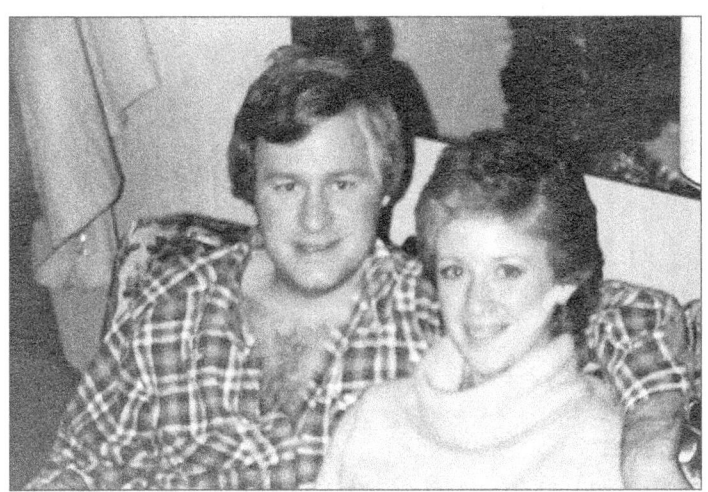

1979: Lisa and Robin dating.

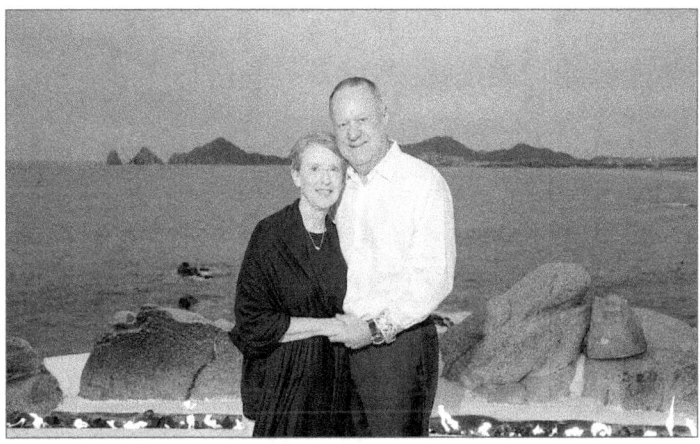

January 24, 2020: Cabo San Lucas. Lisa felt pain in her back while she slept during this trip. She visited their PCP, Dr. Aronoff, a couple of weeks later.

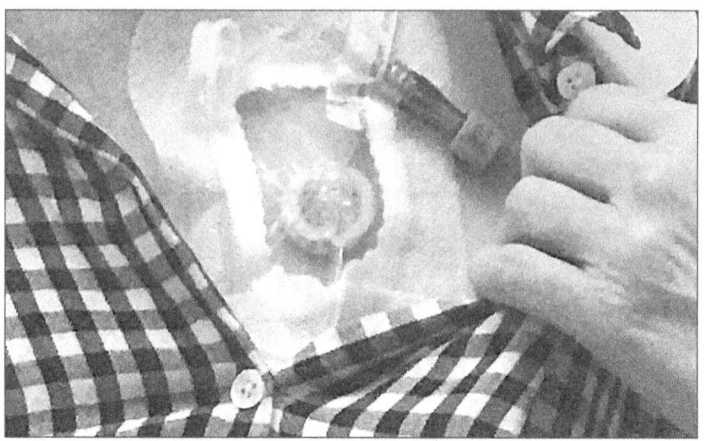

Lisa's port implanted in March 2020.

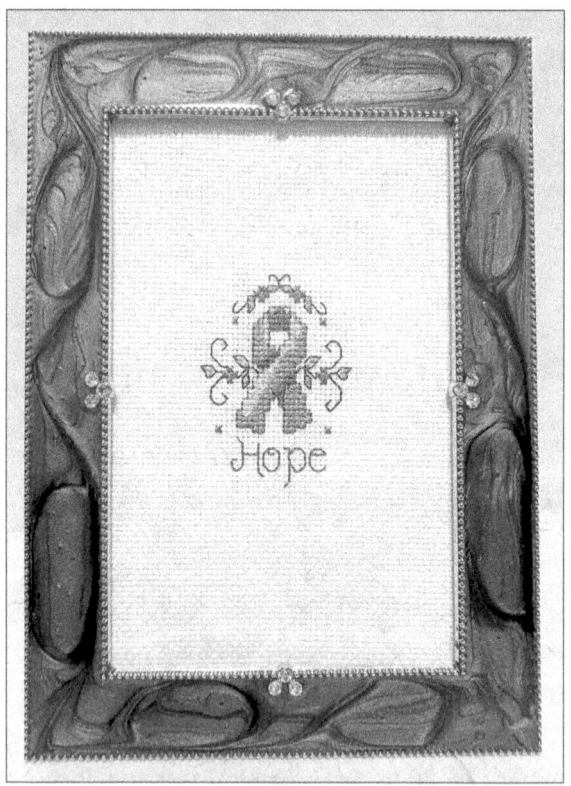

Needlepoint by Amy, Robin's sister, for
Lisa before chemo to give her hope!

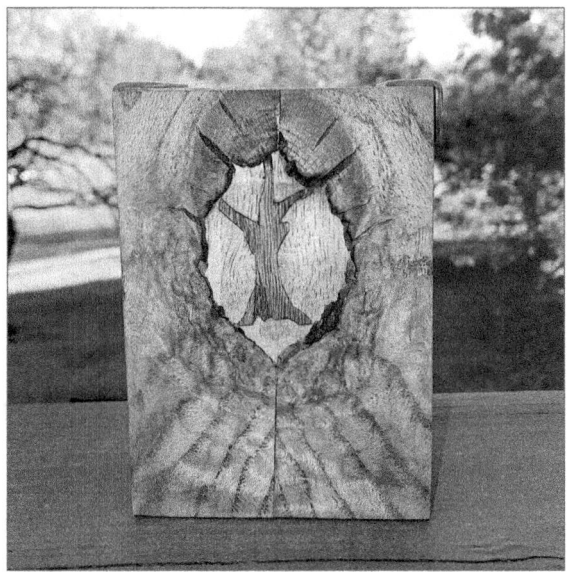

Beautiful box from Lisa's brother-in-law Bill.
It gave her strength.

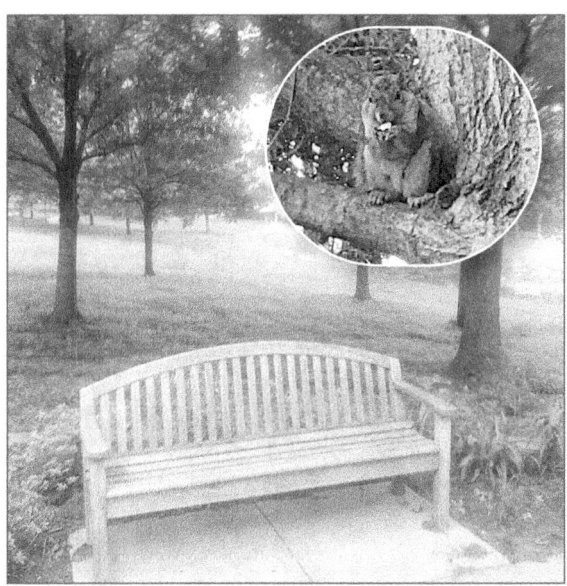

Spring 2020: The bench where Robin waited for Lisa
when he wasn't allowed to accompany her during the
pandemic. He had a friendly squirrel keep him company.

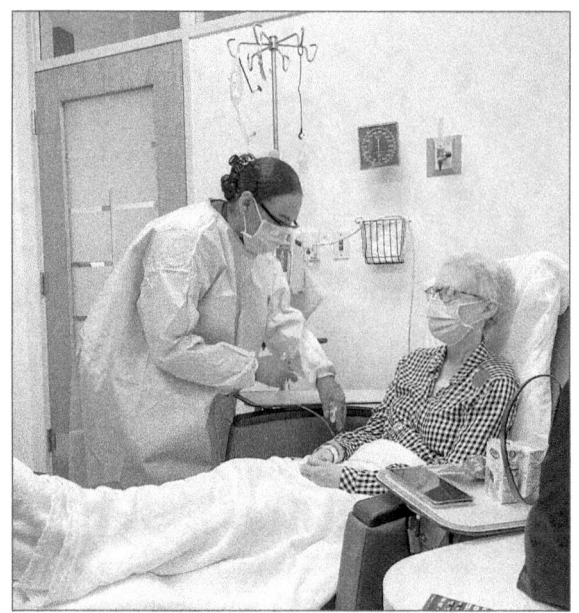

Neoadjuvant chemotherapy in Lisa's
private room at UTSouthwestern.

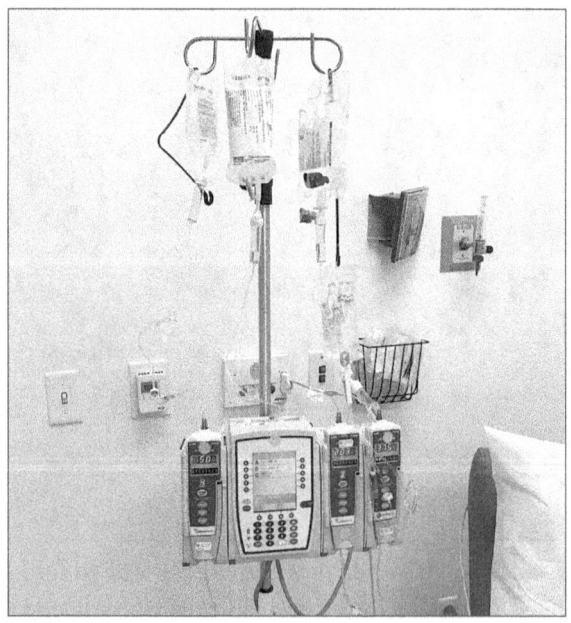

Chemo bags for Lisa.

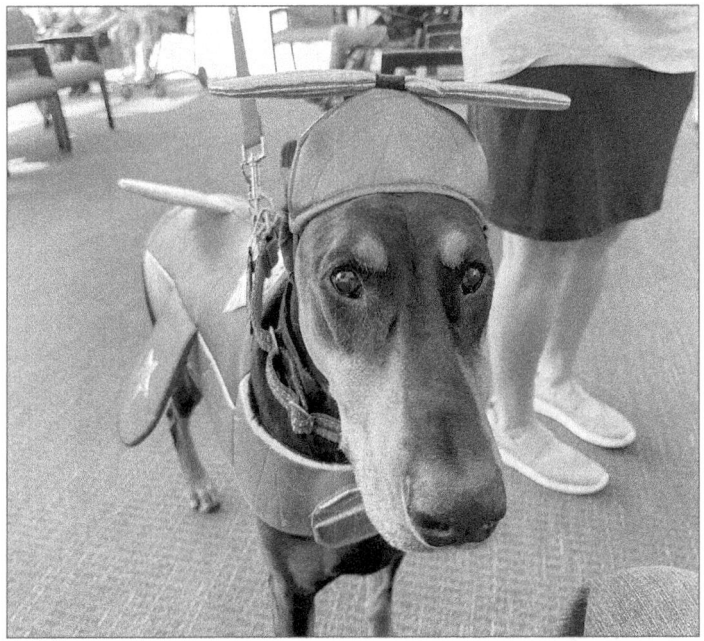

Therapy dog at UTSouthwestern spreading good vibes!

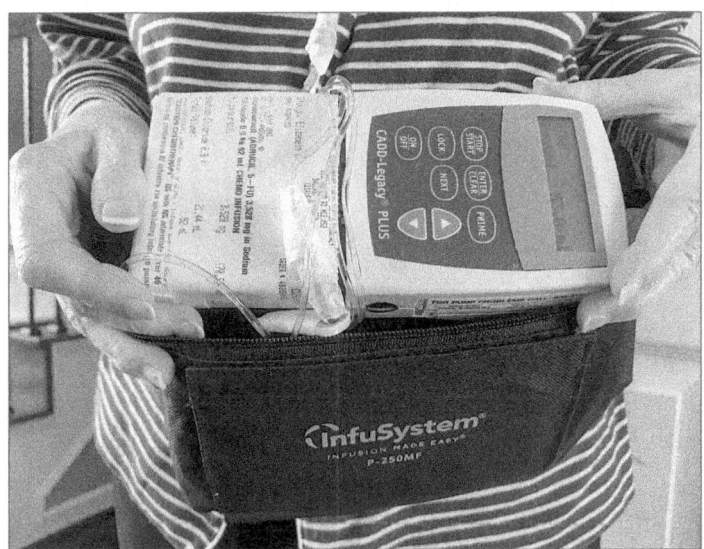

Fluorouracil 5FU chemotherapy: This is the pump
that delivered the 5FU. Lisa wore this for 46 hours
to complete each chemotherapy treatment.

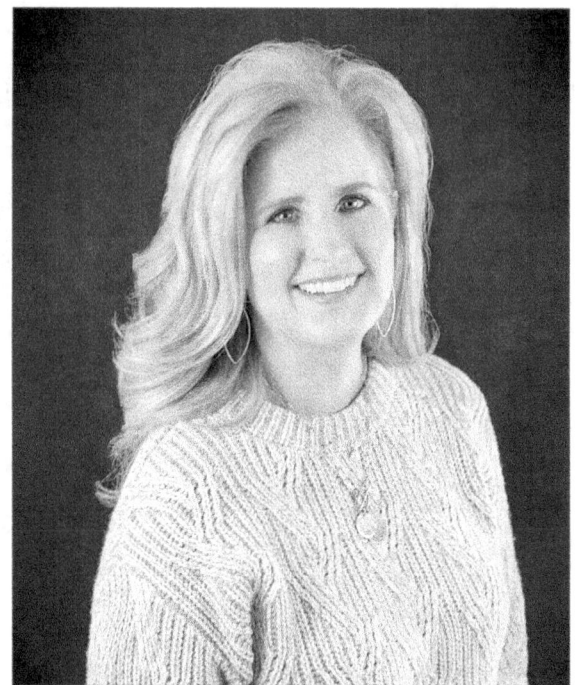

The Stough's great friend and designer, Allison Gimpel, was Lisa's only in-house contact during her treatments.

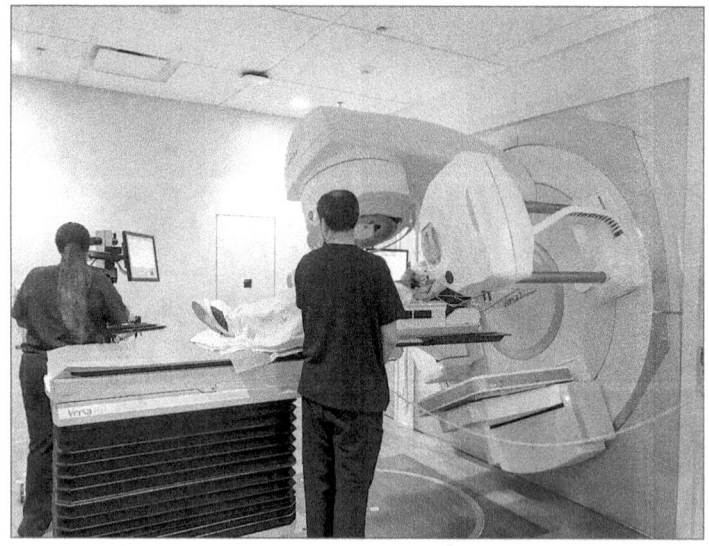

June 2020: Radiation treatments.

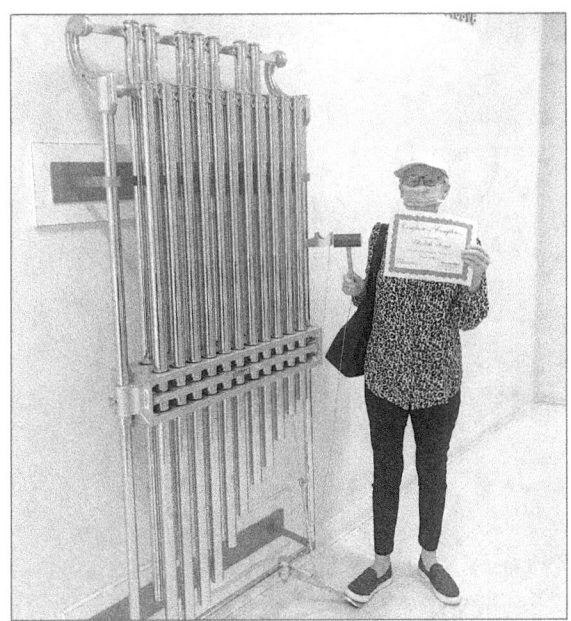

July 1, 2020: Lisa ringing the bells after
completing her radiation therapy.

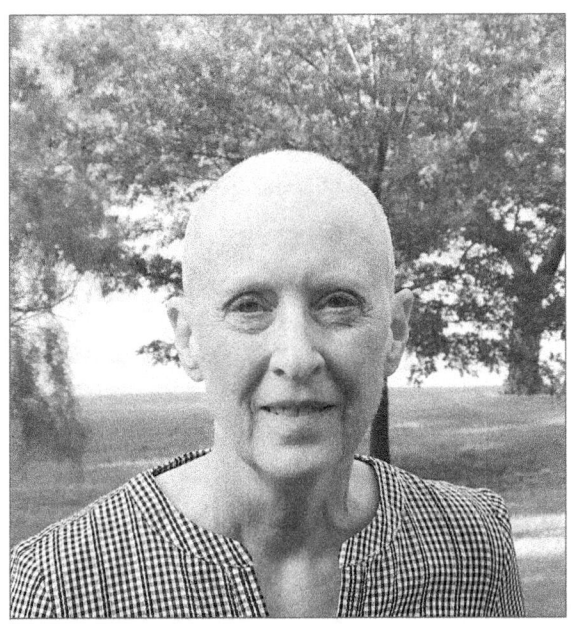

July 8, 2020: Less than a month before Lisa's surgery

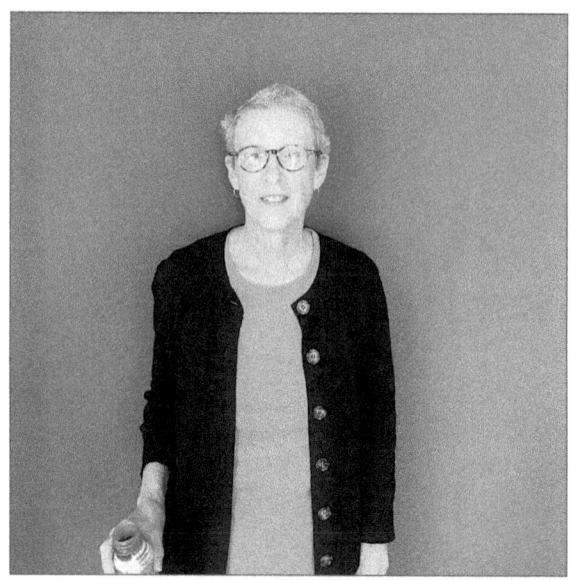

September 17, 2020: About six weeks after Lisa's surgery. Those were very difficult days.

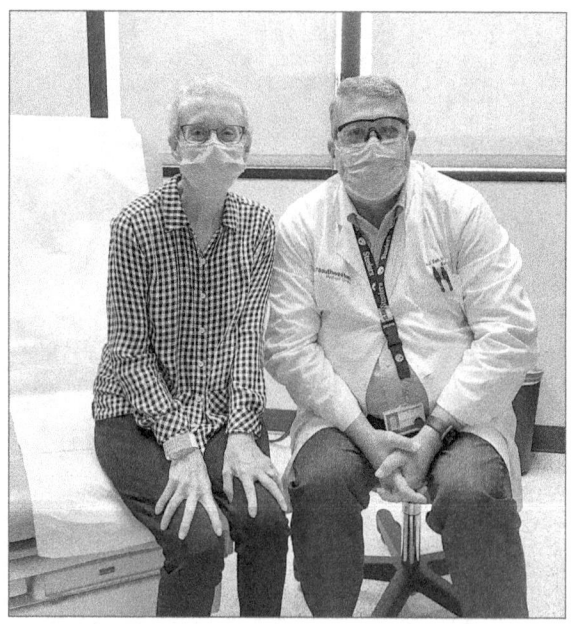

September 25, 2020: Lisa's surgeon Dr. Zeh. Almost two months after her surgery.

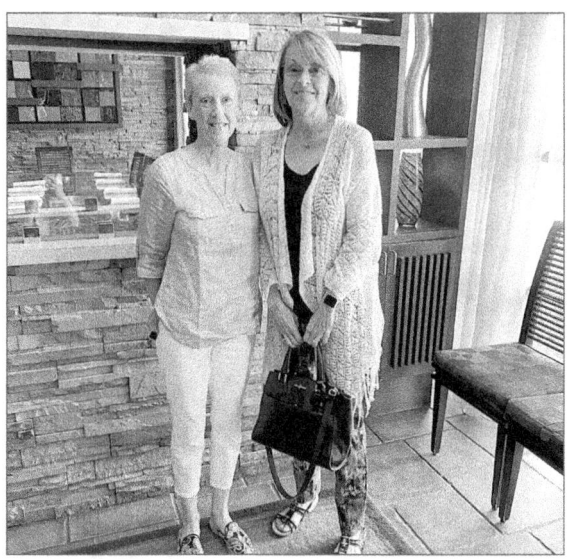

April 12, 2021: Lisa and her good friend Sallie.
Other than doctors, Sallie was her first contact
outside the house since treatments ended.

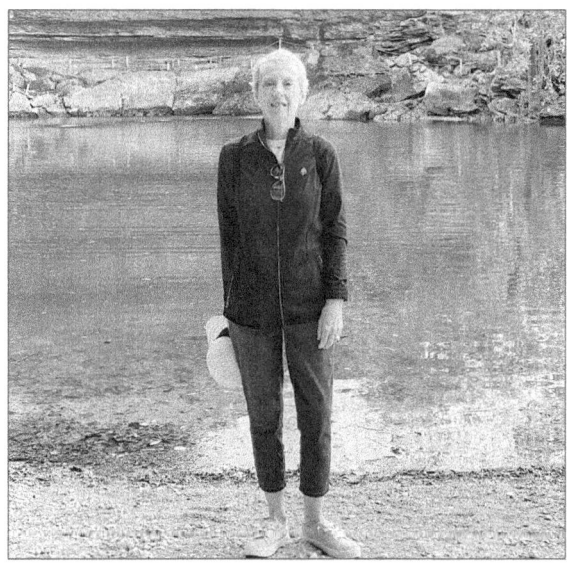

May 5, 2021: A short hike to Hamilton Pool near
Austin was Lisa's first road trip. She felt good,
just frail and gray and 95 lbs. at this point.

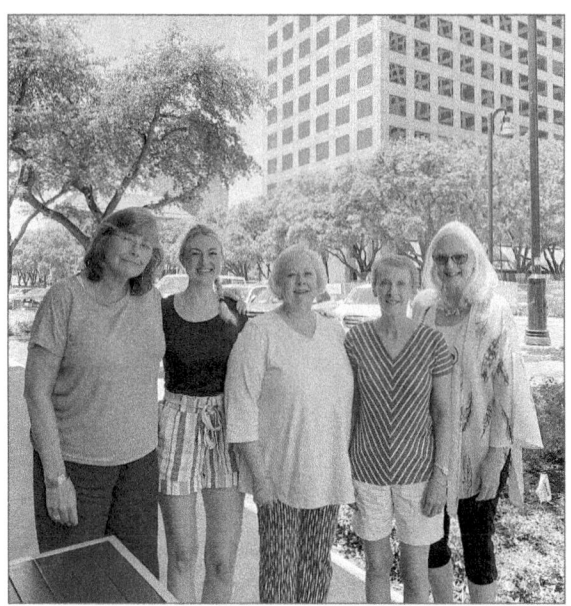

June 2021: Lisa at lunch with former Marsh colleagues and friends. (l to r: Kim, Karla, Ray, Lisa, and Cindy.)

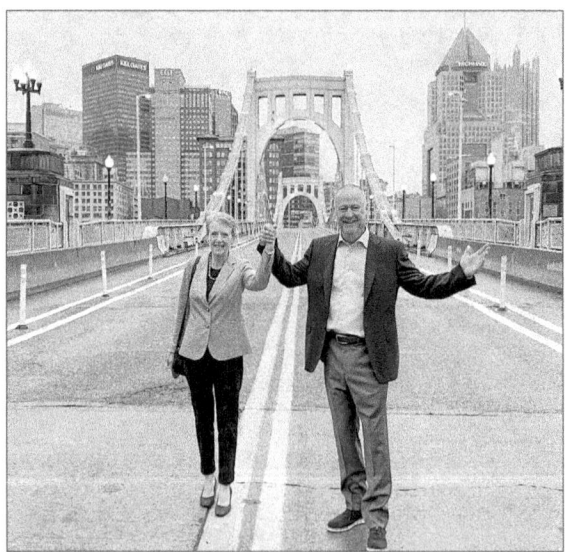

October 22, 2021: Lisa celebrating being a NED with Robin on the Roberto Clemente Bridge in their hometown of Pittsburgh.

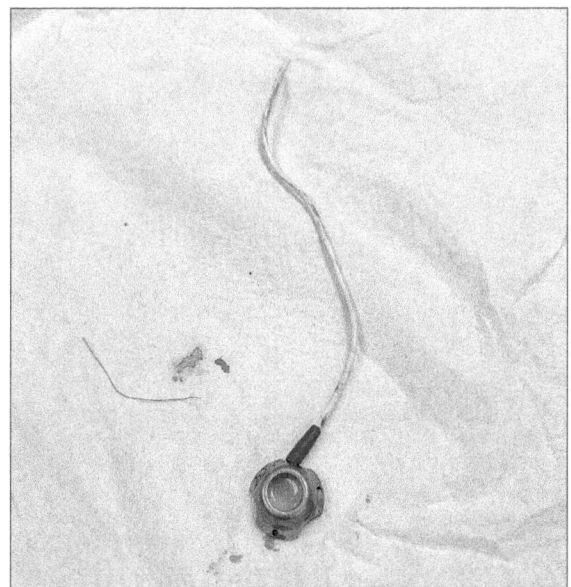

November 15, 2021: Lisa's port and catheter. She
was so excited to have it removed after 20 months.

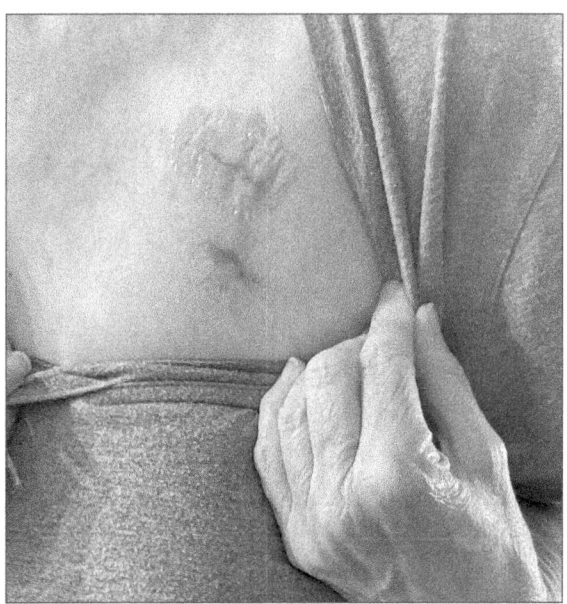

November 2021: Lisa's port scars after the removal.
She had the port for about 20 months.

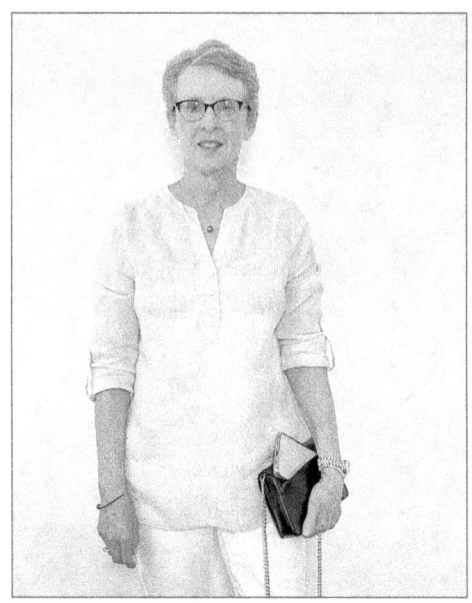

June 2022: Lisa is feeling 100%.

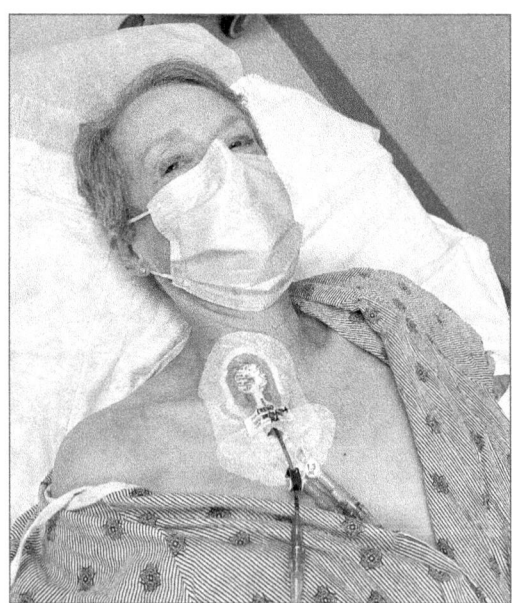

August 16, 2022: Catheter implanted for Lisa's first
Leukapheresis procedure. She endured this procedure
twice for her clinical trial at MD Anderson in Houston.

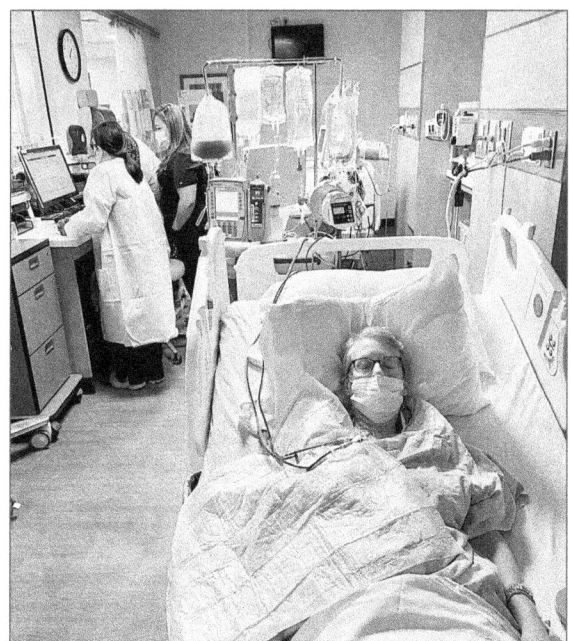

Leukapheresis procedure for Lisa's clinical
trial at MD Anderson in Houston.

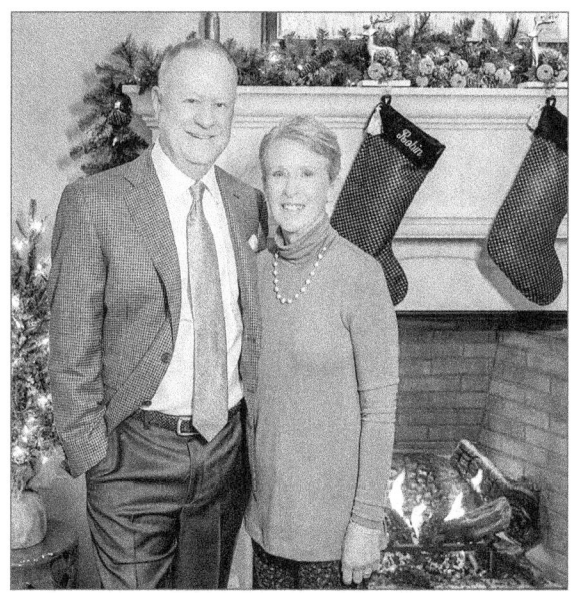

Christmas 2022: Robin and Lisa.

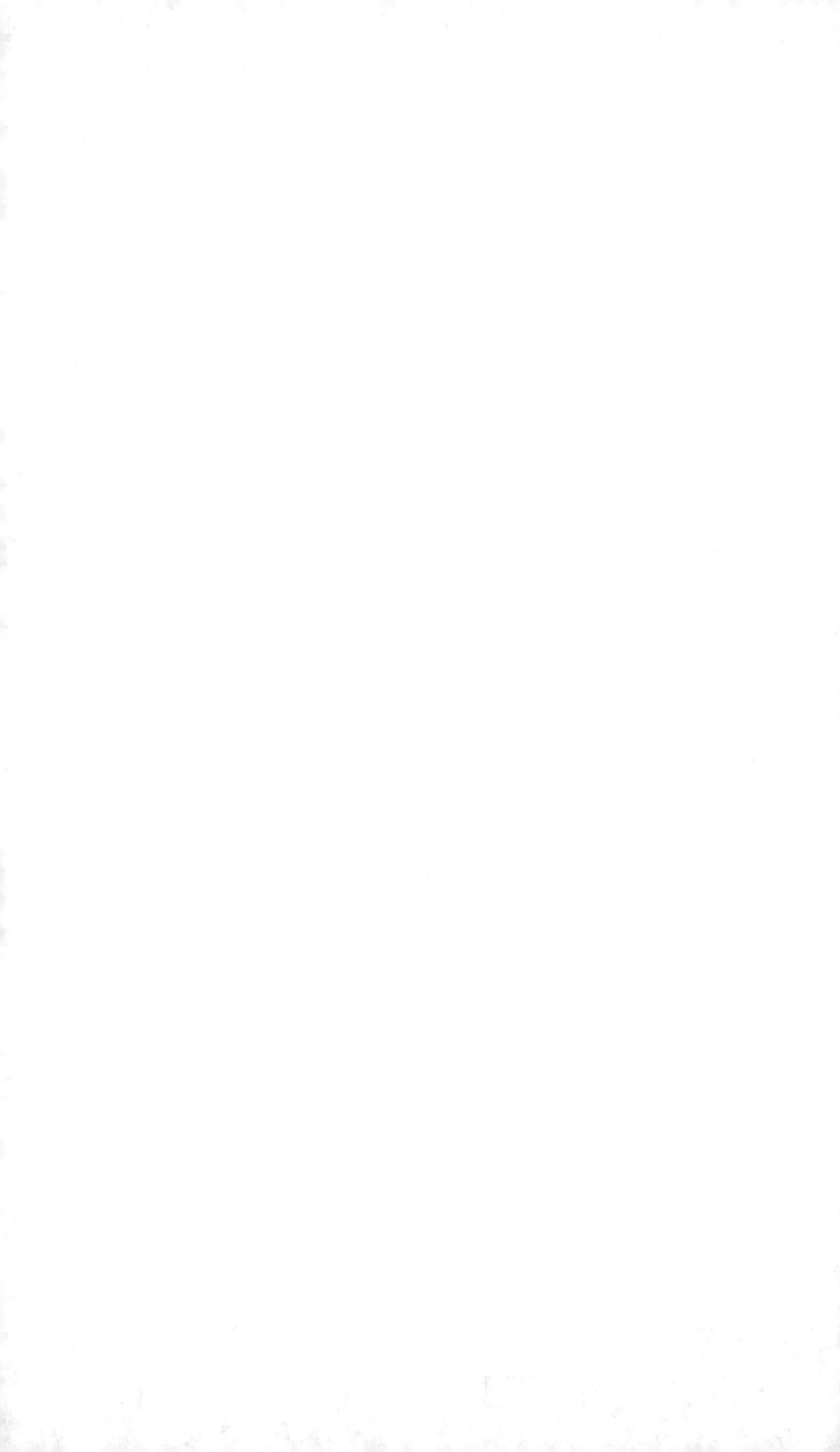

www.ingramcontent.com/pod-product-compliance
Lightning Source LLC
Chambersburg PA
CBHW070847290526

45795CB00001B/20